Basic Pharmacology

Third edition

Editor
R W Foster, BSc, PhD, MB, BS
Reader in Pharmacology

Authors
The pharmacologists of the Department of Physiological Sciences,
University of Manchester, UK, and their teaching collaborators:

A J M Boulton, MD, BS, MRCP
J R Carpenter, BSc, PhD
M J Dascombe, BPharm, PhD
J F W Deakin, PhD, MRCPsych
A J Duxbury, MSc, PhD, DDS, FDS, RCPSGlas
D J S Fernando, MD, BS, MRCP
R W Foster, BSc, PhD, MB, BS
C C Hardy, MD, MRCP
Ariane L Herrick, MD, MRCP
M Hollingsworth, BSc, PhD
G E Mawer, MB, ChB, BSc, PhD, FRCPEd

I D Morris, BPharm, PhD
Barbara J Pleuvry, BPharm, MSc, PhD, MRPharmS
J L Shaffer, MB, BS, MRCP
R C Small, BSc, MSc, PhD, MRPharmS
D G Thompson, MD, FRCP
R D G Tunbridge, MD, FRCP
M Janet Vale, MSc, MRPharmS
A J Watt, BSc, PhD
A H Weston, MSc, PhD
P M Wilkinson, MB, ChB, FRCP

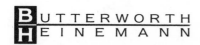

BUTTERWORTH HEINEMANN

Butterworth-Heinemann Ltd
Linacre House, Jordan Hill, Oxford OX2 8DP

 PART OF REED INTERNATIONAL BOOKS

OXFORD   LONDON   BOSTON
MUNICH   NEW DELHI   SINGAPORE   SYDNEY
TOKYO   TORONTO   WELLINGTON

First published 1980
Reprinted 1983, 1985
Second edition 1986
Reprinted 1990
Third edition 1991

British Library Cataloguing in Publication Data
Basic pharmacology. – 3rd ed.
  I. Foster, R. W.
  615

ISBN 0 7506 1414 5

Library of Congress Cataloguing in Publication Data
Basic pharmacology / editor, R. W. Foster: authors, A. J. M. Boulton . . .
  [et al.] – 3rd ed.
    p.   cm.
  Includes bibliographical references and index.
  ISBN 0 7506 1414 5
  1. Pharmacology.   I. Foster, R. W.   II. Boulton, A. J. M. (Andrew James Michael)
  [DNLM: 1. Drug Therapy.   2. Pharmacology.   QV 4 B3109]
RM300.B287   1991
615′.1—dc20
DNLM/DLC   91–26593
for Library of Congress   CIP

Printed in England by Clays Ltd, St Ives plc

Basic Pharmacology

Contents

3 Drug action on peripheral tissues – drugs acting on signalling and transduction mechanisms other than those directly related to receptors for neurotransmitters and hormones 117

4 Endocrine pharmacology 151

5 Drug action on the central nervous system 209

Preface

This third edition of *Basic Pharmacology* retains the overall objectives of the first. It aims to present accounts of drug actions and their mechanisms in a compact, inexpensive and up-to-date form. The book is therefore designed to help students of subjects allied to medicine to appreciate the rationale underlying the uses of drugs in therapeutics.

The authors of this book, the pharmacologists of the Department of Physiological Sciences at Manchester University and their teaching colleagues, have been able to draw on experience developed during many years of teaching pharmacology to students of several different disciplines. Such experience is tempered by other aspects of their work with drugs (prescribing, dispensing, laboratory-based and clinical research).

The book is divided into sections. Each section follows a particular theme and is introduced by the relevant pharmacological general principles. Prompts to revise the relevant anatomical, biochemical or physiological concepts and data are also given. In each section the major groups of drugs relevant to the theme are discussed with detailed expositions of the important 'type' substances. Drugs of lesser importance are placed in proper context.

As outlined in the introduction, this book is addressed to a wide spectrum of readers. We hope that no reader who intends to exploit the properties of drugs will fail to appreciate two key notions.

(1) Selectivity (that is the ability to influence chemically one kind of biological activity without modifying another) is the central theme of pharmacology.
(2) Such selectivity is relative, rather than absolute. This places the onus of responsibility for safe usage firmly on the intending exploiter of the properties of drugs.

The principal changes that this third edition of *Basic Pharmacology* shows from the second are:

(1) updating (as of 1990) of the accounts of mechanisms of drug action;
(2) updating (after *British National Formulary* [*BNF*] 1990, Number 20) of the selection of drugs for discussion; this encompasses not only the

inclusion of new drugs and new mechanisms of drug action but also the deletion of drugs that have become obsolete; on this occasion the deletions outnumber the additions of new drug names;

(3) movement of the section entitled *General pharmacology* from last to first position;

(4) expansion of the chapters on adverse drug interactions, cardiac antidysrhythmic drugs, calcium channel blockers, local hormones, chemotherapy of bacterial infections;

(5) substitution of fully rewritten chapters on adverse effects of drugs, drugs in diabetes mellitus, inflammatory bowel disease, congestive heart failure, asthma, drugs and mental disorders, epilepsy;

(6) provision of new chapters on allergically determined hypersensitivity to drugs;

(7) the provision of additional figures.

Introduction

This book is intended for all who are embarking on the study of pharmacology. Most of its readers will be students of medicine, or of subjects allied to medicine (pharmacy, dentistry, nursing). These students will be studying pharmacology as a subsidiary subject and will require emphasis on the therapeutic exploitation of the properties of drugs. However, other students will regard pharmacology as their main or second subject in biological science. We teach all such students ourselves and have attempted to satisfy their needs in a single text. The text is broadly introductory, covering the first and second years of study by any of the above student groups.

Our various readers will have two things in common: an interest in the uses to which drugs are put, and the fact that they are embarking on the study of pharmacology. Thus, we have provided a textbook that begins at the beginning, assuming only a modicum of chemistry, biology and physiology as prerequisites. The book proceeds in the direction of paramedical or therapeutic, rather than chemical, pharmacology and it is assumed that the student will still be developing his knowledge of biology or physiology.

The principal aim is to explain the basis of the current therapeutic exploitation of drugs. Though some large reference texts already achieve this aim at an advanced level (the most eminent and highly recommended bears the title that most succinctly expresses this aim – *The Pharmacological Basis of Therapeutics* – *see* Suggested further reading) this book is offered to fill the need for a comprehensive yet simple and concise student text.

Drug names

A major problem encountered in the learning of pharmacology is the large and ever-increasing number of drug names. Certainly new students often complain of this. The complaint is not simply about weight of numbers but also about the apparent similarity in the names of drugs from different pharmacological groups. For the inexperienced (for whom drug names are invested with no 'personality') this can lead to misunderstanding and confusion. Therefore, in this book we have defined a rigorous policy on drug names (*see below*). We have limited the number of drugs included, and have attempted an approach to the teaching of pharmacology that places a

premium on understanding, clothing drug names with personality and reducing rote memorization to the essential minimum.

Policy on drug names

We have used the nonproprietary names approved by the British Pharmaco-
poeial Commission and have largely excluded trade names. For readers who
are more familiar with North American terminology the US Pharmaco-
poeial name has been included in square brackets in the text after the first
occurrence of the name. However, only significant Anglo-American differences have been declared; we have not bothered to draw special attention to
systematic differences arising from different spelling conventions (-ph- [-f-],
-oe- [-e-]). Neither did -trophin [-tropin] nor -barbitone [-barbital] seem
likely to mystify our readers.

We were pleasantly surprised by the currently small number of significant
differences, for there was formerly an era of fundamental differences,
witness paracetamol [acetaminophen] and pethidine [meperidine]. Modern
drugs are deliberately being assigned the same name on both sides of the
Atlantic.

Policy on which drugs to include

We have actively sought to limit the number of different drugs described
because our primary objective has been to teach the principles of the
pharmacological basis of therapeutics rather than familiarity with all drugs.
We have therefore a narrower scope than the *BNF*, *MIMS* or the *Data Sheet
Compendium*, which seek full coverage of available drugs – we describe a
limited selection of the most useful drugs. We have followed the advice
offered in the *Notes for prescribers* sections of the *BNF* on the selection of
drugs with maximum available therapeutic efficacy and minimal contam-
inating toxicity. An acknowledged reference drug – described first and
placed out of alphabetical order – is an obvious choice for one of our 'type
substances' (*see below*). This policy is very similar to that adopted by the
WHO Expert Committee reporting on The Selection of Essential Drugs.

Drugs have been categorized according to two criteria:

(1) Drugs listed in *BNF* (1990) and printed in bold type in one of the *Notes
for prescribers* sections are italicized (for example, *nonproprietary
name*).
(2) From each pharmacological group of drugs we have, if possible, chosen
one that typifies the group. If its actions are understood the rest of the
group, too, has been comprehended. We show these substances in bold
type (for example, **nonproprietary name**).

The plan of the book

Each of the eight sections of the book is a reasonably self-contained unit that
expounds a particular pharmacological theme. We have tried to limit the
presentation of material to a single occasion, in its most appropriate location. Cross-references are provided, in preference to succumbing to the
temptation to repeat material, when it is relevant to more than one theme.

Book use that follows the order of the sections will therefore result in minimal following of cross-references leading to new material but the reader intent on acquiring all the contained information on one drug will have to use the index.

The book opens with a section, the theme of which is those general principles that need no specific drug group, physiological system or disease state for their discussion but that can be exemplified from any or all of the other sections.

The drugs that act on peripheral excitable tissues by modulating signalling and transduction mechanisms directly related to receptors for the neurotransmitters acetylcholine and noradrenaline impinge on so many physiological systems that they are most efficiently dealt with as a theme, and comprise our second section. This is a theme presented early in the book because it is in this area that mechanisms of drug action are probably best understood. Also, the system can be used as a model to predict or infer the mechanism of action of drugs in other less well understood areas (for example, central nervous system, CNS).

The third section collects together groups of drugs also acting on peripheral tissues but by modulating signalling and transduction mechanisms other than those directly related to receptors for neurotransmitters and hormones. The fourth and fifth sections – *Endocrine pharmacology* and *Drug action on the central nervous system* – correspond with the system-based subdivision of the subject common in therapeutic texts, though the former section includes Local hormones. Our understanding of drug action in the CNS leans heavily on the concepts of specific interaction with physiological chemical mediators developed in the preceding sections. A second important principle – that of nonspecific depressant action on biological function – also emerges.

So far the section themes have been drug interactions with endogenous systems but in the sixth section consideration is given to the mechanism of drug action on parasites, be they metazoa, microorganisms or neoplastic cells. The emphasis is now on mechanisms by which parasitic cell growth or survival is selectively inhibited.

By now the student has been provided with sufficient information in pharmacology for drugs to be no longer simply names. The theme of the seventh section therefore changes from drug action to drug disposition and metabolism – from what drugs do to the body to what the body does to drugs – so that an appreciation of how these factors influence drug action can be gained.

Our eighth section – *Clinical pharmacology* – illustrates, at least for certain carefully selected disease states, how the principles and concepts of mechanistic pharmacology are exploited in the setting of practical therapeutics.

Policy on unfamiliar words

Words that are unfamiliar to the reader may be part of the technical language of medicine or pharmacology and all such we have defined or explained on their first occurrence. A second category exists in the ordinary stock of the English language – definitions are not provided in the text and the reader is advised to consult a dictionary.

Text revision

Pharmacology, like most other scientific disciplines, develops rapidly and the perennial problem of any text is that of keeping up-to-date. We intend to make regular revisions of this book.

The text has had the benefit of passing through several stages of evolution and refinement. In the form of comprehensive lecture note handouts it was used by Manchester students in its prepublication years and we thank all our previous students who have consciously or unconsciously suggested improvements. We should be happy to receive suggestions for further improvement from users of the book.

Acknowledgements

We thank John Carpenter for preparing the new and altered diagrams, Kay Bond for typing the new sections of manuscript, staff at Butterworth-Heinemann for their care and attention in guiding this book through to publication, John Carpenter for preparing the index and all our colleagues for the time invested in evolving common policies and in proof reading.

Aims and objectives

The aim of this book is to provide the sound pharmacological basis on which could be built a rational approach to therapeutics.

By the end of the book the reader should:

- recognize a selection of the British Pharmacopoeia Commission Approved names of drugs appearing in bold type in the *Notes for prescribers* sections of the *BNF* (latest edition) and be able to group together those drugs that share common pharmacological properties;
- know the pharmacological properties of each drug group that are relevant to its therapeutic uses and adverse effects, with special emphasis on those that can be deduced from a knowledge of the site and mechanism of action;
- know the general principles of the subject and thus be able to assess the described properties and therapeutic claims made for any new drug or group of drugs.

List of abbreviations

These abbreviations are used in multiple locations in the book; there are others, just used in a single chapter, that are defined where first used.

ACE	angiotensin converting enzyme
ACh	acetylcholine
AChE	acetylcholinesterase
ACTH	adrenocorticotrophic hormone, corticotrophin
ADH	antidiuretic hormone
ATP	adenosine triphosphate
AV	atrioventricular
BMR	basal metabolic rate
BNF	*British National Formulary*
BP	blood pressure
C.	*Corynebacterium*
cAMP	cyclic 3'5'adenosine monophosphate
cf.	(lit. *confer*) compare
cGMP	cyclic 3'5'guanosine monophosphate
ChE	cholinesterase
Cl.	*Clostridium*
CL	clearance
CNS	central nervous system
CoA	coenzyme A
COMT	catechol-O-methyl transferase
CSF	cerebrospinal fluid
CTZ	chemosensitive trigger zone
d-	deci (10^{-1})
Da	Dalton
DHF	dihydrofolate
DNA	deoxyribonucleic acid
dopa	dihydroxyphenylalanine
E.	*Escherichia*
EC50	concentration of drug evoking a half maximal effect
ECF	extracellular fluid

e.g.	(lit. *exampli gratia*) for example
epp	end plate potential
epsp	excitatory postsynaptic potential
FEV_1	forced expiratory volume in one second
FSH	follicle stimulating hormone
g	gram
GABA	gamma-aminobutyric acid
GFR	glomerular filtration rate
GH	growth hormone
GMP	guanosine monophosphate
GTP	guanosine triphosphate
H.	*Haemophilus*
h	hour
HCG	human chorionic gonadotrophin
HMG	human menopausal gonadotrophin
5-HT	5-hydroxytryptamine
Hz	Hertz (1 Hertz is 1 cycle per second)
Ig-	immunoglobulin-
im	intramuscular, intramuscularly
IP_3	inositol 1,4,5-trisphosphate
iv	intravenous, intravenously
k-	kilo- (10^3)
Kl.	*Klebsiella*
l	litre
LH	luteinizing hormone
lit.	literally
log	logarithm
LT	leukotriene
μ	micro- (10^{-6})
M.	*Mycobacterium*
m	metre
m-	milli- (10^{-3})
MAC	minimum alveolar concentration for anaesthesia
MAO	monoamine oxidase
MFO	mixed function oxidase
mic	minimum inhibitory concentration
min	minute
mol	mole (gram molecular weight)
mRNA	messenger ribonucleic acid
MW	molecular weight
N.	*Neisseria*
n-	nano- (10^{-9})
NA	noradrenaline
NADPH	nicotinamide adenine nucleotide phosphate (reduced)
NSAID	nonsteroidal anti-inflammatory drug
P.	*Plasmodium*
P-	partial pressure
Pa-	arterial blood partial pressure
PG	prostaglandin
Ps.	*Pseudomonas*

qv.	(lit. *quod vide*) which see
REM	rapid eye movement
RNA	ribonucleic acid
s	second
S.	*Salmonella*
SA	sinoatrial
sc	subcutaneous, subcutaneously
Staph.	*Staphylococcus*
Str.	*Streptococcus*
$t_{\frac{1}{2}}$	half-time, half-life
THF	tetrahydrofolate
Tr.	*Treponema*
tRNA	transfer RNA
TSH	thyroid stimulating hormone, thyrotrophin
UK	United Kingdom
V	apparent volume of distribution
v.	versus
viz.	(lit. *vide licet*) namely
v/v	volume per unit volume
w/v	weight per unit volume

1

General pharmacology

Aims

The theme of this chapter is not drugs but processes.

- Understanding these processes will help your understanding of many drug actions and interactions at the (a) mechanistic, (b) therapeutic and (c) toxic levels.

Mechanisms of drug action

A drug produces its effects by interacting with a biological target that is a chemical component of the body. These chemical components of the body are commonly:

(1) receptors for neurotransmitters, autacoids or hormones;
(2) enzymes;
(3) membranes.

In the following text, drug/receptor interactions are described but similar principles apply to drug interaction with other biological targets – enzymes, uptake pumps and so on.

In the majority of cases this chemical interaction involves the reversible association of drug with receptor, based on a complementary relationship between the structure of the drug and the structure of the receptor.

The relationship between drug concentration and effect

The magnitude of the effect of a drug is usually related to its concentration at its site of action (within certain limits) in a smoothly graded manner. For

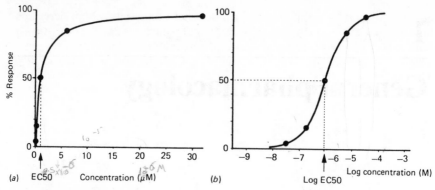

Figure 1.1 Relationship between drug concentration and effect: (a) response v.
concentration; (b) response v. log concentration (the same data are used in both graphs)

example, a piece of intestinal smooth muscle may shorten progressively as
the concentration of a spasmogenic drug is increased. The relationship
between the drug concentration and effect is generally hyperbolic (*Figure
1.1a*). For convenience, pharmacologists generally relate effect to the loga-
rithm of the drug concentration (*Figure 1.1b*), which results in log concen-
tration/effect curves that are sigmoid and contain a useful central portion
(between about 20% and 80% of the maximal effect) where effect is approximately linearly related to the log of the drug concentration.

EC'N' notation

The concentration (or dose) of a drug that evokes a biological effect equivalent to N% of the maximal effect is known as the EC'N' (ED'N'), for
example, EC50 means the concentration of drug evoking a half maximal
effect (*Figure 1.1a*).

Potency

The potency of a drug is a measure of the dilution in which it causes a
specified effect; thus a drug that evokes the specified effect when present in
great dilution is said to be highly potent.

Most commonly the specified effect used in assessment or comparison of
drug potencies is the half maximal effect, thus potency = 1/EC50. The rank
order of potency within a series of drugs is therefore the reverse of the rank
order of their EC50 values and is independent of the absolute magnitude of
their maximal effects. As drugs commonly have EC50 values in the µmol/l
range or less, a convenient way of expressing potency uses the pD_2 scale.
The pD_2 is defined as the negative $\log_{10}$ of the molar EC50 (*cf.* pH, pK_a).
(Strictly speaking, the pD_2 is the $-\log_{10}$ of the equilibrium dissociation
constant but for agonists this is not always easily measurable (*see* page 13).)

Sensitivity

This is the tissue or receptor equivalent of potency (*see above*). In other
words, potency is the property of the drug that describes how little of it is

needed. Sensitivity is the property of the responding system that describes how easily it responds to a drug. The units of measurement are the same in both cases – l/mol (dilution). Desensitization or loss of sensitivity represents a rightward shift of the dose/effect curve, not a reduction in the maximum. Thus in *Figure 1.9*, a shift from curve B to curve A is desensitization. A change from curve C to curve A is not (in fact, it is potentiation).

Selectivity

Selectivity is the central theme of pharmacology and is the phenomenon that allows drugs to be useful. No drug is specific – that is produces only one effect. Selectivity is the term used to describe the ability of a given dose of a drug to act on one system rather than on another. In quantitative terms, selectivity is expressed as the ratio

$$\frac{\text{potency at site A}}{\text{potency at site B}}$$

If site A is the location at which the desired action is mediated and site B that at which an undesired action occurs, then the selectivity ratio is equivalent to the therapeutic index (*see* pages 254 and 340).

Sometimes selectivity is used to describe properties of drugs within a group of drugs. Thus, the group of antagonists at β-adrenoceptors (**propranolol, atenolol**), are highly selective for β-adrenoceptors – that is, they act at β-adrenoceptors at concentrations several orders of magnitude lower than at any other receptor type. However, **propranolol** is sometimes described as a nonselective antagonist at β-adrenoceptors because it acts at subgroups of adrenoceptors, namely β_1- and β_2-adrenoceptors, at essentially the same concentration. **Atenolol**, on the other hand, is 10–100 times more potent at β_1- than at β_2-adrenoceptors and is sometimes described as a selective β-adrenoceptor antagonist.

Summation

Summation is the term used to describe the phenomenon in which two drugs acting together produce a predictable response. If a dose, 2x, of drug A produces the same response as a dose, 2y, of drug B, then summation of drug A and B is said to occur when the response to x + y is the same as that to either 2x or 2y.

This phenomenon occurs with full agonists acting at the same receptor.

It may appear to occur with drugs acting at different receptors and in functional antagonism (page 17) but in both the circumstances, it usually only applies over a narrow range of doses.

Theories of drug action

Drugs may be divided into two general classes on the basis of their mechanism of action:

(1) structurally nonspecific;
(2) structurally specific.

By structure we mean the distribution of charge within a molecule and the spatial distribution of these potential binding sites.

Structurally nonspecific drugs

Certain chemically dissimilar drugs can affect biological activity in a similar manner. The action of these drugs is not related to their precise three-dimensional structure. These drugs are said to be structurally nonspecific. It is the characteristic of structurally nonspecific drugs that:

(1) small (or even large) changes in structure have negligible effects on activity;
(2) they do not display stereoselectivity;
(3) drugs with widely different structure share a common pharmacological action.

The only example of structurally nonspecific drugs of pharmacological interest is the general anaesthetic agents. General anaesthesia may be brought about by a wide variety of chemically dissimilar compounds including inert gases (xenon), halogenated hydrocarbons (**halothane**), cyclic hydrocarbons (*cyclopropane*), ethers (diethyl ether), alcohols (ethanol), oxides of nitrogen (**nitrous oxide**).

The pharmacological activity of the general anaesthetic agents is not attributable to a common three-dimensional structure but rather to a physical property.

Figure 1.2 compares the potency of a range of anaesthetic agents having widely different structures with their lipid solubility (expressed as a partition coefficient). A close correlation exists implying that the drugs are general anaesthetic agents because they are lipophilic. The site of this lipid phase is discussed on page 245.

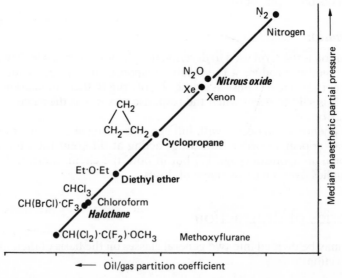

Figure 1.2 The high correlation in mice between potency as a general anaesthetic agent and oil/gas partition coefficient despite very varied structure (both scales are logarithmic)

Structurally specific drugs

Structurally specific drugs have the following characteristics:

(1) they produce their effects at low doses;
(2) minor changes in structure have major effects on activity;
(3) they commonly show stereoselectivity.

The pharmacological activity of structurally specific drugs results from an interaction between drug molecules and receptors, which have precise three-dimensional structures. Drug molecules must satisfy different structural requirements for each kind of receptor. The interaction between drug and receptor must be considered from two aspects:

(1) the distribution of charge within the molecule;
(2) the spatial distribution of these centres of charge.

Charge distribution

Structural components that convey centres of charge in drug molecules are ions and dipoles.

Ions – examples are weak acids and bases (which account for the vast majority of drugs) resulting in the charged $-NH_3^+$ and $-COO^-$ substituents. Note the importance of pH and pK. Less common are the quaternary nitrogen compounds $-NR_4^+$.

Dipoles – in a chemical bond between two atoms of different electronegativities the electron distribution will be uneven. The greater the difference in electronegativities the greater the dipole moment. Common atoms in drug molecules (and their receptors) in ascending order of electronegativity are H, P, C, S, N, Cl, O, F. Thus the $-OH$ group has a strong dipole moment, $-CH$ a weak moment.

The same principles must be applied to the structure of the drug target – revise the structures of proteins, sugars, lipids and nucleic acids.

The complementary structures of drug and receptor then result in the formation of various kinds of bond.

Polar bonds

Ion–ion bonds

This kind of bond has a strength of the same order as that of a covalent bond.

Ion–dipole, dipole–dipole

Such bonds are very common in drug interactions; they are weaker than ion–ion bonds.

Covalent bonds

The familiar covalent bond is unusual in drug/receptor interactions. Examples are the covalent bond formed in alkylation of the receptor by some cytotoxic drugs, and the phosphorylation of the cholinesterase enzyme. Since the process is irreversible, such bonds are relatively unimportant in therapeutics but are of importance in toxicology.

Hydrogen bonds

The hydrogen bond is an electrostatic attraction between a proton and the unshared electrons of an atom (usually O). It is a weak bond but of enormous biochemical importance – without it water would not exist as a liquid and it is the one bond that essentially determines the shape of proteins and nucleic acids. Only the hydrogen atom can be involved in such a bond because it possesses no inner electron shell, which would otherwise contribute a repulsive influence.

Common drug substitutents that may be involved in hydrogen bonding are —OH and —NH—.

Coordinate bonds

Chelates

This is a coordinate bond between electron donor atoms (commonly N, O and S) and a metal. Two or more atoms donate pairs of electrons holding the metal ion in a ring. Chelate formation is important in drugs used to treat metal poisoning (**desferrioxamine**), in receptor binding (the catechol group of agonists at adrenoceptors) and drug toxicity (the binding of tetracyclines with calcium).

Van der Waals forces

In neutral molecules (hydrocarbon chains, phenyl substituents), centres of positive and negative charge do not always correspond and the substituent behaves like a little magnet. Typical attraction might occur between a benzene ring of a drug and a benzene ring of an amino acid component of the receptor. The bond is highly dependent on very close proximity of the participating substituents.

Drug shape

The above summarizes why parts of molecules carry charge which determines how drugs can associate with their receptors. The other consideration is the shape that holds these centres of charge in a conformation that complements that of the receptor.

Many drug molecules are based on a rigid framework on which essential substituents are placed. Good examples are the phenanthrene structure of **morphine**, the steroid nucleus and the phenothiazine ring structure.

Exercise: Study the shape of the steroid nucleus. Compare the structures of oestradiol and testosterone.

Note how many neurotransmitters are flexible structures on which essential substituents are arranged. The neurotransmitter can then adopt different conformations thereby effecting neurotransmission at stereochemically different receptors.

Exercise: Write down the structures of acetylcholine (ACh) and 5-hydroxytryptamine (5-HT). Identify the important parts of the molecule that could be involved with receptor association. Note how these centres of charge can be arranged in different conformations.

When a flexible neurotransmitter can effect transmission at more than one receptor, more selective agonist activity can often be achieved by synthesizing stereochemically more rigid derivatives.

One such derivative may hold the essential components of the neurotransmitter in one fixed conformation, a different rigid analogue holding the same components in a different shape.

Compare the structures of ACh, nicotine and muscarine.

Isomerism

Optical isomerism

If the four substituents around a carbon atom differ, they can be arranged in one of two ways, which are mirror images of each other. If three of these substituents are involved in receptor binding, it is clear that if one of these conformations can associate with a rigid receptor, the other cannot (*Figure 1.3*).

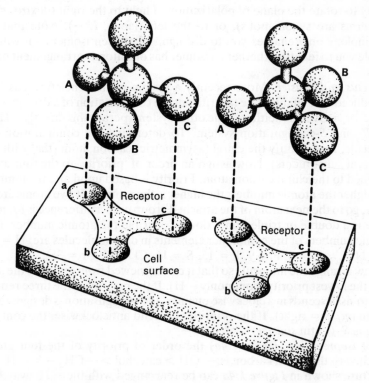

Figure 1.3 Failure of optical isomer to fit a 3-point binding site

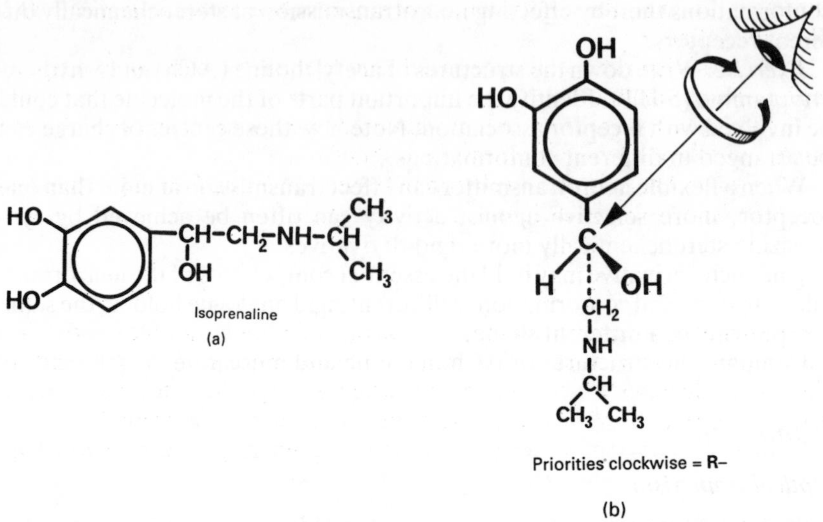

Priorities clockwise = R–

(b)

Figure 1.4 The conformation of isoprenaline: (a) structure of isoprenaline; (b) priorities clockwise = *R*-

Laevo and dextro. Such isomers were originally distinguished by their ability to rotate the plane of polarization of light to the right (dextro, *d*, +; the terms are synonymous), or to the left (laevo, *l*, −). Note that this terminology only enables you to distinguish between isomers – it will not enable you to identify whether an isomer has one atomic arrangement or the other.

Rectus and sinister. More recently a system of nomenclature has been introduced that enables one to write out the configuration of a drug given its name, or vice versa (neither of the other systems permit this directly). This is the *R*- and *S*-configuration system. To determine the configuration of a molecule, first identify the chiral (asymmetric) carbon atom (that with four different substituents). Now assign an order of 'priority' to the four atoms attached to the chiral carbon atom. Priority is based upon atomic number – the higher the atomic number, the higher is the priority. If two atoms are the same, go to the next atom of the attached group until a difference is found. If there is a double or triple bond, double or triple the atomic number. (The atomic numbers of the commoner elements in drug molecules are: H = 1, C = 6, N = 7, O = 8, F = 9, P = 15, S = 16, Cl = 17, Br = 35).

Now arrange the molecule so that it can be viewed from opposite the atom with the lowest priority (commonly —H). If the priority of the three remaining atoms descends in a clockwise manner, the configuration is designated *R*- (Latin *rectus* = right). If the priorities descend anticlockwise, the configuration is *S*- (Latin *sinister* = left).

For *isoprenaline* (*Figure 1.4a*) the order of priority of the four groups attached to the chiral carbon is: —OH > catechol > —CH$_2$— > —H. The structure shown in *Figure 1.4a* can be rearranged with the —H away from the eye (*Figure 1.4b*). The priorities will then be seen to fall in a clockwise direction – that is, the conformation of *isoprenaline* shown in *Figure 1.4a* is *R*-isoprenaline.

In fact, this isomer rotates polarized light to the left, so its full description is *R*-(−)-isoprenaline.

If a drug has more than one chiral centre (*ephedrine* has two), the *R/S* configuration at each centre must be defined.

Reminder: There is no correlation between the *R* and *S*, and (+) and (−) systems. They tell you different things about the molecule.

Cis–trans *isomerism*

Two pairs of similar substituents can be arranged about a double bond in one of two ways. When the same (or similar) substituents are on the same side of the bond, the isomer is designated *cis*, when on opposite sides, *trans*. Draw the two isomers of *stilboestrol*, and compare each with oestradiol.

Similar isomers can occur about a cyclopropane ring – *tranylcypromine*.

Preferred conformation

Although flexible molecules can theoretically exist in a wide range of conformations, a molecule is most stable in one preferred conformation. An indication of preferred conformation has been achieved by X-ray crystallography but nowadays can be computed.

Generally the preferred conformation of a drug is in a fully extended shape. The shape of *isoprenaline* as drawn in *Figure 1.4a* is extended. (An 'unfavoured' conformation would be with the side-chain rotated so that the amino group lies above the benzene ring). The long side-chain of a tricyclic antidepressive drug (page 224) would lie distant from the rings.

Steric hindrance

The substitution of a substituent (usually bulky) close to a critical part of a drug molecule can have a profound effect on the stability and/or pharmacology of a drug.

Such substitution may:

(1) render a drug resistant to enzymic breakdown (*cf.* ACh and methacholine; **benzylpenicillin** and **flucloxacillin**);
(2) turn a substrate for an enzyme into an enzyme inhibitor (*cf.* phenylethylamine and **phenelzine** or *tranylcypromine*);
(3) alter the selectivity of an agonist (*cf.* noradrenaline (NA) and *isoprenaline*);
(4) turn an agonist into an antagonist (*cf. adrenaline* and **propranolol** [the bulky substituent is the second benzene ring]; **morphine** and **naloxone**).

Chemical structure and drug disposition

Changes in drug structure alter the disposition of drugs as well as their pharmacodynamic properties. For example, the removal of the hydroxyl substituents from a catecholamine not only results in a drug that cannot interact directly with adrenoceptors but also results in a drug that can enter the central nervous system (CNS) easily (amphetamine). The quaternization of **atropine** not only restricts it to the periphery but also conveys some activity at nicotinic receptors.

Receptor mediation of drug effects

A drug receptor has two fundamental properties:

(1) the ability to recognize and bind or associate with certain structurally similar drug molecules;

(2) the ability to initiate a biological response when an appropriate drug molecule is associated with it.

Modern techniques of molecular biology have revealed the precise structures of many kinds of cell surface receptors. All are proteins and on the basis of their three-dimensional structure and function, they can be classified into two distinct groups – 'fast' and 'slow' receptors (*Figure 1.5*).

'Fast' receptors are part of transmembrane, ion-selective channels or ionophores. Binding of the drug to the receptor causes a conformational change in the ionophore that alters the permeability of the membrane to a particular ion (Na^+, Ca^{2+}, K^+, Cl^-).

'Slow' receptors have an amino acid sequence that includes seven highly lipophilic segments that are believed to be oriented in the cell membrane. Responses mediated through 'slow' receptors take longer to appear because the response is secondary to the activation or inhibition of an intracellular enzyme (e.g. adenylyl cyclase $\rightarrow$ cAMP; phospholipase C $\rightarrow$ inositol trisphosphate). The second messenger produced by the enzyme forms part of a cascade of intracellular events, usually leading to a change in the cytoplasmic Ca^{2+} concentration. 'Slow' receptors (recognition units) are linked to their enzymes (catalytic units) by a family of GTP-dependent proteins known as G-proteins (regulatory units).

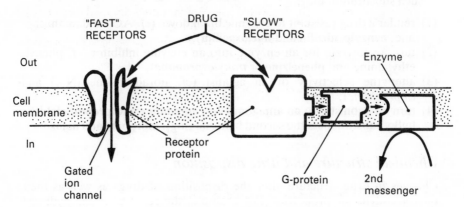

Figure 1.5 'Fast' and 'slow' receptors

Whether they are 'fast' or 'slow', drug receptors are in some ways analogous to the active centres of enzymes and the carriers of biological transport mechanisms (*Table 1.1*).

Table 1.1 Comparison of drug receptors with other biological binding sites

Biological binding site	Interaction	End effect
Drug receptor	Attachment of drug	Triggering of response
Active centre of enzyme	Attachment of substrate	Chemical alteration of substrate
Carrier molecule of transport mechanism	Attachment of substrate	Transport of substrate

Active and passive biological responses: agonists and antagonists

A drug-induced response from a living cell is active if a change in ongoing activity occurs even when the cell is isolated from all external biological control factors (neurotransmitters and hormones). Active responses may be either excitatory (depolarization of the membranes of excitable cells, muscle contraction, increased glandular secretion) or inhibitory (hyperpolarization of the membranes of excitable cells, muscle relaxation, reduced pacemaker frequency).

In contrast, passive responses are observed when a drug acts to remove the effects of some external biological factor regulating cellular function.

A drug that induces an active response by activating receptors is known as an agonist, whether the response is an increase or decrease in cellular activity. Some drugs behave like agonists but act through an intermediary and do not themselves activate the receptor responsible for the response. They are commonly referred to as indirectly acting agonists (for example, tyramine, page 99).

Of the drugs that attach to a particular receptor site:

(1) agonists form a drug/receptor complex that triggers an active response from the cell;
(2) antagonists form a drug/receptor complex that does not evoke an active response from the cell. Antagonists simply prevent attachment of agonists to the receptor. The response to the antagonist is therefore passive – blockade of the effects of an agonist.

The binding of drugs to receptor sites

The binding of drugs to their receptor sites can be described in terms of the law of mass action:

$$\text{drug} + \text{receptor} \underset{k_{-1}}{\overset{k_1}{\rightleftharpoons}} \text{drug/receptor complex}$$

Let initial molar concentration of drug $= [D]$

Let initial (that is total) concentration of receptors $= R$

When a drug is added to the system the initial concentration of the drug/receptor complex is zero but with time (progress of the reaction) rises towards an equilibrium level. What are the concentrations of each of the reactants when the reaction is at equilibrium?

Let us assume that:

(1) the drug is present in such excess that its concentration is not significantly reduced by maximal formation of the drug/receptor complex;
(2) one molecule of drug combines with one molecule of receptor;
(3) the concentration of receptor molecules combined with the drug at equilibrium is r.

Then, at equilibrium:

Molar concentration of free drug $= [D]$
Concentration of occupied receptors $= r$
Concentration of unoccupied receptors $= R-r$
The rate of the forward reaction $= k_1 [D] (R-r)$

where $k_1 =$ association rate constant.

The rate of the back reaction $= k_{-1} r$

where $k_{-1} =$ dissociation rate constant.

When equilibrium is reached these two rates are equal:

$$k_1 [D] (R-r) = k_{-1}r$$

Rearranging:

$$k_{-1}/k_1 = K_d = [D] (R-r)/r \tag{1.1}$$

where K_d is known as the equilibrium dissociation constant.

The equation is often rearranged and presented in terms of receptor occupation:

$$r = [D].R/(K_d + [D])$$

Both of these are equations for a rectangular hyperbola, that is, a curve relating two variables (in the case of equation 1.1, $[D]$ and $(R-r)/r$) that vary in such a way that their product (K_d) is constant, (noting that R is constant as well). All rectangular hyperbolae can in fact be described by just two values:

(1) the maximal value of the dependent variable (r)
(2) a constant, called the location parameter, that fixes the position of the curve on the axis of the independent variable ($[D]$).

In this case, the maximal value that r can have is R, when all the receptors are occupied. The value of the location parameter is K_d, the equilibrium dissociation constant, which has the same units as $[D]$, that is, those of concentration: mol/l.

Some pharmacologists use the equilibrium association constant or 'affinity' instead of the dissociation constant. This term is simply the reciprocal of K_d.

$$K_a = 1/K_d = r/([D] (R-r))$$

The units of K_a are l/mol (dilution rather than concentration).

It can easily be shown that K_d is the concentration of drug ($[D]$) that causes half the receptors to be occupied, that is, when $r = R/2$.

The triggering of responses by agonists: modern receptor occupancy theory

Our knowledge of the mechanism by which an agonist triggers an active biological response is still incomplete. Modern receptor occupancy theories propose that drugs have a property that governs their ability to trigger an active biological response once they have combined with a receptor. Different terms for this property have been used in the past but the most useful term now is 'intrinsic efficacy'.

It is envisaged that agonist drugs with high intrinsic efficacy can evoke the maximal effect of which the biological system is capable. Such drugs are known as full agonists and may be able to elicit the maximum possible effect without occupying all the receptors. In such circumstances the receptors not occupied by the drug are known as 'spare receptors' or 'receptor reserve'.

An agonist drug with low intrinsic efficacy cannot evoke the maximal response of which the biological system is capable, despite occupying all available receptors. An agonist drug of this kind is known as a partial agonist. By competing for the same receptors, a partial agonist can antagonize a full agonist. Partial agonists that are therapeutically exploited include those acting at opioid receptors (page 235).

Pure antagonists have zero intrinsic efficacy.

The process by which an agonist triggers a response can be envisaged as a two-step process, the first being the binding of the drug to the receptors, governed by the concentration of the drug and its equilibrium dissociation constant. The second step is transduction of this binding into a response from the tissue, depending upon the number of receptors occupied and the intrinsic efficacy of the drug.

The modern usage of the term 'intrinsic activity' should not be confused with intrinsic efficacy. Intrinsic activity is used simply to describe the maximal effect a partial agonist can produce as a fraction (or %) of the theoretical maximum that can be induced via a particular kind of receptor. Thus in *Figure 1.6*, if drug A is a full agonist (intrinsic activity of 100%), drug B has an intrinsic activity of 60%.

Although concentration/response curves usually have the same shape as concentration/binding curves (that is, hyperbolic) the positions of the curves on the concentration axis differ. This is because the location parameter of the concentration/response curve (the potency of the drug) is determined by two factors:

(1) the K_d;
(2) the intrinsic efficacy.

A drug can therefore be potent either because it has a low K_d or because it has a high intrinsic efficacy.

Clinical or therapeutic efficacy, often abbreviated to 'efficacy', describes the ability of a treatment to effect a 'cure' in a patient. The term must not be confused with 'intrinsic efficacy'.

Antagonism

Antagonism is the name given to the interaction between two drugs when the biological effect of the two drugs together is smaller than the expected

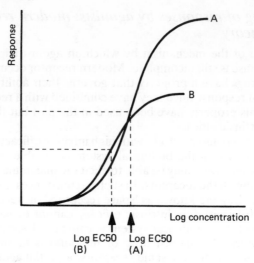

Figure 1.6 Drug B is more potent than drug A but has lower intrinsic activity

sum of their individual effects.

The many mechanisms by which antagonism can occur may be divided into two principal kinds:

(1) where the concentration of agonist at its site of action is reduced by the antagonist (it alters agonist disposition, pharmacokinetic antagonism, page 39);

(2) where the concentration of agonist at its site of action is not reduced by the antagonist. This kind (pharmacodynamic antagonism) may be due to direct or indirect mechanisms.

Direct mechanisms of pharmacodynamic antagonism

The agonist and antagonist have the same receptors. Antagonists, by attachment to the receptors themselves, prevent attachment of agonist molecules to the receptors. There are two main kinds of pharmacodynamic antagonism: competitive and noncompetitive.

Competitive antagonism

The agonist and antagonist compete for the same receptors. Both agents combine with the receptor in a readily reversible fashion, so the proportion of receptors occupied by each agent at equilibrium is related to their relative concentrations and their equilibrium dissociation constants. The proportion of receptors occupied by the competitive antagonist at equilibrium can be reduced by increasing the concentration of agonist. This means that, in the continued presence of the antagonist, the same response can be achieved by providing a higher concentration of agonist.

The effects of a competitive antagonist on the shape and position of the log concentration against effect curve of an agonist are shown in *Figure 1.7*. Increasing the concentration of antagonist causes progressive parallel shifts of the log concentration effect curve of the agonist to the right along the log

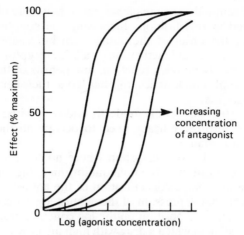

Figure 1.7 Competitive antagonism

concentration axis. The slope of the curve is unchanged and the maximal effect is undiminished.

The magnitude of the antagonism is expressed as the antilog of the rightward displacement of the curve: that is, the equieffective agonist concentration (or dose) ratio.

The increment in shift is a simple function of the increment in competitive antagonist concentration.

Competitive antagonism is sometimes described as 'surmountable' antagonism, a term that implies both that the antagonist dissociates from the receptors and that the full maximal response can be restored. However, note that even when the maximal response has been restored by increasing the concentration of agonist (that is the antagonism has been 'surmounted') the antagonism is still present and its extent can be expressed by the increased concentration of agonist needed to cause the same response as in the absence of antagonist.

Examples of competitive antagonism include **atropine** antagonism of ACh at muscarinic cholinoceptors; **tamoxifen** antagonism of oestradiol at oestrogen receptors; **naloxone** antagonism of *diamorphine* at opioid receptors.

Measuring potency is more difficult for a competitive antagonist than for an agonist as antagonists do not cause responses. However potency (*see* page 2) is still a dilution and the 'standard effect' is the rightward shift in the agonist concentration/effect curve (equieffective concentration or dose ratio). The pA scale for expressing the potency of antagonists is analogous to the pD_2 scale and the pA_2 is defined as the negative $\log_{10}$ of the molar concentration of antagonist that causes a two-fold rightward shift of the agonist concentration/effect curve (that is, a dose ratio of two). Under certain circumstances the pA_2 is the $\log_{10}$ of the K_d for the antagonist.

Noncompetitive antagonism

Again the agonist and antagonist occupy the same receptors but in this case the antagonist forms a chemical (usually covalent) bond with the receptor that is not easily disrupted. As time passes, more and more of the receptors become inactivated in this fashion. Increasing the concentration of the agonist may delay the onset of the antagonism but cannot prevent the eventual outcome – the total inactivation of all the receptors.

As there is effectively no back reaction, antagonists of this kind do not follow ordinary equilibrium kinetics; this has led to their being called 'nonequilibrium' antagonists.

In a biological system that is only modestly endowed with receptors, even agonists with high intrinsic efficacy need to occupy all the receptors to produce a maximal response.

Figure 1.8a shows a biological system where no spare receptors exist. Increasing the concentration of the nonequilibrium antagonist (or increasing exposure time to a single concentration of the antagonist) results in a progressive proportional depression of the agonist log concentration/effect curve, without changing its position on the log concentration axis.

However, in a system in which a drug with high intrinsic efficacy can elicit a maximal response when occupying only a small fraction of the receptors, nonequilibrium antagonists cause a parallel, rightward shift of the curve that cannot be reversed by even prolonged washing. This is eventually followed by depression of the maximum, once the 'spare' receptors have been inactivated (*Figure 1.8b*). This behaviour gives the illusion of nonequilibrium antagonists being competitive at first but then becoming noncompetitive.

Providing no spare receptors are available, a noncompetitive antagonist reduces the maximal response that can be attained, no matter what agonist concentration is used. The antagonism is therefore said to be 'insurmountable'. The reversibility of noncompetitive antagonism depends on the kind of chemical bond that is formed between the receptor and the antagonist. Some noncompetitive antagonists can be removed from the receptor by

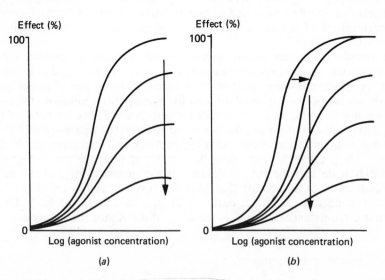

Figure 1.8 Noncompetitive antagonism: (a) biological system with no spare receptors; (b) biological system having spare receptors

prolonged washing or the use of a chemical reactivator. Other noncompetitive antagonists have truly irreversible actions, for example: **phenoxybenzamine** at α-adrenoceptors.

No convenient scale exists for expressing the potency of noncompetitive antagonists as so many patterns of antagonism exist.

Indirect mechanisms of pharmacodynamic antagonism

The agonist acts indirectly to cause the release of or to potentiate a second agent – this second agent acting as the final mediator of the observed response. The antagonist (which can be of the competitive or noncompetitive kind) occupies the same receptor as the mediator.

Examples of indirect antagonism include: **atropine** antagonism of nicotine on the guinea pig ileum (contraction mediated by ACh released from postganglionic parasympathetic nerves); **propranolol** antagonism of tyramine on the isolated heart (stimulation mediated by NA released from postganglionic sympathetic nerves).

Functional antagonism

This is the term applied to the situation in which two different agonists evoke opposing responses from a single biological system by activating different receptors. For example, one agonist causes active contraction of a piece of smooth muscle and a second agonist causes active relaxation. If two such agonists are administered together then the net response will be smaller than either of their individual effects.

The term 'antagonism' may be a misnomer since the phenomenon could well represent the algebraic sum of the individual agonist actions and, if so, would fall outside the definition of antagonism just provided. Examples of functional 'antagonism' include: reversal of histamine-induced contraction of bronchial smooth muscle by **salbutamol**; reversal of vasodilatation induced by ACh by *adrenaline*.

Identification and classification of drug receptors

Major receptor types are usually easily identifiable and are classified in terms of the transmitter they recognize (ACh acts at cholinoceptors, NA acts at adrenoceptors). However, it often appears that major receptor groups comprise a number of subgroups (muscarinic and nicotinic cholinoceptors, α- and β-adrenoceptors). The existence of such subgroups is asserted on the observation of two or more rank orders of potency when a selection of structurally related drugs is tested on different systems.

Such subclassifications are justified only if potentially distorting influences have been eliminated so that pharmacological differences are not erroneously assigned to receptor differences when in fact such factors as differential metabolism may be sufficient to explain the selectivities of the drugs. Sometimes selective antagonists exist which help in the confirmation of receptor classification.

Examples of drug receptors that have been identified in this way are presented in *Table 1.2*.

Table 1.2 Drug receptors

Receptor designation	Cross reference
Skeletal muscle nicotinic cholinoceptor	*Table 2.2*
Neural tissue nicotinic cholinoceptor	*Table 2.4*
M_1- and M_3-muscarinic cholinoceptors	*Table 2.6*
α_1- and α_2-adrenoceptors	*Table 2.11*
β_1- and β_2-adrenoceptors	*Table 2.13*
H_1 and H_2 histamine receptors	*Table 4.16*
5-HT_2 receptors	Page 197
PG receptors	*Tables 4.18* and *4.19*
Opioid receptors	Page 232

Potentiation

This is the phenomenon in which one drug (usually devoid of activity itself) makes another drug more potent. In *Figure 1.9*, curve B represents potentiation, whereas curve C does not. Potentiation is measured as the leftward shift in the log concentration/effect curve or equieffective concentration (or dose) ratio.

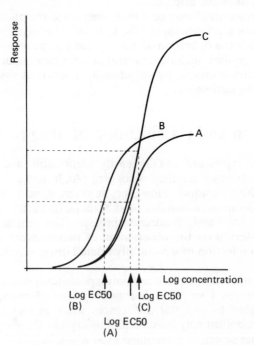

Figure 1.9 A change from curve A to curve B represents potentiation; to curve C does not

Adverse effects of drugs

Because drugs are not the 'specifics' sought by the ancient mind, the risk of adverse effects is inseparable from their therapeutic use.

Incidence

In hospital practice, adverse effects of drugs (not including acute poisoning *qv.*) are responsible for 3% of admissions to acute care beds (0.3% to all beds), occur in 10–20% of patients, prolong hospital stay in 2–10% of patients in acute medical beds and may be responsible for 0.1% of deaths in medical wards.

In general practice, adverse effects of drugs are responsible for 2–3% of consultations and may occur in up to 5% of patients.

Predisposing factors

Adverse effects of drugs occur most often in female patients aged over 60 or under 1 month, with a previous history of adverse drug reaction, or hepatic disease or renal disease.

Systems affected

The bodily systems or functions most often adversely affected by a drug reaction are the gut, skin, mental alertness and plasma K^+ concentration.

Drugs responsible

The drugs most commonly responsible for adverse drug reactions vary with the practical setting (occurring in hospital, causing admission, on death certificates) but include: antibiotics, anticoagulant drugs, antihypertensive drugs, *chloramphenicol*, **digoxin**, diuretic drugs, glucocorticoids, insulin, K^+-salts, NSAIDs, opioids, tranquillizers and **warfarin**.

Definitions

Adverse drug reaction

An adverse drug reaction is a harmful, or seriously unpleasant, effect occurring at a dose intended for therapeutic (prophylactic or diagnostic) effect and that calls for reduction of dose or withdrawal of the drug and/or forecasts hazard from future administration.

Causation

The features of an adverse drug reaction that suggest a cause and effect relationship between the drug administration and the adverse reaction are:

(1) the time sequence between drug taking and occurrence of the adverse reaction is reasonable;

(2) the reaction corresponds to the known pharmacology of the drug;
(3) the reaction ceases on stopping the drug;
(4) the reaction returns on restarting the drug.

Secondary adverse effects

These form a subset of adverse drug reactions that have an indirect causation.

Examples:
Superinfection (antibiotic associated colitis, AAC) under the conditions of altered bowel flora due to a broad spectrum antibacterial drug.
Vitamin K deficiency due to an altered bowel flora after a broad spectrum antibacterial drug.
Digoxin intolerance in hypokalaemia due to a diuretic drug.

Adverse drug event

In epidemiological and drug surveillance studies, an adverse drug 'event' is any harmful incident occurring during drug treatment, whether or not believed to be caused by the drug.

Side-effect

A side-effect is an unwanted but unavoidable consequence of drug administration (less harmful or unpleasant than an adverse drug reaction) arising because the unwanted action is just as integral as the therapeutic effect to the properties of the drug.

Examples:
Sedation due to *phenobarbitone* in the treatment of epilepsy.
Vomiting due to **digoxin** in the treatment of atrial fibrillation.
Vomiting due to **morphine** in the treatment of pain.
Hypokalaemia due to a diuretic drug in the treatment of oedema.

Toxic effect

A toxic effect is one that occurs by direct action upon the cells by which the effect is expressed, at high dosage, and produces tissue damage.

Examples:
Paracetamol overdosage causing liver damage.
Gentamicin overdosage kills cochlear hair cells.

Intolerance

Intolerance implies a low dose threshold (or high sensitivity) in the production of the normal pharmacological action of the drug.

Idiosyncrasy

Idiosyncracy implies an individual patient's inherent qualitatively abnormal reaction to a drug (usually due to genetic abnormality).

In some cases the adverse effects of drug treatment arise when there is an inappropriate combination of drugs (*see* Adverse drug interactions, page 37).

Classification

Two kinds of adverse drug reaction are recognizable (*see Table 1.3*).

Table 1.3 Distinction between the two kinds of adverse drug reaction

Label	Type A Augmented Anticipatable	Type B Bizarre (Idiosyncrasy)
Predictability	Good	Poor
Dose-dependency	Usual	Uncommon
Potential reactors	Every recipient	Only a fraction of recipients
Morbidity	High	Low
Mortality	Low	High
Relative incidence	75–80%	20–25%

Predictability refers to that arising from both:

(1) the doctor's knowledge of the pharmacology and toxicology of a drug;
(2) the results of preclinical animal testing during drug development.

Type A: Predictable adverse effects

The adverse effect is anticipatable; that is predictable from the pharmacology of the drug, the size of the dose and the pathology of the patient.

Examples:
Postural hypotension caused by the loop diuretics is a manifestation of salt and water depletion arising from an excess of the desired or therapeutic effect.

AV blockade caused by **digoxin** may imperil a patient with disease of the conducting pathways of the heart yet it is the basis of the therapeutic action in atrial fibrillation.

The adverse effect is an augmentation of the normal effects of the drug. A common reason for augmentation is overdosage. This may be caused by the administration of an excessive amount by accident or design. In other circumstances the dose is standard but the elimination processes are impaired or the patient is particularly sensitive.

Overdosage

This may be accidental, as when a child receives tablets intended for an adult, or when a doctor, pharmacist or nurse makes an error in prescribing, dispensing or administration. The consequences for the recipient and for the professional reputations of those responsible may be very serious.

Intolerance due to impaired elimination

Standard doses produce an excessive concentration at the site of action. The renal or hepatic elimination of drugs may be impaired.

Renal. The GFR is disproportionately low in the newborn baby, particularly when delivered very early preterm (before 28 weeks in gestational age or below 1 kg in weight). The GFR is reduced by advanced cardiac failure, hypothyroidism, old age and shock. All these states predispose to accidental overdosage with water soluble drugs if the prescriber does not anticipate the problem.

Examples:
Drugs predominantly eliminated by the kidney (aminoglycoside antibiotics, **digoxin**).
Drugs that produce pharmacologically active metabolites (**carbamazepine, diazepam**, *hydralazine, isosorbide dinitrate*, **metronidazole**).
Shock reduces subcutaneous perfusion with blood with the inevitable distortions of drug absorption after sc administration.

Hepatic. Impaired hepatic perfusion (congestive heart failure) or advanced hepatocellular disease (cells lost, sick or by-passed) can also lead to accidental overdosage because of impaired drug metabolizing capacity for fat soluble drugs. Hypoalbuminaemia impairs the drug-binding capacity of plasma. In thyroid disease the metabolic drug clearance parallels the BMR.

Examples:
Drugs susceptible to extensive first pass metabolism (*see* page 327) show an increased bioavailability (**lignocaine, morphine** and **propranolol**).
More slowly metabolized drugs show an increased $t_\frac{1}{2}$ (**diazepam**, *phenobarbitone* and *theophylline*).

Intolerance due to increased sensitivity

A standard dose produces a standard concentration at the site of action but this produces an excessive response. This arises when the pathology of a patient confers special sensitivity to adverse drug effects.

Examples:
Propranolol at conventional dosage seriously aggravates airway obstruction in asthma, which is also characterized by hyper-reactivity to cholinomimetics.
Gentamicin aggravates muscle weakness in myasthenia gravis.
Morphine causes a life-threatening retention of secretions in severe chronic bronchitis.
Potassium depletion confers excessive sensitivity to **digoxin**.
In encephalopathy all CNS depressants produce coma.
A malfunctioning respiratory centre (raised intracranial pressure, severe pulmonary insufficiency) produces intolerance to all CNS depressant drugs.
Myocardial infarction predisposes to dysrhythmias with **digoxin** and sympathomimetic drugs.
Infectious mononucleosis predisposes to rash with **ampicillin**.
Prostatic enlargement predisposes to urinary retention with diuretic drugs, sympathomimetic agents or antagonists at muscarinic cholinoceptors.

Pain predisposes to confusion when a sedative is administered without an analgesic agent.

Type B: Unpredictable adverse effects

The patient may be intolerant because he/she is hypersensitive (allergic) or may have a genetically determined abnormal response (idiosyncrasy). The adverse effect may be one factor only in a causal sequence, as in teratogenesis, or the cause/effect link may be obscured by a long interval, as in carcinogenesis.

Hypersensitivity

The allergic patient may have received the drug before without the prescriber's knowledge and may have produced tissue sensitizing (reaginic) IgE antibodies (*see* Allergically determined hypersensitivity to drugs, page 24). Even a single subsequent dose of the drug can then result in an adverse effect ranging from mild urticaria to bronchospasm and to acute circulatory collapse (anaphylactic shock). There may be cross hypersensitivity to closely related drugs (different penicillins) or more distantly related drugs (cephalosporins and penicillins).

Hypersensitivity may have a cellular basis as in the systemic lupus erythematosus-like syndrome that sometimes develops after exposure to *hydralazine*. Although not a predictable consequence of excessive dosage, the risk is dose related and there is also a genetic predisposition (slow acetylator status).

Allergic causation

The features of an adverse drug reaction that suggest an allergic cause are:

(1) the symptomatology does not correlate with the known pharmacological properties of the drug;
(2) there is no graded dose/effect relationship;
(3) the symptomatology resembles classic protein allergy;
(4) an induction period is required on primary exposure but not re-exposure;
(5) the reaction disappears on cessation of drug exposure; it reappears on re-exposure to a small dose;
(6) it occurs in only a minority of recipients;
(7) desensitization may be possible.

Further actions

Avoid further use of the causative drug and its congeners. Make an appropriate and obvious entry on the patient's case folder. Tell the patient to tell other prescribers of his hypersensitivity.

Idiosyncrasy

Genetically determined adverse effects (*see* Pharmacogenetics, page 27) vary in frequency with different racial groups. The possibility of detection of the patient's idiosyncracy by a screening test sometimes exists (atypical cholinesterase, induction of aminolaevulinic acid synthetase, slow acetylator status) but the cost and delay in treatment are unacceptable except in patients believed to be particularly at risk.

Teratogenesis

Adverse effects on the embryo (*see* Developmental toxicity, page 33) are seldom so characteristic or so frequent as with thalidomide. More typical is an increase in the incidence of common congenital abnormalities, as reported with anticonvulsant drugs. Dietary deficiency, other drugs and genetic factors probably all contribute to the outcome.

Carcinogenesis

The incidence of many malignant tumours is influenced by reproductive history. Carcinoma of breast, for example, is more common in women who married late, bore no children and had a late menopause. It is very likely therefore that drugs that modify reproductive function (the contraceptive steroids) will also alter the incidence of tumours of the reproductive organs. History gives one glaring example – carcinoma of the vagina in the teenage offspring of mothers given large doses of exogenous oestrogens in early pregnancy. Long-term epidemiological studies will no doubt reveal less dramatic changes in the incidence of tumours.

Antineoplastic drugs and immunosuppressant drugs used to prevent transplant rejection increase the risk of developing malignant tumours. The detection of adverse effects that can be greatly delayed demands prolonged surveillance of patients at risk.

Intolerance due to low efficiency of disposal occurs under 1 month of age to *chloramphenicol* (grey baby syndrome) and over 65 years of age to *chlorpropamide*, and tricyclic antidepressives.

Advice

Safety lies in knowledge of both the drug and the disease and an awareness of the possibilities. The incidence and severity of adverse drug reactions can be dramatically reduced by the exercise of skill in the choice and use of drugs by knowledgeable prescribers.

Allergically determined hypersensitivity to drugs

Allergy is characterized by a group of qualitatively similar unusual responses involving an antigen/antibody reaction, after a previous uneventful exposure of which the patient may be unaware. Allergy commonly affects the skin, respiratory tract, gut, blood cells and blood vessels as target organs.

Examples:
Anaphylactic reaction to a penicillin.
Haemolytic anaemia due to *methyldopa.*

Patients with a history of allergic disease (*see below*) develop drug allergy more readily than others. Patients with one allergically based adverse drug reaction are about four times more likely to have another than those with none.

Production of the sensitized state of the patient

In most cases the drug molecules themselves are too small to induce antibody formation. However, these small molecules or their metabolites behave as haptens, that is they bind covalently to body proteins and these complexes then function as antigens inducing the formation of antibodies directed against the particular hapten and its close chemical relatives.

The sensitization involves the engulfing and detection of the hapten/protein complex by mononuclear cells located in the lymphoreticular organs (thymus, spleen, bone marrow, lymphoid tissue) close to the site of exposure to the antigen. The antigen is presented to, and is recognized as foreign by, a T-lymphocyte that multiplies to produce a memory clone of T-helper lymphocytes and that programmes the proliferation and differentiation of B-lymphocytes into plasma cells committed to the production of an antibody specific for the hapten.

Classification

Allergy-based diseases are classified mechanistically into four kinds, of which three commonly underlie allergic drug reactions.

Type I: Immediate/anaphylactic

The antibody responsible for immediate hypersensitivity is an IgE (or reagin). Atopy is an inherited predisposition to exaggerated development of immunoglobulin E (IgE) antibody in response to various antigens (allergens), such as the large MW constituents of house-dust, dandruff, liquorice, tomato, cow's milk and egg white. A previous medical history of allergic diseases (seasonal rhinitis, eczema, food allergy, asthma of early onset) and a family history of any of these disorders suggest atopy.

The Fc region of IgE has a high affinity for cell surface receptors on circulating basophil leucocytes or tissue mast cells. Hence IgE molecules are cleared from the circulation by being bound to these cells. This results in cellular sensitization that shows itself when subsequent exposure to the antigen results in the antigen becoming bound to the IgE, initiating the release of chemical mediators of tissue anaphylaxis from the basophils or mast cells (*Figure 1.10*).

The release of chemical mediators from storage granules (degranulation) is a consequence of the allergen/IgE combination making the membrane more permeable to Ca^{2+}. This triggers the release of intracellular Ca^{2+} (modulated by cAMP concentrations) and the aggregation of microtubules results in the movement of granules to the membrane and extrusion of preformed mediators (histamine, chemotactic factors, lysosomal enzymes) and the synthesis of other mediators (kinins, arachidonic acid derived PGs and especially LTs). These mediators produce tissue anaphylaxis by evoking:

(1) local arteriolar vasodilatation;
(2) increased protein permeability of postcapillary venules and oedema;
(3) contraction of smooth muscle (other than vascular);
(4) secretion from mucosal glands;
(5) leucocyte infiltration;
(6) sensitization and irritation of afferent nerves.

Because the antibody is bound, the localization of the tissue anaphylaxis developing in response to an initially free antigen depends upon the route of administration of the hapten. Localized reactions produce urticaria in the skin and extrinsic asthma in the lungs. Systemic administration results in anaphylactic shock. This commonly develops within minutes and lasts about 2 h.

Penicillins and cephalosporins are common haptens but a huge variety of other drugs produce these reactions.

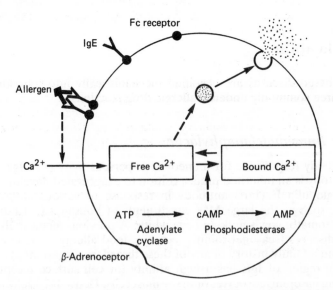

Figure 1.10 Influences upon the mast cell in tissue anaphylaxis and sites of drug action

Treatment of anaphylactic shock

Reduction of the action of some mediators:

(1) by functional antagonism with *adrenaline* 0.5–1 mg im (0.5–1 ml of 1 mg/ml or 1 in 1000), repeated at 3 min then every 10 min – this combats, especially, the increased protein permeability of postcapillary venules;
(2) by competitive antagonism of histamine with *chlorpheniramine* 10 mg iv.

Prevention of the formation of some mediators is best achieved with *hydrocortisone sodium succinate* 100 mg im/iv.

Type II: Cytolytic/autoallergy

Hapten binds to a cellular surface protein so the allergen is tissue bound and the IgG and IgM antibodies circulate. When antibodies attach to cell-bound drug, complement is fixed and lysis occurs.

Examples:
Granulocytopenia – *chloramphenicol*, sulphonamides, thioamides and gold compounds.
Thrombocytopenia – *quinidine* and *quinine*, gold compounds and sulphonamides.
Haemolysis – *methyldopa* and penicillins and cephalosporins.
Aplastic anaemia – gold compounds.
Hepatitis and cholestatic jaundice – **carbimazole** and **chlorpromazine.**
Collagen disease-like lupus erythematosus – *hydralazine* and *procainamide*.

Type III: Complex mediated

Large complexes form from the binding of soluble antigen to circulating IgG antibodies. These deposit in vascular endothelium, activate complement and produce a vasculitis resembling serum sickness. This is a mechanism in sulphonamide and penicillin allergies.

Type IV: Delayed/cell mediated

Both the allergen and the antibody are tissue bound. Killer T-cells are activated and tissue cell death is induced. This mechanism is probably responsible for some adverse skin reactions to drugs (general toxic erythema, fixed drug eruption), a common reaction to penicillins, aminoglycosides, local anaesthetics or antihistamines applied to the skin.

Genetically determined idiosyncracy to drugs (pharmacogenetics)

When the adverse effect is part of the drug's normal (but not necessarily its main) action, its size, and therefore severity, depends on the dose.

However, the response is neither qualitatively nor quantitatively unusual. Consequently the treated population displays a unimodal frequency distribution of the toxic response. All individuals will show the response if given enough of the drug so that when the number of individuals showing toxicity (frequency) is plotted against the minimum toxic dose, a smooth, continuous, bell-shaped curve, with a single peak (mode) is obtained (*Figure 1.11a*). This kind of distribution arises because sensitivity to the drug is the result of the expression of many genes (multifactorial).

When an abnormal reaction to a drug is determined by the expression of a

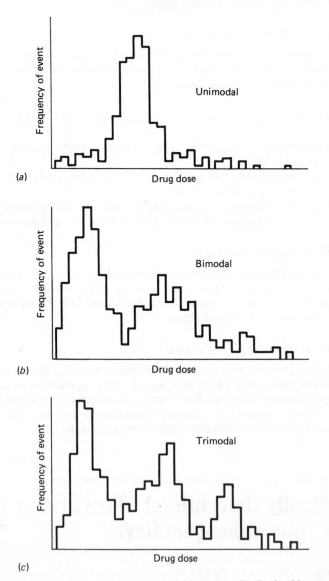

Figure 1.11 Typical uni-, bi- and trimodal frequency distribution histograms

single allele (the synthesis of an atypical enzyme) the frequency distribution curve is discontinuous, that is, multimodal (*Figures 1.11b* and *1.11c*), the phenotype of each individual depending upon the genetic contributions of the parents.

Autosomal recessive (Figure 1.12)

Isoniazid acetylation

In North America and Europe approximately half of the population inactivate **isoniazid** slowly. In other populations the figure may be as low as 20% or as high as 90%. This is due to heterogeneity in the gene responsible for directing the synthesis of hepatic *N*-acetyltransferase. The atypical enzyme acetylates **isoniazid** more slowly than the normal enzyme. There are three possible genotypes – those homozygous (rapid/rapid), those heterozygous (slow/rapid) and those homozygous (slow/slow). These genotypes give rise to two phenotypes – rapid acetylators and slow acetylators (*Figure 1.12*). When given to slow acetylators at dose rates suitable for rapid acetylators, **isoniazid** accumulates to toxic concentrations, often resulting in peripheral neuropathy. Other drugs that are acetylated and that therefore accumulate in patients with the atypical acetylation enzyme include *hydralazine*, **phenelzine**, *sulphasalazine*, *dapsone*, *nitrazepam* and *procainamide*.

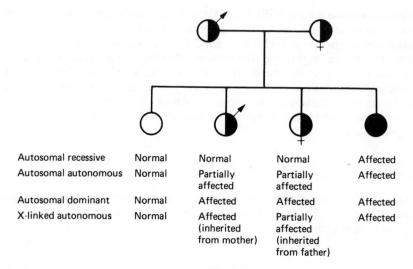

Autosomal recessive	Normal	Normal	Normal	Affected
Autosomal autonomous	Normal	Partially affected	Partially affected	Affected
Autosomal dominant	Normal	Affected	Affected	Affected
X-linked autonomous	Normal	Affected (inherited from mother)	Partially affected (inherited from father)	Affected

Genotype:

O Normal - normal (homozygous for normal gene)

● Affected - affected (homozygous for affected gene)

◑ Normal - affected
   or   } (heterozygous for affected gene)
Affected - normal

Figure 1.12 Typical distribution of phenotype with genotype under various modes of inheritance

Hereditary methaemoglobinaemia

In hereditary methaemoglobinaemia, NADH methaemoglobin reductase is deficient. This enzyme does not of itself inactivate any drugs but it is the main route for regenerating haemoglobin from methaemoglobin (*see Figure 1.13*). Consequently the methaemoglobinaemia produced by certain oxidizing drugs (nitrites, nitrates, *prilocaine*, sulphonamides) is severe and prolonged in individuals with this condition. Methylene blue is useful as a reducing agent to regenerate haemoglobin.

Impaired drug hydroxylation

Debrisoquine hydroxylation is impaired in about 9% of people in the UK (20–90% in some other populations). A hepatic mono-oxygenase is deficient or defective. Adverse effects may arise from the loss of metabolizing capacity or the altered profile of metabolites. Other drugs affected include *nortryptyline*, **phenytoin** and **tolbutamide**.

Autosomal autonomous (Figure 1.12)

Suxamethonium apnoea

Suxamethonium occasionally (1:2500) produces unduly prolonged respiratory muscle paralysis, necessitating artificial ventilation, as there are atypical forms of the enzyme cholinesterase (ChE). Atypical ChE is due to an abnormality in a single gene. In heterozygotes the trait is partially expressed so that there are individuals with intermediate ChE activities (trimodal frequency distribution curve, *Figure 1.11c*). The 'dibucaine' test (page 91) identifies individuals with the atypical form of ChE – the enzyme in blood from normal subjects is more easily inhibited by cinchocaine than is the atypical enzyme.

Steroid glaucoma

Topical ophthalmic glucocorticoids produce an abnormally large intraocular pressure rise in 1:75 of patients, who have a high incidence of family history of wide angle glaucoma.

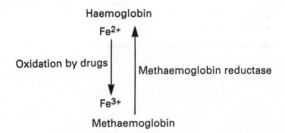

Figure 1.13 Modulation of the balance between haemoglobin and methaemoglobin

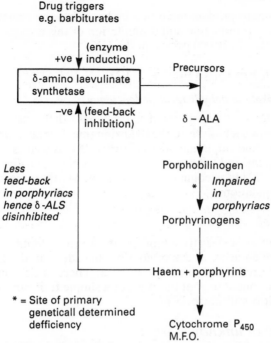

Figure 1.14 Porphyrin metabolism relevant to acute intermittent porphyria

Autosomal dominant (Figure 1.12)

Malignant hyperthermia

In the rare condition of malignant hyperthermia the ability of skeletal muscle to sequester Ca^{2+} in the sarcoplasmic reticulum is impaired. **Halothane** and **suxamethonium** depolarize the cell and trigger the intracellular release of Ca^{2+}, which persists too long in the cytosol producing contracture, greatly increased metabolic heat production and lactic acidosis. *Dantrolene* interferes with the Ca^{2+} release from the sarcoplasmic reticulum and reduces the mortality in malignant hyperthermia.

Acute intermittent porphyria

Acute intermittent porphyria is a condition in which sufferers have an inborn error of their haem synthesis pathway (*see Figure 1.14*) at the level of porphobilinogen utilization. They are generally free from symptoms but acute attacks can be triggered by drugs, especially the barbiturates but also by other hypnotics, **griseofulvin,** gonadal steroids, sulphonamides, sulphonylureas and most anticonvulsants. Symptoms include abdominal pain, motor neuritis, anxiety and psychosis and the urinary excretion of large amounts of porphobilinogen and delta-aminolaevulinic acid. It is unlikely that any of these drugs was responsible for triggering George III's episodes but attacks can also be precipitated by ethanol and infections. Attacks are sometimes fatal. A common step in drug-triggered attacks is a sudden increase in the activity of the liver mitochondrial enzyme, delta-aminolaevulinic acid synthetase, the first step in the porphyrin synthetic pathway. This is normally subject to product inhibition by haem but the common action of the drug triggers is induction and disinhibition of this enzyme. The gene is carried by about 1 in 10 000 people in the UK.

X-linked autonomous (Figure 1.12)

Glucose-6-phosphate dehydrogenase deficiency

People with glucose-6-phosphate dehydrogenase deficiency respond idiosyncratically with haemolysis to the oxidizing (electrophilic) drugs *nalidixic acid*, salicylates and sulphonamides (*Figure 1.15*), as well as to the antimalarials **chloroquine** and **primaquine**. The deficiency occurs in about 3% of people in the UK but is commoner in African, Mediterranean and South-East Asian populations.

Multifactorial

Another example of a drug triggering an attack in a susceptible person is the precipitation of an acute attack of gout by thiazide diuretics in individuals with a genetic predisposition to the disease. There is clear evidence of a hereditary component in gout but it is not a simple trait carried by a single gene (that is, it is multifactorial).

Idiosyncrasy of unknown origin

Aplastic anaemia

Approximately 1 in 100 000 patients treated with *chloramphenicol* develops fatal aplastic anaemia. Individuals who are at risk cannot be identified in advance. For a list of other drugs that produce aplastic anaemia *see Table 1.4*.

Table 1.4 Potential to produce aplastic anaemia

Definite	Probable
Chloramphenicol	Sulphonamides
Sodium aurothiomalate	**Phenytoin**
Organic arsenicals	**Tolbutamide**
	Chlorpropamide

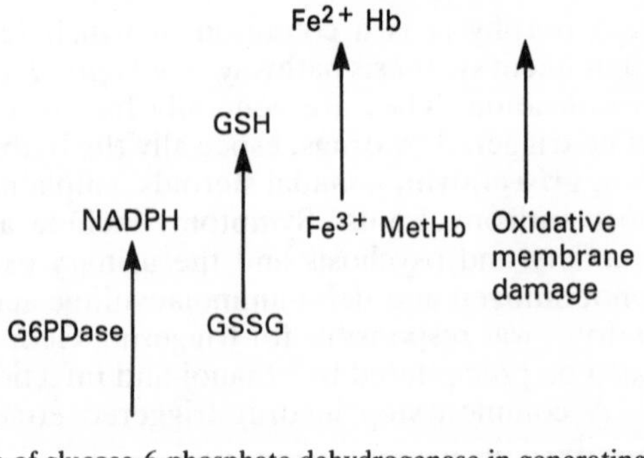

Figure 1.15 Role of glucose-6-phosphate dehydrogenase in generating the glutathione necessary to protect red cells from damage by oxidizing drugs

Mydriatics produce an attack of glaucoma in patients with a shallow angle (1:500).

Developmental toxicity

Drug treatment during pregnancy and lactation is unique in that a second individual will receive some of the drug. It can be more difficult to determine the toxicity of drugs in these individuals than in the mother. Drugs taken at the end of pregnancy can exert their predictable reversible effects on the newborn – respiratory depression with *pethidine*, sedation with benzodiazepines, goitre with **carbimazole.** These effects are likely to last longer in the newborn than the mother due to the newborn's slower elimination of drugs, particularly when liver metabolism is the predominant route.

Many drugs have been shown to be toxic to the developing fetus in animal studies but their effects in humans cannot be directly extrapolated. Therefore drug treatment during pregnancy should be avoided if possible.

A knowledge of the stages of development *in utero* can provide a logical basis for understanding the permanent adverse effects of drugs on such development.

Human development

Development *in utero* can be conveniently separated into three stages (*see Figure 1.16*):

(1) preimplantation;
(2) embryonic;
(3) fetal.

Preimplantation stage

Fertilization (fusion of haploid oocyte and spermatozoon) occurs in the oviduct to form a zygote. This progressively divides to form a ball of cells. A blastocyst, formed soon after this ball has passed into the uterus, embeds in the endometrium.

Embryonic stage

Implantation occurs 1 week after fertilization or about 3 weeks after the commencement of the last menstrual period and pregnancy will not usually be confirmed until some 4 weeks after implantation. Any restriction of the use of a drug during pregnancy should, therefore, apply to all women of reproductive age.

In the human embryo, organogenesis starts soon after implantation. During this stage differentiation of cells is occurring and primordia of organ systems are being formed.

Fetal stage

By about 9 weeks after conception, the major organ systems have been formed. Fetal development consists of growth in size, finer differentiation and functional maturation. Some development of major organ systems occurs during this stage – major brain growth occurs around birth in the human. Obviously, much human development takes place after birth.

Drug effects on development

Developmental toxicity is the study of factors and mechanisms producing abnormalities of development. It can be assumed that virtually all drugs distribute to the fetus. The physicochemical properties of drugs dictate their rate of distribution but at a steady-state fetal plasma and tissue concentrations are likely to be similar to those of the mother (page 317).

Possible adverse effects of drugs on development include:

(1) embryonic or fetal death;
(2) major structural malformation;
(3) growth retardation;
(4) functional defects.

The nature of any adverse effect principally depends on the drug and on the time of administration in relation to the stage of development. For example, thalidomide produced limb deformities (phocomelia) and internal organ deformities. The critical period was 3–5 weeks after conception, that is during the period of organogenesis. Thalidomide used towards the end of pregnancy had no effect on development. A comparison of maternal and embryonic timings is shown in *Figure 1.16*. It should be recognized that there is a spontaneous occurrence of altered embryonic/fetal development – in the absence of drugs natural abortion occurs in one in five pregnancies.

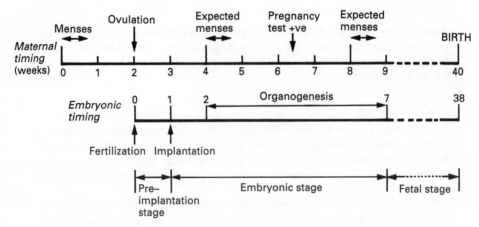

Figure 1.16 Relative timings of maternal and embryonic events from conception to birth

Drug effects on development

Anticonvulsant drugs

The incidence of malformations is increased in babies born to mothers with epilepsy. There is also a further increase when the mother has received anticonvulsant drugs. Some of the malformations are minor or self correcting (hypoplasia of the nails). Cleft lip and palate have been associated with **phenytoin** and neural tube defects with **sodium valproate** but no anticonvulsant drug can be exonerated.

When the epileptic manifestation is mild (simple partial seizures) it may be appropriate to stop the drug before conception. Uncontrolled tonic/clonic seizures by contrast are probably more harmful than anticonvulsants.

Cytotoxic drugs

Present cytotoxic drugs show only a narrow degree of selective toxicity towards neoplasms relative to normal cells. These drugs act particularly on rapidly proliferating cells and could be expected to produce embryo- and fetotoxicity. The group includes antimetabolites (**methotrexate,** *mercaptopurine*) and alkylating agents (**cyclophosphamide,** *chlorambucil, busulphan*). If used during the first trimester (one-third) of pregnancy miscarriages or malformations frequently, but not inevitably, result. Following their use in the second and third trimesters growth retardation often occurs.

Despite these observations there have been many successful pregnancies in renal transplant and other patients receiving immunosuppresant drugs including *azathioprine*, which is converted to mercaptopurine *in vivo*.

Exposure of either parent to cytotoxic drugs before fertilization does not seems to increase the incidence of mutations in their children.

Vitamin A analogues

Vitamin A analogues are used for the systemic treatment of some severe skin diseases, *isotretinoin* for acne and *etretinate* for psoriasis. These compounds produce a high incidence of ear and eye defects, cleft lip and palate and craniofacial dysmorphology. Contraceptive measures should be taken for at least 1 month before, during and after treatment with these compounds.

Antithyroid drugs

Neonatal hypothyroidism and even cretinism is possible but is rarely seen following the use of antithyroid drugs (**carbimazole**). Thyroid gland enlargement present at delivery is usually temporary.

Stilboestrol

Use of high doses of *stilboestrol* in pregnancy led to the development of a kind of vaginal carcinoma in a small proportion of postpubertal offspring.

Tetracyclines

Tetracyclines are readily deposited, by calcium chelation, in developing teeth and bone in the third trimester and postnatally, leading to discoloration and occasionally hypoplasia.

Warfarin

There may be an association between **warfarin** use in the first trimester and a variety of structural malformations including facial deformities and optic nerve atrophy and perhaps mental retardation. Patients are therefore generally advised to avoid conception until it is practicable to withdraw **warfarin.** Excessive 'moulding' of the skull during delivery produces intracranial bleeding. Oral anticoagulant drugs are therefore withdrawn in late pregnancy and replaced by sc **heparin,** which does not cross the placenta.

General anaesthetic agents

A higher incidence of spontaneous abortions and deformities in the offspring of females who work in operating theatres is presumed to be due to inhalation of general anaesthetic gases in the atmosphere.

Ethanol

There are several reports of a higher incidence of growth retardation, microcephaly, limb and heart deformities and mental deficiency in the offspring of chronic alcoholic mothers. Deficiency of maternal diet probably contributes. A withdrawal syndrome may occur in babies born to alcoholic mothers.

Tobacco smoking

This is associated with smaller neonates and a higher incidence of perinatal complications.

The justifiability of treating a pregnant woman with a drug having one of these adverse effects depends on:

(1) the nature and incidence of the effect;
(2) the severity of the disease;
(3) the therapeutic value of the drug to the mother.

As an example, the use of anticonvulsant drugs is generally justified as, despite evidence of an increased incidence of fetal malformations associated with their use, their therapeutic benefit is high. In contrast, the use of antagonists at H_1 histamine receptors (*cyclizine*) or antagonists at muscarinic cholinoceptors (**hyoscine**) to treat vomiting of early pregnancy is generally not justified. There is little evidence of any serious adverse effects of these drugs on development but the condition can usually be treated by nondrug methods.

Adverse drug interactions

Many patients receive multiple drug therapy and one component may modify the activity of another, either enhancing or reducing it. Such an interaction may be beneficial, for example, antihypertensive drugs in combination but this chapter is concerned with the problems posed by two or more drugs acting simultaneously to cause an unwanted response, that is, an adverse drug interaction.

Definitions

The 'interacting' drug modulates the activity of a 'target' drug. Expressed in potency terms this modulation may take the form of potentiation (page 18) or antagonism (page 13). Described, alternatively, in terms of the modulation of the effects of the target drug, these may be enhanced (increased, augmented) or impaired (reduced, diminished). Summation (page 3) describes the effect of two drugs acting together that equals the anticipated sum of their effects acting alone.

Classification

Adverse drug interactions are of two basic kinds:

(1) pharmacodynamic interactions can occur between drugs having similar or opposing pharmacological effects and give rise to summation or antagonism (competitive or functional). The concentration of each drug, at its site of action, is unaltered by the interaction;

(2) pharmacokinetic interactions arise because one drug interferes with the disposition of another and give rise to potentiation or antagonism. The concentration of the target drug at its site of action is modified by the presence of the interacting drug.

Epidemiology

In UK hospital practice more than 40% of patients receiving any drugs at all are taking six or more. In them the incidence of unwanted effects is seven times higher than in those taking fewer than six drugs. The factors that lead to multiple drug prescriptions are also those that predispose to adverse drug effects – old age and severe illness.

**Table 1.5 Relationship between the number of drugs pre-
scribed and the number of potential interactions (pairs)**

Drugs prescribed	Potential interactions
1	0
2	1
3	3
4	6
5	10
6	15
7	21

The total number of known or predicted adverse drug interactions is huge. Discussion here is limited to the more clinically relevant – those that have important repercussions for the patient. These involve modulation of the activity of a target drug having:

(1) a steep dose effect relationship;
(2) a small therapeutic index.

Then small degrees of antagonism cause loss of therapeutic effectiveness and small degrees of potentiation produce toxicity.

Commonest drugs responsible

Oral anticoagulant drugs, cardiac glycosides, antidysrhythmic drugs, sympathomimetic drugs, antihypertensive drugs (diuretics, antagonists at β-adrenoceptors, calcium entry blockers), anticancer drugs, antiepileptic drugs, oral hypoglycaemic drugs, oral contraceptives, alcohol, NSAIDs, Li^+, antidepressive drugs, antipsychotic drugs.

Pharmacodynamic interactions

Pharmacodynamic interactions are common. They represent the majority of adverse interactions and are, in most instances, predictable.

Classification

Pharmacodynamic interactions can be subdivided on the site of action of the interacting drug, which may be:

(1) near the site of action of the target drug;
(2) distant from the site of action of the target drug – the interaction depends on a secondary effect exerted through some common necessary link.

Near the site of action of the target drug

Result in summation

Examples:
Ethanol increases the sedative effect of all CNS depressant drugs (antihistamines, benzodiazepines, neuroleptic drugs).
Aminoglycoside antibiotics increase the muscle weakness produced by antagonists at the nicotinic cholinoceptor of skeletal muscle (page 77).
Aspirin in high doses reduces the prothrombin concentration and increases the anticoagulant effect of **warfarin** (page 207).

Result in antagonism

Examples:
Simultaneous prescription of agonists and antagonists at same receptor.
Antagonists at muscarinic cholinoceptors prevent the increase of gastric motility due to *metoclopramide*.

Distant from the site of action of the target drug

Result in summation

Examples:
Propranolol masks the adrenergically mediated symptoms and homeostatic mechanisms, and increases the severity of insulin hypoglycaemia.
Phenothiazines cause orthostatic hypotension and summate with antihypertensive drugs.
Diuretics cause K^+-depletion and increase the dysrhythmogenicity of **digoxin**.

Result in antagonism

Examples:
NSAIDs or glucocorticoids cause salt and water retention and antagonize antihypertensive drugs.

Pharmacokinetic or dispositional interactions

This classification of possible sites of such interaction follows the order of their discussion in the *Drug disposition and metabolism* section, pages 307–328.

Outside the body (by chemical reaction)

Examples:
If **suxamethonium** and **thiopentone sodium** solutions are mixed in the same syringe the former is rapidly hydrolysed by the strong alkalinity of the latter.
If **phenytoin sodium** is injected into glucose (5% w/v) solution for iv infusion, which has a low pH, the phenytoin anion is partly precipitated as the less soluble acid.

At the site of entry

Before absorption

By forming an insoluble complex. Antacids (calcium, magnesium or aluminium salts) or iron salts with tetracyclines.

By altering gastric emptying. Food has a variable effect. Opioids and antagonists at muscarinic cholinoceptors slow gastric emptying and *metoclopramide* increases it. **Levodopa** and **digoxin** peak blood concentrations are affected but total absorption is usually unchanged. Absorption from liquid formulations is little affected.

By alteration of gut flora. Broad spectrum antibacterial drugs reduce the size of the colonic bacterial population. A reduction in vitamin K synthesis can lead to potentiation of oral anticoagulant drugs. **Ethinyloestradiol** is normally metabolized to the glucuronide conjugate, which undergoes hydrolysis in the gut resulting in enterohepatic recycling. Thus, reduction in hydrolytic activity, normally produced by gut bacteria, can cause therapeutic failure of the oral contraceptive drugs (*see Figure 7.7,* page 323).

During absorption

Monoamine oxidase inhibitors potentiate tyramine by inhibition of the enzyme in the gut wall and in the liver.

During distribution (by competition for plasma protein binding sites)

Displacement from serum albumin binding occurs at the onset of concomitant exposure to a drug of higher affinity or of equal affinity in higher dose. The effect of this interaction is short-lived because the displaced drug is metabolized, or there is increased tissue binding, and a new steady state is achieved with elimination equal to the dose ingested, that is, the same effect is achieved at a lower total drug concentration in plasma. The physician must resist the temptation to treat the reduced plasma concentration (total concentration is reported in drug monitoring assays) by dosage increase – it is the concentration free in plasma water that is significant.

This is the basis of a clinically relevant interaction only when the interacting drug has a high affinity for the acid binding site and the target drug is extensively bound to the same site (**warfarin** 99%, **tolbutamide** 98%) and has a low therapeutic index. Free plasma concentration increases a lot only if the volume of distribution is small (**warfarin** 8 l/70 kg, **tolbutamide** 7 l/70 kg) in relation to plasma volume.

In both of the above cases the displacing drug also interferes with metabolism (*see below*).

Examples:
Salicylic acid with **warfarin.**
Sulphonamides with **tolbutamide.**
Sodium valproate with **phenytoin.**

Alteration of drug metabolism

Stimulation of drug metabolism

A number of factors increase the rate at which endogenous (steroid hormones) and exogenous (drugs, foodstuffs) substances are metabolized by hepatic oxidation. The capacity for metabolism is greater in smokers, alcoholics (without advanced cirrhosis), in those exposed to hydrocarbons and in patients taking a wide variety of lipid soluble drugs. This increased rate of drug oxidation is due to enzyme induction (associated with an increase in enzyme activity, cytochrome P_{450} concentration, liver weight and microscopically visible smooth endoplasmic reticulum) and can occur after a few days or weeks of exposure to the inducing agent. Induction is generally nonspecific so that oxidation of other drugs in addition to that of the inducing agent is promoted.

Table 1.6 lists drugs that induce mixed function oxidase (MFO). Most anticonvulsant drugs (but not **sodium valproate**) and most hypnotics and sedatives (but not benzodiazepines) are included. Regular consumption of more than 100 mg daily is required for induction to occur. Consequences are more rapid inactivation of target drugs and more rapid activation of target prodrugs.

Table 1.6 Drugs inducing MFO and MFO target drugs

Inducing agents	Target drugs inactivated by oxidative metabolism
Carbamazepine	Glucocorticoids
Ethanol	Oral contraceptive steroids
Griseofulvin	*Theophylline*
Phenobarbitone	**Warfarin**
Phenytoin	
Rifampicin	

More rapid inactivation (Table 1.6). Therapeutic failure of a target drug arises from its greater metabolic clearance.

There are two occurrences that can reveal this interaction: the onset and offset of induction. A patient in steady state with a target drug inactivated by oxidative metabolism commences concurrent treatment with an inducing agent (*Figure 1.17*). As induced enzyme concentration builds up the steady state plasma concentration of target drug declines over a few days with associated therapeutic failure.

Compensation for the higher clearance by prescribing a higher dose rate allows therapeutic control to be regained.

Cessation of administration of the inducing agent and declining clearance of the target drug leads to accumulation of the latter over 2–3 weeks and the associated occurrence of toxic effects.

Common settings are the onset and offset of drug treatment of either tuberculosis or epilepsy in a patient under long-term treatment with oral contraceptives or **warfarin.**

More rapid activation. Toxicity of a target prodrug arises from the more

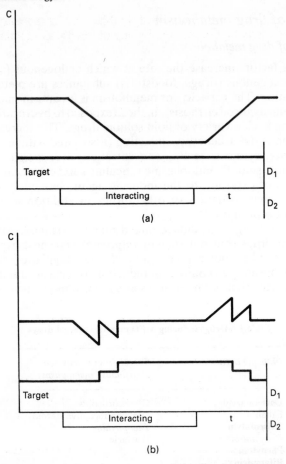

Figure 1.17 Drug interactions based upon enzyme induction: (a) the faster onset and slower offset of the reduced plasma target drug concentration caused by addition of an interacting inducer of MFO; (b) a response to the anticipated onset of therapeutic failure, increasing the target drug dose rate – remember to reduce it again when the interacting drug is withdrawn

rapid production of the active drug. The duration of action is shortened. **Paracetamol** overdosage produces more severe toxic effects when the patient has been taking an inducing agent.

Inhibition of drug metabolism

In general, inhibition of drug metabolism, and the interactions based on it, shows more selectivity than induction. Onset often occurs within 1 or 2 days.

Deliberate. The desired therapeutic response to some drugs is mediated by inhibiting the metabolism of endogenous or exogenous substances. The administration of other drugs, in their presence, can then produce an adverse response. One interacting drug potentiates all alternative substrates.

Incidental. The metabolism of some drugs is inhibited in an unpredictable manner by others. Dosage reduction is usually all that is needed but changing to a different drug may be desirable. One therapeutically vulnerable substrate may be potentiated by any of several interacting drugs.

Examples:

Enzyme system	Inhibitor	Metabolism inhibited
MAO	**Phenelzine**	Tyramine
	Tranylcypromine	
Aldehyde dehydrogenase	Disulfiram	Ethanol
	Chlorpropamide	
	Metronidazole	
Xanthine oxidase	**Allopurinol**	*Azathioprine*
		Mercaptopurine
MFO	**Phenelzine**	*Pethidine*
	Cimetidine	**Phenytoin**
	Isoniazid	**Phenytoin**
	Sodium valproate	**Phenytoin**
	Sulphonamides	**Tolbutamide**
	Cimetidine	**Warfarin**
	Erythromycin	**Warfarin**
	Sulphonamides	**Warfarin**
	Theophylline	**Warfarin**

Again, you need to be aware of, and compensate for, the changing interaction at the offset of inhibition as well as that at the onset.

Pharmacokinetic interaction near the site of target drug action

The active transport of released noradrenaline back into the noradrenergic neurone is a site of competitive drug interaction. Tricyclic antidepressive drugs:

(1) prevent the antihypertensive action of noradrenergic neurone blocking agents (*guanethidine*) (page 97);
(2) potentiate *adrenaline* administered with a local anaesthetic (page 121).

A part of the potentiation of sympathomimetic amine substrates by MAO inhibitors arises at the level of the noradrenergic nerve terminal (page 10) in addition to the liver and gut mucosa.

Alteration of renal excretion

Diuretics (particularly thiazides but also loop diuretics) cause Na^+ depletion and the proximal tubules of a patient taking **lithium carbonate** retain more Li^+.

Loop diuretics reduce the GFR and therefore the renal clearance of **gentamicin.**

Competition for renal excretory mechanisms

Most drugs are eventually filtered and excreted by the kidney, the 'purpose' of Phase I and Phase II metabolism being to increase water solubility (polarity). Active tubular secretion of anions and cations is a potential site for interactions of therapeutic relevance (salicylate with **methotrexate**).

Prescribing advice

'Every time a physician adds to the number of drugs a patient is taking he may devise a novel combination that has a special risk.' (Laurence and Bennett, 1987).

Keep the number of drugs you prescribe to a minimum. Select, of the alternatives, the best known to you. When adding a drug to the regimen, consider all the new pairings. Take care when injecting drugs into the giving set of iv infusion.

Abuse of drugs

Drug abuse is the taking of a drug or a dose of drug different from that advised by authoritative medical opinion.

In addition to the well publicized aspects of drug dependence, drug abuse also involves such practices as excessive self medication with proprietary preparations (analgesics, vitamins, cold 'remedies'), the bulk addition of antibiotics to animal foodstuffs in factory farming, the use of some drugs in sport in an attempt to improve performance, over prescribing and misprescribing by the medical profession, the unnecessary sale of 'nostrums' by pharmacists, noncompliance by the patient and much else. In this brief coverage so many facets cannot be encompassed. The following points are intended to provide some factual information and to encourage discussion.

Dependence

Dependence is defined in terms of the consequences of stopping drug taking. If the consequences are psychic or mental (craving, behavioural changes), this is psychic or mental dependence (habituation). Drugs that cause psychic dependence include nicotine (as in tobacco), centrally acting sympathomimetics (amphetamines, ephedrine), caffeine and cannabis.

If the consequences are physical, this is physical dependence (addiction). Although withdrawal of caffeine or nicotine can give rise to physical effects, these are minor and the drugs are not usually included amongst those that cause physical dependence. Only two groups of drugs cause true physical dependence:

(1) opioid analgesics (page 234) – withdrawal syndrome includes diarrhoea, abdominal cramps, sweating, vomiting;
(2) structurally nonspecific drugs and anxiolytics (page 251) – withdrawal syndrome includes confusion, disorientation, convulsions.

The severity of the syndrome depends both on the drug and the frequency of drug taking. **Diazepam** or ethanol require years of regular taking before dependence is detectable, *diamorphine* (heroin) requires a few days.

Withdrawal after six consecutive injections of *diamorphine* may produce only a mild syndrome, but withdrawal after 1 year may be fatal.

The molecular mechanism of dependence is unknown. Any theory must explain both tolerance (which is a prerequisite of dependence) and the nature of the withdrawal syndrome.

The following should be regarded as a model rather than an actual mechanism of action (*Figure 1.18*).

Consider a part of the brain in which there is a balance between an excitatory and an inhibitory transmitter (E and I). Assume the drug of dependence (D) acts as a mimic of transmitter I. The balance is altered to a state of inhibition or depression as a result of the primary effect of the drug.

If the drug effect persisted, the body would try to compensate and a method of compensation could be to increase excitatory activity. This could be by an increase in E (as shown), or by receptor proliferation or other mechanisms of supersensitivity. The balance is restored although the drug is still present (tolerance). If the drug is withdrawn a new imbalance occurs that produces symptoms opposite to those of the drug (the withdrawal syndrome). It will then require some time (during treatment of the withdrawal syndrome) before the biological adaption reverts to normal.

Two other points are pertinent:

(1) there is a grey area between psychic and physical dependence; characteristics are best defined for each drug group;
(2) people are creatures of habit. Dependence can occur to almost anything done habitually. A person accustomed to walking round the block before retiring will not sleep so well (a behavioural response) if deprived of the habit. Linked to this is dependence on an environment (social dependence), which can be a very potent behavioural influence.

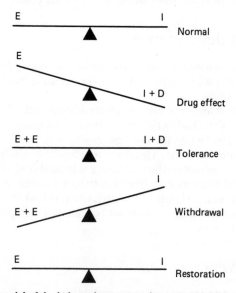

Figure 1.18 A model of the balance between excitatory and inhibitory transmitters: tolerance and withdrawal

Drug-related deaths

Nearly 2000 people die by poisoning each year in England and Wales. This is half the number reported 5 years ago. Commonly, more than one drug appears on the death certificate and it is difficult to list exact poisoning figures. *Table 1.7* shows approximate numbers. Appearance in the list is a function of both toxicity and availability.

Table 1.7 Drug causes of acute fatal poisoning

Approximate number of acute fatal poisonings in England and Wales (1987)	1821
Carbon monoxide	1268
Analgesics – total including antirheumatic drugs (salicylates alone 94)	692
Ethanol	110*
Benzodiazepines	57
Barbiturates	8
Solvents	7

* = excludes deaths from chronic abuse related to liver cirrhosis.

Major changes that have occurred during the last two decades are a large decrease in barbiturate deaths (previously responsible for about two-thirds of all drug deaths) and the virtual disappearance of domestic gas as a cause of death.

In the opposite direction there has been a steady increase in deaths due to ethanol, benzodiazepines and other psychoactive drugs. The net effect has been a steady decline in the poisoning statistics during the past 20 years.

If chronic poisoning is considered, tobacco, which causes cardiovascular and lung damage, puts all other drugs in the shade (estimated 75 000).

Incidence of dependence

As with acute fatal poisoning, the incidence of drug dependence is a function of availability. Ethanol is responsible for the greatest incidence of physical dependence (500 000).

Before 1960 the number of known opiate addicts in the UK had remained constant at about 300. During the 1960s there was a massive increase, which levelled at about 2000 when the law concerning availability was changed. In the late 1970s there was a sharp increase to a figure of about 7500 (in 1984). These are 'notified' addicts – the real figure is probably several-fold greater.

Whatever social reasons may have contributed to the increase in dependence in recent years, a significant contribution is that there are now large supplies of inexpensive diamorphine and cocaine of high purity available on the black market.

The drug laws

An assortment of laws control the availability, prescribing, storage and labelling of drugs in the UK.

Before 1970 the act that covered the drugs of abuse was the Dangerous Drugs Act, which had little pharmacological basis. It covered the opiates, cannabis and cocaine.

During the 1960s there was an unexpected increase in illicit drug taking and the law was changed progressively in an attempt both to stem this and to cope with the changes in drug taking habits. This culminated in the Misuse of Drugs Act of 1971, which covered the original 'Dangerous Drugs' and those that had become fashionable – the centrally acting sympathomimetics (amphetamines and some other anorectic drugs), the hallucinogens (LSD), and the barbiturate-like drug methaqualone. At that time the absence of barbiturates from the Act was a notable anomaly.

Since 1985 the barbiturates too have become 'controlled drugs'.

(1) The controlled drugs are grouped into four classes (A, B, C and D) dependent on abuse potential; **morphine** is more rigidly controlled than **codeine.**

(2) Control of a drug may vary dependent on its formulation; **morphine** injection is in Class A, kaolin and morphine mixture is exempt.

Some points for discussion

Drugs have always been a part of society. Many primitive societies revolved around (usually hallucinogenic) drug cults (religions). Ethanol was established in Roman and Greek cultures and has remained so in those that succeeded them throughout Europe and the Americas. Cannabis is established in some Asian societies. Because drugs are a part of society drug laws cannot always be rational (some would argue that tobacco should be banned and ethanol put on prescription, or even controlled).

Society's attitude towards drug toxicity changes. Apart from obvious differences between what was deemed acceptable in medieval times and that acceptable now, recent changes have been:

(1) the virtual disappearance of amphetamines and barbiturates compared to their widespread use and acceptance 30 years ago;
(2) gradual (and unpredictable) changes in society's attitude to cannabis;
(3) the disappearance of several new NSAIDs from the market with the re-evaluation of those of similar toxicity that have been on the market for 30 years.

Medication with legally obtained drugs occurs on a vast scale. Sales of antipyretic analgesics suggest a national intake of one tablet per person per day. Twenty million prescriptions for anxiolytics are dispensed each year (assume about 60 tablets or capsules per prescription).

It is estimated that half the number of prescription items are unnecessary (overprescribing).

The likelihood of a patient taking a preparation as instructed can be remote (noncompliance): 5% of all prescriptions are not even handed to a pharmacist to be dispensed. The more complicated the instructions, the greater the noncompliance. This can have serious consequences in certain conditions (notably epilepsy, page 419). Bacterial resistance can be encouraged by erratic taking of antibiotics.

The influence of drug promotion (advertising, representatives) on doctors' prescribing in western countries becomes dominant a few years after doctors qualify, by which time the cost of such promotion roughly equals the cost of medical education. Whilst the volume of medical information (biased and unbiased) is indeed vast, the existence of concise independent assessments of new drugs (*Prescribers' Journal, Drug and Therapeutics Bulletin*) simplifies the problem of keeping up to date.

The cost of prescriptions has risen to such a level that physicians are now required to restrict the drugs that they prescribe within the NHS to a 'limited' list. The content of that list is essentially that which medical schools have been teaching for years.

Ignorance (not only on the part of the lay public) remains one of the most important contributions to drug abuse. People fail to appreciate that drugs are more or less selective poisons. Lay people commonly categorize strychnine as a poison, penicillin as a medicine, diamorphine as a drug and ethanol as none of these. Cannabis has appeared in all categories. This lack of respect for drugs as poisons contributes much to drug abuse and is also at the root of many well-meant irresponsible habits such as handing over prescribed drugs to neighbours (irrespective of disorder or drug) or children (parent's anxiolytics for child's school examinations). This is the province of health education. Pharmacists are in an ideal position to act as health educators but general practitioners are regrettably seldom involved.

Drug design, development and testing

Most new drugs are discovered, and all are developed, by pharmaceutical companies. The vast financial investments that these companies must make in order to develop a new drug is protected by a 20 year patent. During this time only the patent holding company or other agreed, licensed companies, can make and sell the drug. Such patents cover only the particular chemical structure and not a general principle of drug action. It currently takes about 10 years from first synthesis of a new drug until its appearance on the market with a Product Licence issued by the Committee on the Safety of Medicines (CSM). The average research and development cost for a new drug is of the order of £90m (£120m if expenditure on failures is included), all of which must be recouped in the remainder of the drug's patent-protected life.

A company will only decide to embark upon a research programme if it can predict sufficient sales to cover the research and development costs. Most rewarding are those programmes leading to the development of a drug to treat a relatively common condition for which no other successful treatment exists – filling a gap in the therapeutic armamentarium. Another approach is to develop another drug to treat a condition for which other treatments already exist. This is more likely to be profitable if the new drug has a novel mechanism of action, although often 'me too' drugs are developed by modifying the molecular structure of existing drugs until a novel structure is found that still has the desired pharmacological properties: to succeed, such a drug must have certain advantages. Higher potency alone is not an advantage. A better drug must show one or all of the following features:

(1) increased selectivity; that is a higher therapeutic index, which is achieved either by increasing therapeutic potency or by reducing toxic potency or both;
(2) occasionally decreased selectivity; the introduction of a second desirable property – neuromuscular blocking action in a general anaesthetic agent;
(3) better pharmacokinetics – longer or shorter duration of action, depending upon the indications for use;
(4) more convenient formulation – tablets for oral dosing are usually preferable to a solution for injection;
(5) cheaper.

This approach has been called 'molecular roulette' and has led to the introduction of many very similar drugs. For example, there are now 16 antagonists at β-adrenoceptors on the UK market sold under 38 trade names. This excludes preparations that contain more than one drug and different formulations of the same product. Despite unnecessary replication, many novel drugs have been discovered 'accidentally' during games of molecular roulette.

Pharmacological activity is detected by means of batteries of pharmacological tests commonly known as 'screens'. Preliminary screens are intended to detect all compounds that have the desired action. Such screens should ideally produce more 'false positive' than 'false negative' results. Promising compounds then pass to a series of more detailed pharmacological tests intended to confirm and extend the findings of the preliminary screen. The first chemical showing the desired activity is often referred to as the 'lead compound'.

Once promising activity has been found in a compound many lines of attack are followed simultaneously. These centre around a medicinal chemistry laboratory, which studies the relationships between chemical structure and pharmacological activity. The hope is that the 'ideal' structure can be predicted, synthesized, tested and eventually sold as an effective drug. Additional studies involve full pharmacological evaluations, both quantitative and qualitative, dispositional and metabolic studies in animals and preliminary toxicological evaluation in animals.

Once preliminary toxicity tests in animals show that the compound is unlikely to be toxic in man, short-term, healthy volunteer (Phase I) studies are carried out. These are intended to provide quantitative and qualitative information on the absorption, metabolism and excretion of the drug and its pharmacological effects. The volunteers are young and healthy, and able to give their informed consent to participate. They are usually men as this eliminates the risk of damaging an unrecognized pregnancy (page 34). Volunteers are usually paid for their services but it is considered bad practice to offer such large sums that caution is outweighed by financial considerations. The risk of death or serious harm occurring to the volunteer in such studies is comparable to that involved in flying with a commercial airline.

From healthy volunteer studies, likely dosage regimens in clinical practice can often be predicted. Major differences in metabolism between experimental animals and man may also be detected.

When healthy volunteer studies and more detailed pharmacological and toxicological tests have produced favourable results, application can be made to the CSM for a clinical trials certificate. Only when the clinical trials and detailed toxicity tests have been successfully completed and confirm that the drug has the intended therapeutic efficacy and is acceptably safe can application be made to the CSM for a product licence. Once granted, this enables the manufacturer to promote and sell the new compound under its trade name, for use in certain specified conditions. The CSM attempts to monitor the occurrence of adverse effects and the evidence of therapeutic efficacy for the whole of a product's life on the market. The most critical phase in this postmarketing (that is postproduct licence) surveillance is the first few years, when sales are expected to be highest. Should unacceptable adverse effects be detected, the CSM can modify either the indications for use of the drug, the contraindications to the use of the drug or its recommended dose. They may even recommend withdrawal of the product licence.

Toxicity testing

Testing new drugs for adverse effects begins with toxicity tests in animals. Whenever possible, nonanimal tests replace those in animals, both on humane grounds and because it is usually possible to reduce the variability associated with tests not based on whole animals. However, tests designed to detect unforeseeable toxicity generally require that the drug be given to intact animals. Such preclinical predictive toxicity tests of new drugs fall into three major categories:

(1) acute toxicity evaluation;
(2) subacute toxicity evaluation;
(3) chronic toxicity evaluation.

Acute toxicity tests ask the questions how poisonous (lethal) is the drug in the short term and by what mechanisms does it kill? The best known acute toxicity parameter is the LD50 – the median lethal dose. In addition to providing information about the dosage levels needed for other toxicity tests, acute toxicity testing provides information about the likely effects of accidental or self-administered overdoses once the drug is marketed. Few licensing authorities still require LD50 tests to be carried out on new drugs. Subacute toxicity tests are of intermediate duration, usually around 12 weeks, and involve giving animals doses that are near the limits of tolerance on the assumption that the frequency of occurrence of a rare adverse effect increases with the cumulative dose given to the test population. Chronic toxicity tests involve giving doses of the new drug for prolonged periods of time – commonly 2 years. The dose levels used are chosen to be representative of normal (and likely maximal) therapeutic doses in man.

All three kinds of test are performed using at least two species of animals, typically rats, mice, guinea-pigs or rabbits. Other species (dogs, cats, monkeys) are employed when the chemical fate of the drug more closely resembles that in man. Throughout toxicity tests, animals are examined frequently for behavioural changes and general well-being in addition to which, as many body functions as possible are monitored. At intervals, sample groups of animals are killed and examined post-mortem in detail. This includes biochemical analysis of body fluids and histological examination of every organ and tissue. At the end of the tests, all surviving animals are subjected to this procedure. A prime concern is to detect toxicity that is selective for a particular organ (bone marrow, kidney, liver).

Special testing techniques are used to detect adverse effects on reproductive function in both male and female animals and particularly the effects of the drug on embryonic and fetal growth and development – teratogenicity testing. Testing for carcinogenicity forms part of the chronic toxicity trial but is backed up by nonanimal tests, most of which are based upon the ability of known carcinogens to cause mutations in certain strains of bacteria (for example, the Ames test).

Clinical trials

The assessment of new drug action on human beings is conventionally divided into four phases.

Phase I: Volunteer studies

Human pharmacology is assessed in a small number of healthy volunteers (often male students). The dose is gradually increased until an effect can be measured. These studies, which require Ethics Committee approval, assess immediate responses to the new drug but it is not usually possible to perform long-term studies on these subjects. Sometimes, as with antitumour drugs, the first human tests are done on patients.

Phase II: Patient studies

A few patients, intensively studied in an open uncontrolled manner, are used to see if the desired pharmacological effect is achieved in pathological states. For example, does the drug lower BP in patients with hypertension? These studies are usually carried out within a hospital environment.

Phase III: Clinical trials

More patients are assessed less intensively. Controlled clinical trials compare the new drug with placebo and with established therapy (if any). The indications for the drug and its place in the therapy of a condition are identified as are dosages and methods of administration.

Phase IV: Postmarketing surveillance

After the drug has been granted a marketing licence, assessment of its long-term value continues. Does it alter the underlying disease process? Why are some patients nonresponsive? What is the drug's potential for misuse or abuse? Are there any clinically relevant drug interactions? Are there important unusual adverse effects? Are there any novel indications? Is the recommended dose appropriate? In a sense this phase lasts throughout the drug's life.

Risk versus benefit

At all stages in drug development unwanted effects are searched for and a risk *versus* benefit analysis is constantly being performed. For example, an effective but toxic agent is unsuitable for treating a minor illness (upper respiratory tract infection) but acceptable if successful against a currently untreatable neoplasm.

Trial design

Most trials attempt to disprove the null hypothesis that the new agent is no better than a placebo or the established treatment. Initially, the trials are uncontrolled – subjects or patients are identified and the drug administered. The trial is open – both the investigator and the subject know a new substance is being given. There is great potential for subjective bias amongst both patients and investigators but it is useful to know that a beneficial response can occur. To obtain objective data a trial is performed comparing the drug with either an inert substance (placebo) or conventional therapy. The administration is controlled – the order of giving the two substances is regulated usually by using a random order and is also double blind – neither the investigator nor the patient knows which of the two substances is being administered at any one time.

Aims

Should be as simple and as few as possible. Clearcut end points must be set before the trial begins. For example, after 6 weeks of therapy can drug X heal more duodenal ulcers than **cimetidine**?

Placebo

This is pharmacologically inert (usually starch) but many beneficial and unwanted effects can be demonstrated in a 'blind' subject, possibly mediated through endorphins and enkephalins. Tablet size, shape and colour and the method of administration each influence the response. Placebos should therefore be indistinguishable from the trial drug. Similarly the doctor's expectations influence both the patient's response and the doctor's assessment. For this reason the investigator must also be unable to distinguish drug from placebo or drug A from drug B.

Trial type

The commonest is a group comparison. Patients are randomly allocated to one or other treatment. Large numbers are needed to overcome problems of unsuspected bias (for example, more smokers in one group than another). If such interfering factors are known then bias can be avoided by ensuring even distribution of the kinds of patient between the two treatment groups (stratification).

Another problem is that the trial compares populations as a whole rather than individuals. An alternative design is the crossover trial in which each patient receives both treatments but in random order. Thus, each patient acts as his own control. This design is not applicable in many diseases as the first treatment radically alters the disease state (pneumonia is cured). It is necessary to incorporate a 'washout' period to avoid the effects of the initial treatment carrying over into the second period but it does require fewer patients than a group comparison.

Ethical considerations

All trial designs should be scrutinized by a local Ethics Committee of doctors, scientists and lay people not involved in the study. The likely discomfort to the patient and the anticipated risks are discussed. The use of a placebo may be unethical when an effective remedy is available. Prior to a trial a patient must be informed of the possible risks involved and written consent obtained. The patient must be able to withdraw at any time without detriment to the quality of the medical care provided.

Patient exclusions

Pregnant women, children, the elderly (unless specifically indicated), the acutely ill and patients with an allergic (atopic) history are not included. In volunteer studies those with abnormal findings on initial assessment are also excluded, as are patients with other diseases than that under study.

Dosage

Phase II studies should determine whether the drug has a flat dose response curve requiring a fixed dose or whether the dose must be varied according to effect or body weight.

Assessment

Objective measurement is the ideal but is not always feasible. If subjective assessment is unavoidable (for example, the effect of an analgesic) then use of visual analogue scales reduces observer bias. Unwanted effects must be actively sought as they may not be volunteered. Patient compliance in drug taking can be assessed by measurement of blood concentrations. An alternative method is to provide a varied excess of tablets for the known interval between assessments and to count the unused tablets at each visit.

Analysis

Using the null hypothesis, treatment groups or individuals are compared using a number of statistical methods (for example, χ^2, paired t-test, analysis of variance). Further details are beyond the scope of this textbook. Two common errors in trials are:

(1) type 1 errors – the two treatments are not different in reality but the trial says they are – the usual reason is poor trial design;
(2) type 2 errors occur when the trial says that there is no difference between the two treatments when in fact they are different; this fault is usually due to insufficient numbers of patients in the trial.

2

Drug action on peripheral excitable tissues – drugs acting on signalling and transduction mechanisms directly related to receptors for the neurotransmitters acetylcholine and noradrenaline

Aims

In common with other sections of this book, the drugs chosen for discussion are included in preparations listed by the *BNF* or constitute pharmacological tools of particular importance. For each drug mentioned you should know:

- its mechanism of action and the changes it evokes in effector cell activity both *in vitro* and *in vivo*;
- its interactions with other pharmacological agents;
- something of its therapeutic or scientific usage – and the rationale behind that usage;
- something of its undesirable effects.

Consideration of these four items will not give you a complete understanding of the pharmacology of a given drug. By reference to other sections of this book, you should seek knowledge of the drug's handling by the body (absorption, disposition and elimination) and whether it has actions on physiological systems that are outside the scope of this section.

Introduction

Studies of drug effects exerted upon the peripheral nervous system or the cells that it innervates can provide an excellent introduction to mechanisms of drug action, the rationale behind the use of drugs as investigative tools or as therapeutic agents and the methods by which the properties of drugs are measured. Furthermore, such studies will provide a working base from which to approach the pharmacology of other body systems.

Clinical applications

Many of the drugs described in this section are clinically useful. They may be used:

(1) to modify physiological processes and thus permit an operative or other procedure, for example, **tubocurarine** (page 76)
(2) as aids in the diagnosis of disease, for example, *edrophonium* (page 91)
(3) in the symptomatic treatment of disease, for example, **propranolol** (page 114)

It is important to realize that (with the exception of some antibiotics, *Table 2.3*) the agents mentioned in this section cannot be used to effect radical cure of disease.

Anatomy and physiology of the (efferent) peripheral nervous system and its effectors

Before we can understand how drugs produce their effects in the body we must have a thorough understanding of the anatomy and physiology of the relevant organ systems.

The nervous system can be subdivided as shown in *Figure 2.1*.

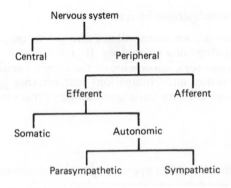

Figure 2.1 Subdivision of the nervous system

The central nervous system (CNS) comprises the brain and spinal cord. The peripheral nervous system lies outside the skull and vertebral column and comprises 12 pairs of nerves that emerge from the brain stem (cranial nerves) plus 31 pairs of nerves that emerge from the spinal cord (spinal nerves).

Peripheral neurones that carry impulses towards the CNS are called afferent neurones. Those that carry impulses away from the CNS are called efferent neurones.

Some cranial nerves consist only of afferent neurones, some of both afferent and efferent neurones and some only of efferent neurones. For the major part of their length, the spinal nerves consist of both afferent and efferent neurones and are thus called mixed spinal nerves. However, between its main trunk and the spinal cord, each spinal nerve breaks into a dorsal and a ventral root. Afferent neurones enter the spinal cord via the dorsal root whilst efferent neurones emerge via the ventral root (*see Figure 2.5*).

The efferent peripheral nervous system can be subdivided into somatic and autonomic components.

The somatic division of the efferent peripheral nervous system comprises neurones that emerge from the spinal cord (via the ventral roots of spinal nerves) to provide excitatory innervation of skeletal muscle (*Figure 2.5*). The region where a somatic motoneurone closely approaches a skeletal muscle cell is known as the skeletal neuromuscular junction. Acetylcholine (ACh) is the chemical transmitter at this junction (*Figure 2.2*).

The autonomic division of the efferent peripheral nervous system provides excitatory or inhibitory innervation to cardiac muscle, smooth muscle and exocrine glands (its effector cells). The autonomic nervous pathway between the CNS and the effector cells comprises two neurones. The axon of the first neurone in the pathway emerges from the CNS (either in the course of a cranial nerve or via the ventral root of a spinal nerve) and terminates a short distance from the cell body of the second neurone in the pathway.

The region where an axon terminal of the first neurone closely approaches

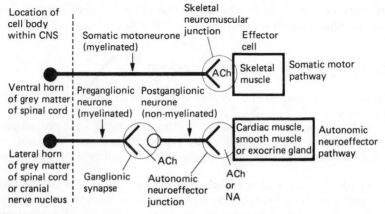

Figure 2.2 Comparison of a somatic motor pathway with an autonomic neuroeffector pathway

a dendrite or cell body of the second is called a synapse. In many cases the synapses of autonomic pathways occur together in the course of a peripheral nerve. The collection of cell bodies in this region gives rise to a swelling of the nerve known as a ganglion. Hence the first neurone in an autonomic pathway is called the preganglionic neurone and the second cell is called the postganglionic neurone. ACh is the chemical transmitter at all autonomic ganglionic synapses (*Figure 2.2*).

The region where the axon of the postganglionic neurone closely approaches its effector cell is called an autonomic neuroeffector junction. The chemical transmitter at this junction may be ACh or noradrenaline (NA [norepinephrine]) depending on the particular pathway under consideration (*Figure 2.2*).

The autonomic division of the efferent peripheral nervous system is subdivided into parasympathetic and sympathetic components according to the point of outflow of preganglionic neurones from the CNS.

The parasympathetic nervous system

A plan of the parasympathetic nervous system and its effectors is presented in *Figure 2.3*. Parasympathetic outflow comprises both cranial and sacral elements.

Cranial parasympathetic outflow is carried in cranial nerves III (oculomotor), VII (facial), IX (glossopharyngeal) and X (vagus). Sacral parasympathetic outflow is carried in the spinal nerves of sacral segments 2, 3 and 4 of the spinal cord.

Many parasympathetic ganglia are located close to, or are embedded within, the wall of the effector organ. Such ganglia are called terminal ganglia. In general parasympathetic preganglionic neurones are long while postganglionic neurones are short.

The distribution of parasympathetic innervation in the body is relatively limited – to certain effectors located within the head and to viscera within the thorax, abdomen and pelvis. The parasympathetic system does not innervate effectors located in the skin, limbs or body wall.

In every case ACh is the chemical transmitter between postganglionic parasympathetic neurones and their effector cells.

The sympathetic nervous system

Diagrams of the sympathetic nervous system and its effectors are presented in *Figures 2.4–2.7*.

Sympathetic outflow from the CNS is thoracolumbar – the preganglionic neurones emerge from the CNS in the ventral roots of the spinal nerves of the first thoracic to third lumbar segments of the spinal cord inclusive (*Figure 2.4*).

Sympathetic preganglionic fibres briefly join the course of the mixed spinal nerve but soon branch away to form white communicating rami (side branches of the spinal nerve), which enter the chains of paravertebral ganglia. These chains of ganglia lie on either side of the vertebrae. There are

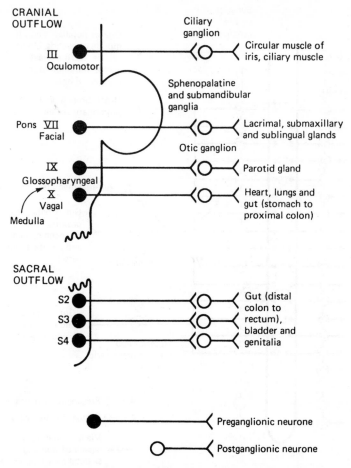

CRANIAL
OUTFLOW

Ciliary
ganglion

III
Oculomotor
Circular muscle of
iris, ciliary muscle

Sphenopalatine
and submandibular
ganglia

Pons VII
Facial
Lacrimal, submaxillary
and sublingual glands

Otic ganglion

IX
Glossopharyngeal
Parotid gland

X
Vagal
Heart, lungs and
gut (stomach to
proximal colon)

Medulla

SACRAL
OUTFLOW

S2
S3
S4
Gut (distal
colon to
rectum),
bladder and
genitalia

Preganglionic neurone

Postganglionic neurone

Figure 2.3 The parasympathetic nervous system and its effectors. Parasympathetic outflow is
bilaterally paired; only one side is illustrated

22 ganglia in each chain. Each ganglion in a paravertebral chain is connected
to the ones above and below by nerve trunks.

Only 15 of the ganglia in each chain are supplied by white communicating
rami. The three cervical ganglia at the top of the chain and the four sacral
ganglia at the bottom of the chain only receive input from the CNS by
neurones running upwards or downwards through the chain of ganglia by
way of the interconnecting nerve trunks.

The sympathetic pathways supplying effectors located in the head and
thorax are shown in *Figure 2.5*. The ganglionic synapse of these pathways
occurs within the chain of paravertebral ganglia.

The sympathetic pathways supplying effectors located in the abdomen
and pelvis are shown in *Figure 2.6*. In these pathways the preganglionic fibre
enters the chain of paravertebral ganglia but passes straight through without
synapsing. The synapse with the postganglionic neurone occurs in a prevertebral ganglion. In contrast to the paravertebral ganglia, the prevertebral
ganglia are not bilaterally paired. They are ill-defined structures that form

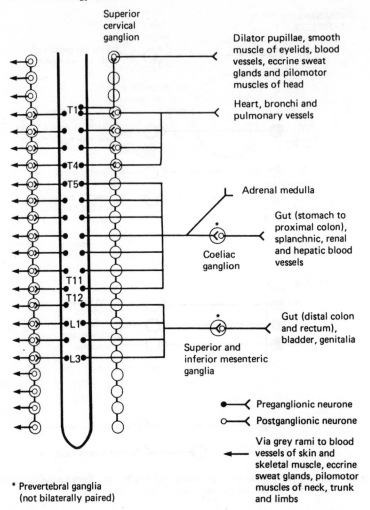

Figure 2.4 The sympathetic nervous system and its effectors. Most pathways illustrated are bilaterally paired

part of a neural plexus ventral to the abdominal aorta and its major branches. The coeliac and mesenteric ganglia are major components of this plexus. The adrenal medullae are embryologically and functionally equivalent to sympathetic prevertebral ganglia.

The sympathetic pathways supplying the blood vessels of skin and skeletal muscle, and the eccrine sweat glands and pilomotor muscles of the neck, trunk and limbs are shown in *Figure 2.7*. The preganglionic neurone of these pathways forms a synapse with the postganglionic neurone within a paravertebral ganglion. The postganglionic neurone rejoins the course of the mixed spinal nerve (via the grey communicating ramus) for distribution to the effectors.

In contrast to the parasympathetic system, postganglionic sympathetic

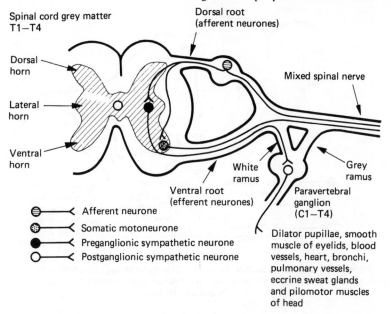

Figure 2.5 Sympathetic outflow from the CNS. Synapse in paravertebral ganglion; distribution to sympathetically innervated structures in head and thorax

neurones are distributed almost universally throughout the body. With only a few exceptions (page 93), NA is the transmitter substance between post-ganglionic sympathetic neurones and their effector cells.

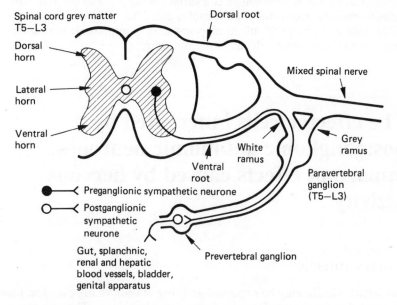

Figure 2.6 Sympathetic outflow from the CNS. Synapse in prevertebral ganglion; distribution to sympathetically innervated structures in abdomen and pelvis

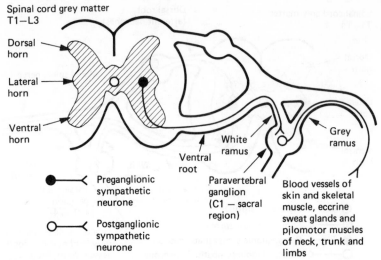

Figure 2.7 Sympathetic outflow from the CNS. Synapse in paravertebral ganglion; distribution through mixed spinal nerves to sympathetically innervated structures in neck, trunk and limbs

The autonomic neuroeffector junction

Postganglionic autonomic neurones branch and ramify within the effector organ to form a complex autonomic ground plexus. The number of autonomic neurones that approach an effector cell and the closeness of their approach varies greatly. Furthermore, the membranes of autonomic effector cells do not have regions that are specialized for the neuroeffector transmission process – the entire cell surface is sensitive to the action of the neurotransmitter (contrast with the motor end plate of skeletal muscle, page 73). Hence it is often difficult to pinpoint sites of autonomic neuroeffector transmission, even using electron micrography.

The effector cells innervated by postganglionic autonomic neurones: important effects caused by nervous activity

Ciliary muscle

The ciliary muscle may be regarded as a ring of smooth muscle. The lens is suspended at the centre of the ring by means of ligaments. The ciliary muscle receives only parasympathetic innervation. ACh released from postganglionic

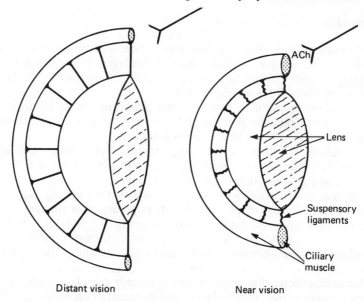

Figure 2.8 Control of accommodation by the ciliary muscle; oblique view of sagittal section through ciliary muscle, suspensory ligament and lens

neurones evokes ciliary muscle contraction and the eye is accommodated for near vision (*Figure 2.8*).

Accommodation can be altered voluntarily – but normally the ciliary muscle is automatically regulated to keep the most distinct image of the object of fixation imposed on the retina. Activity of the ciliary muscle also aids pumping of aqueous humour from the canals of Schlemm (*Figure 2.9*) into the veins. Interference with ciliary muscle control may thus not only paralyse accommodation (cycloplegia) but may also predispose to an elevation of intraocular pressure (glaucoma).

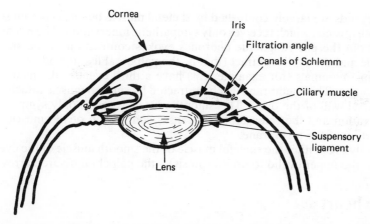

Figure 2.9 Flow of aqueous humour from the ciliary body, through the anterior chamber of the eye; transverse section through eye

The iris

The iris contains pigment cells that give the eye its characteristic colour and render the iris opaque. The iris contains two layers of smooth muscle – the sphincter pupillae (fibres arranged concentrically around the pupil) and the dilator pupillae (fibres arranged radially).

The sphincter pupillae receives only parasympathetic innervation and ACh released from the postganglionic neurones causes contraction of the muscle fibres. The pupil thus constricts (miosis).

The dilator pupillae receives only a sympathetic innervation and NA released from the postganglionic neurones causes contraction of the muscle fibres. The pupil thus dilates (mydriasis).

Changes in the activity of the parasympathetic pathway supplying the sphincter pupillae are responsible for the pupil diameter changes associated with the light reflex. An increase in the intensity of light falling on the retina induces a reflex increase in parasympathetic discharge to the sphincter pupillae. The pupil constricts and reduces the amount of light entering the eye.

Parasympathetic discharge to the sphincter pupillae is also increased when viewing a near object. The pupillary constriction results in utilization of only the central portion of the lens. The spherical and chromatic aberration of the lens is thus minimized and its depth of focus is increased.

Paralysis of the sphincter pupillae can lead to photophobia and also a narrowing of the angle (filtration angle) between the base of the iris and the inner surface of the cornea. This may predispose to impaired drainage of aqueous humour into the canals of Schlemm and hence to a rise in intraocular pressure (glaucoma) (*Figure 2.9*).

The dilator pupillae plays little part in the light reflex. Sympathetic discharge in response to fright or other emotional states may evoke mydriasis.

The eyelids

The eyelids are largely controlled by skeletal muscle but also contain some smooth muscle, which receives only sympathetic innervation. The release of NA from the postganglionic neurones evokes contraction of the smooth muscle and the eyelids retract (that is, the palpebral fissure widens).

Some mammals (for example, cat) have a third eyelid – the nictitating membrane. This membrane can be retracted by smooth muscle attached to the nasal wall of the orbit. This smooth muscle receives only sympathetic innervation and the release of NA causes contraction of the muscle and retraction of the membrane.

Paralysis of either the skeletal muscle or the smooth muscle of the eyelids allows the upper eyelid to droop (ptosis) – the palpebral fissure narrows.

The heart

The heart receives both parasympathetic and sympathetic innervations.

Parasympathetic neurones innervate the sinoatrial (SA) node (cardiac pacemaker). The release of ACh from parasympathetic nerve terminals reduces the discharge rate of the node and the heart rate falls (bradycardia or negative chronotropic effect).

Parasympathetic neurones also innervate the atrioventricular (AV) node. This is located on the right side of the interatrial septum and gives rise to a bundle of specialized conducting cells (Purkinje fibres), which carry the cardiac excitation wave across the AV septum and distribute the excitation wave to the ventricles. The release of ACh from parasympathetic neurone terminals depresses conduction through the AV node.

The ventricular myocardium (which performs most of the cardiac pumping work) does not receive a parasympathetic innervation.

Sympathetic neurones innervate all regions of the heart. The release of NA from these neurones increases the discharge rate of the SA node and the heart rate rises (tachycardia or positive chronotropic effect). It also increases conduction through the AV node and its associated Purkinje fibres and increases the force of contraction (positive inotropic effect) of the ventricular myocardium.

In a healthy young human adult heart rate is normally dominated by vagal tone when the subject is at rest. With increasing age, vagal tone becomes less dominant. During exercise, sympathetic tone may dominate the heart irrespective of the subject's age.

Respiratory smooth muscle

The smooth muscle of the respiratory tract receives both parasympathetic and (sparse) sympathetic innervation. ACh release from parasympathetic neurone terminals evokes contraction of respiratory smooth muscle (bronchoconstriction) while NA release from sympathetic neurones evokes relaxation (bronchodilatation).

In a healthy young subject the bronchial airways are almost maximally dilated even when the subject is at rest. The activation of sympathetic pathways during exercise does not therefore evoke much more bronchodilatation. The parasympathetic pathway to respiratory smooth muscle is reflexly activated in response to the inhalation of irritant substances or particles.

Gastrointestinal smooth muscle

The propulsive smooth muscle of the gut receives both parasympathetic and sympathetic innervation. The release of ACh from parasympathetic neurones causes smooth muscle contraction (stimulates propulsive activity) whilst NA release from sympathetic neurones causes relaxation (inhibits propulsive activity).

Under normal circumstances the propulsive smooth muscle of the gut is dominated by parasympathetic tone.

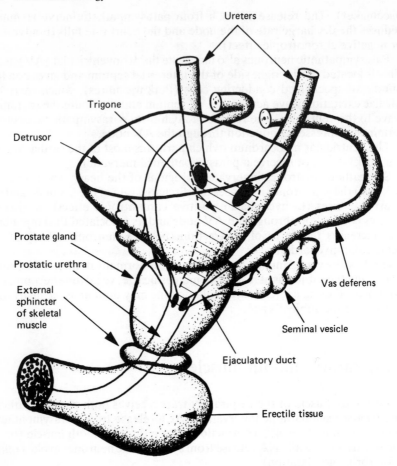

Ureters

Trigone

Detrusor

Prostate gland

Prostatic urethra

External
sphincter
of skeletal
muscle

Vas deferens

Seminal vesicle

Ejaculatory duct

Erectile tissue

Figure 2.10 Male genitourinary tract

The urinary bladder

The urinary bladder comprises a capsule of smooth muscle whose function is
the storage and periodic evacuation of urine. The smooth muscle of the
bladder comprises the detrusor (the greater part of the capsule) and the
trigone (that part bounded by the ureteric orifices and the bladder neck). An
external sphincter of skeletal muscle surrounds the bladder neck (*Figure
2.10*).

The detrusor receives parasympathetic innervation only. Bladder dis-
tension is the normal stimulus for micturition (passage of urine), which is
normally started at will. The release of ACh from parasympathetic neurone
terminals causes contraction of the detrusor and closure of the ureteric
orifices. The bladder neck is shortened and widened as it is pulled upwards.
This causes a fall in urethral resistance and allows the passage of urine.

The activity of skeletal muscle is involved to a variable degree in voluntary
micturition. The first event may be a relaxation of the external sphincter

round the bladder neck, accompanied by contraction of the diaphragm and abdominal muscles. As intra-abdominal pressure rises, urine may start to flow before detrusor activity reaches its peak. However, continence and voluntary micturition are possible in the absence of skeletal muscle activity.

The trigone and bladder neck receive only sympathetic innervation but the role of this sympathetic innervation in continence and micturition is negligible.

In males the release of NA from sympathetic nerve terminals during ejaculation causes a contraction of the trigone and bladder neck that prevents the reflux of seminal fluid into the bladder.

Seminal vesicle and vas deferens

The seminal vesicle and vas deferens (*Figure 2.10*) receive only sympathetic innervation. NA release evokes contraction of the smooth muscle of these organs and hence ejaculation of spermatozoa into the prostatic urethra. Ejection of seminal fluid from the urethra (emission) is dependent on the clonic contraction of skeletal muscle.

Vascular smooth muscle

The smooth muscle of blood vessels is arranged circularly around the lumen. Most blood vessels receive sympathetic innervation only. The release of NA from the sympathetic neurone terminals causes contraction of vascular smooth muscle and hence vasoconstriction. The brain stem vasomotor centre governs the tonic discharge of the sympathetic neurones innervating blood vessels and the resultant vascular muscle tone is one of the factors responsible for the maintenance of blood pressure (BP).

Arterioles of skeletal muscle

The arterioles of skeletal muscle receive a noradrenergic, sympathetic innervation controlled by the vasomotor centre as described for other vascular muscle. In addition they receive a second sympathetic innervation. The postganglionic neurones in this pathway, although anatomically sympathetic, release ACh as their transmitter, which causes vasodilatation of the skeletal muscle arterioles. This vasodilator pathway is activated in response to emotional shock (and so produces fainting) or in response to exercise (anticipated or current).

Arterioles of external genitalia

The arterioles of the erectile tissue of the external genitalia receive only parasympathetic innervation. The release of ACh from the parasympathetic

Table 2.1 The effector cells innervated by postganglionic autonomic nerves: the important effects on them of nervous activity

Sympathetic nervous activity	Organ	Parasympathetic nervous activity
	Eye	
No effect	Ciliary smooth muscle	Contracted
No effect	Circular smooth muscle of iris	Contracted
Contracted	Radial smooth muscle of iris	No effect
Contracted	Smooth muscle of eyelids and nictitating membrane	No effect
No effect	*Lacrimal and salivary glands*	Secretion
	Heart	
Increased firing rate	SA node	Reduced firing rate
Reduced refractory period	AV node	Increased refractory period
Reduced refractory period and increased automaticity	Conducting tissue	No effect
Increased contractile force	Ventricular myocardium	No effect
	Respiratory tract	
Relaxed	Airway smooth muscle	Contracted
No effect	Bronchial glands	Secretion
	Gut, stomach to rectum	
Inhibited	Propulsive smooth musculature	Stimulated
No effect	Alimentary and pancreatic exocrine glands	Secretion
	Urinary system smooth muscle	
No effect	Detrusor	Contracted
Contracted	Bladder neck and trigone	No effect
	Genital apparatus	
Contracted	Smooth muscle of seminal vesicles and vas deferens	No effect
No effect	Blood vessels of erectile tissue of external genitalia	Dilated
	Blood vessels	
Constricted	All	No effect
Dilated*	Those in skeletal muscle involved in fainting and exercise	No effect
	Skin	
Contracted	Pilomotor smooth muscles	No effect
Secretion*	Eccrine sweat glands	No effect

* Cholinergic transmission occurs at this site.

neurone terminals causes relaxation of the vascular muscle with resultant engorgement of the organ with blood (aided by reduced drainage due to venous compression).

Pilomotor muscles

Pilomotor muscles are responsible for the attitude of the hair shaft. They receive only a sympathetic innervation. NA release from the sympathetic neurone terminals evokes muscle contraction and the hair shaft erects. In furry animals the pilomotor muscles play an important role in thermoregulation – in man their role is vestigial (gooseflesh).

Eccrine sweat glands

The eccrine sweat glands receive only a sympathetic innervation. The postganglionic neurones of this pathway, although anatomically sympathetic, release ACh as their transmitter and thereby evoke sweat secretion. The eccrine sweat glands play an important role in thermoregulation by removing excess body heat as the latent heat of vaporization of sweat.

Other exocrine glands

The lacrimal glands, salivary glands, mucous glands of the respiratory tract, gastric oxyntic glands and digestive glands of the alimentary canal in general receive parasympathetic innervation. The release of ACh from parasympathetic neurone terminals in each case stimulates glandular secretion.

Table 2.1 summarizes the autonomic effectors and the important effects on them of nervous activity.

The pharmacology of cholinergic axons and their terminals

Revise

- The anatomy of somatic motoneurones (page 57) and anatomy of parasympathetic nerves (pages 57, 59).
- The effects of stimulating parasympathetic nerves (*Table 2.1*).

Cholinergic neurones synthesize, store and release ACh as their transmitter.
   They include:

(1) all preganglionic autonomic neurones (parasympathetic and sympathetic);
(2) all postganglionic parasympathetic neurones;
(3) a few postganglionic sympathetic neurones;
(4) all somatic (lower) motoneurones;
(5) some neurones lying entirely within the CNS.

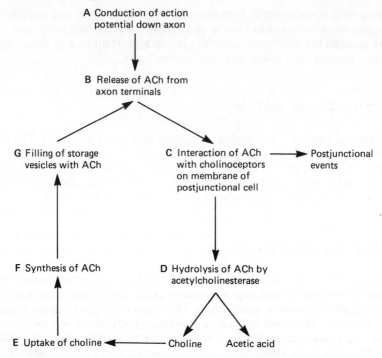

A Conduction of action
potential down axon

B Release of ACh from
axon terminals

G Filling of storage
vesicles with ACh

C Interaction of ACh ⟶ Postjunctional
with cholinoceptors   events
on membrane of
postjunctional cell

F Synthesis of ACh

D Hydrolysis of ACh by
acetylcholinesterase

E Uptake of choline ⟵ Choline   Acetic acid

Figure 2.11 Cholinergic neurotransmission

Cholinergic transmission

This process is basically similar at all sites in the body. It can be represented
by *Figure 2.11*.

Drugs that act on cholinergic axons and their terminals (drugs that interfere with stages A, B, E, F and G in *Figure 2.11*) will similarly modify
cholinergic transmission at all sites. The clinical usefulness of such agents is
thus limited by the diversity of their effects in the intact animal. Nevertheless
some drugs in this group (for example, the local anaesthetics) remain useful
because their sphere of action in the body can be restricted by the method of
administration.

Neuronal action potential conduction

Action potential conduction down the cholinergic axon may arbitrarily be
regarded as the first stage in the transmission process. It can be prevented
(and hence cholinergic transmission will be prevented) by local anaesthetics
(page 117) and tetrodotoxin (page 124) but these agents are not selective for
cholinergic neurones.

Release of ACh from axon terminals

In the absence of action potential traffic in cholinergic nerves, the random
migration of storage vesicles to the axon surface occasionally results in the

release of ACh into the cleft. Although the amount of transmitter released spontaneously is small, it can still influence the membrane of the post-junctional cell if the cleft is narrow. The miniature end plate potentials of twitch skeletal muscle (*Figure 2.13*) and the spontaneous postsynaptic potentials of ganglia (*Figure 2.19*) result from the spontaneous release of ACh.

Since spontaneous release does not depend on the arrival of action potentials it is unaffected by tetrodotoxin.

When action potentials invade terminal axons, membrane permeability changes occur, resulting in Na^+, Cl^- and Ca^{2+} entering the cells and K^+ emerging. The influx of Ca^{2+} triggers migration of many transmitter storage vesicles to the cell surface and release of ACh by exocytosis. The empty vesicular membranes are probably recycled within the cell and refilled with newly synthesized transmitter.

Transmitter release in response to nerve action potentials is prevented by local anaesthetics and tetrodotoxin.

As transmitter release by this mechanism requires influx of Ca^{2+} it is reduced if the extracellular fluid (ECF) is deficient in this ion or contains a high concentration of Mg^{2+}.

After treatment of a tissue with triethylcholine, action potentials release acetyltriethylcholine (a false transmitter) from cholinergic axon terminals (page 72). Triethylcholine interferes with the response to both spontaneous and action potential induced release of transmitter.

Botulinus toxin is an exotoxin produced by *Clostridium (Cl.) botulinum*, which also prevents both action potential-induced and spontaneous release of ACh from all cholinergic axons. Death in botulism results from respiratory paralysis.

Interaction of ACh with postsynaptic or postjunctional cholinoceptors

ACh in the cleft reversibly forms complexes with receptors (cholinoceptors) on the outer surface of the postsynaptic or postjunctional membrane. Some function of this interaction (page 13) determines the nature and size of the change in ionic permeability of the postsynaptic or postjunctional cell membrane. It may also trigger the synthesis of intracellular second messengers (inositol trisphosphate).

There are three types of cholinoceptor, which differ both in their affinities for drugs and in their anatomical location. Hence this is the stage in the transmission process that offers the pharmacologist the greatest opportunity for selective interference (pages 72–89).

Hydrolysis of ACh

The enzyme acetylcholinesterase (AChE) can hydrolyse (and thus inactivate) ACh to form choline and acetic acid. Drugs that inhibit the activity of AChE are the anticholinesterases (page 91).

Uptake of choline

Choline (dietary, synthesized from ethanolamine and methionine or formed from the hydrolysis of ACh) is taken up actively by neurones.

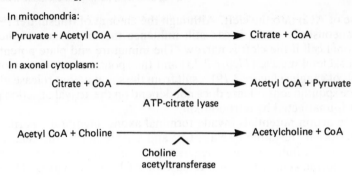

Figure 2.12 Synthesis of ACh

Hemicholinium blocks the choline pump and thus produces delayed block of cholinergic transmission (preformed ACh must be used up). Hemicholinium has no clinical application. Triethylcholine competes with choline for transport into the neurone.

Synthesis of ACh (Figure 2.12)

Some newly synthesized ACh is immediately hydrolysed by acetylcholinesterase of the axonal membrane. That which is taken up into the membrane-bound storage vesicles is protected from hydrolysis. This ACh is stored in the vesicles as a concentrated solution.

Triethylcholine competes with choline for the synthetic mechanism and acetyltriethylcholine is synthesized and stored. Since acetyltriethylcholine can be released from the nerve terminal but is much less potent on cholinoceptors than ACh it is said to function as a false transmitter. Triethylcholine thus produces delayed block of cholinergic transmission. Triethylcholine has no clinical application.

The pharmacology of the cholinoceptors of skeletal muscle

The receptors were originally designated 'nicotinic' since nicotine could readily mimic the action of ACh at these sites. Nicotinic cholinoceptors of skeletal muscle are characterized by the orders of drug potency shown in *Table 2.2*.

How do these agonists or antagonists (page 11) at the nicotinic cholinoceptor influence the development of tension by skeletal muscle? The answer depends to a certain extent upon the kind of muscle cell considered.

Table 2.2 Orders of drug potency at the nicotinic cholinoceptor of skeletal muscle

Agonists		
ACh		
Carbachol	> >	Muscarine
Nicotine		Methacholine
Suxamethonium (succinylcholine)		
Antagonists		
Tubocurarine		
Gallamine	> >	**Atropine**
Pancuronium		Hexamethonium
α-Bungarotoxin		

Note: Compounds to the left of the > > symbol are potent but not equally so; those to the right are so impotent that they may be regarded as inactive at this site.

Focally innervated (twitch) skeletal muscle

The majority of mammalian skeletal muscle cells are of this kind. Each muscle cell forms only one region of close association with a somatic moto-neurone terminal. Here the muscle cell membrane is specialized to form the motor end plate. Under normal circumstances this is the only part of the muscle cell membrane that has nicotinic cholinoceptors on the exterior surface.

The motoneurone axon branches near its terminal and each branch in-nervates a single muscle cell. The group of muscle cells innervated by a single axon is termed the 'motor unit' and the whole motor unit responds when an action potential is transmitted down the axon.

Functionally the skeletal muscle cells may be subdivided into fast fati-guable (white or glycolytic) and slow fatigue-resistant (red or oxidative) kinds. There may also be intermediate kinds. Most muscles contain some of both kinds of muscle cell. However the neuromuscular transmission process and its susceptibility to drugs do not appear to differ significantly between these kinds of muscle cell.

Although the end plates depolarize in a graded manner in response to increasing concentrations of ACh, the muscle cells exhibit 'threshold behav-iour'. That is, if the end plate depolarizes rapidly through a 'threshold of excitability' an action potential is triggered and this potential normally propagates to the cell extremities without decrement and is the electrical event that is associated with the Ca^{2+} fluxes necessary for shortening of the myofibrils. Action potential firing (and the presence of a well developed T-tubule system and sarcoplasmic reticulum) allows the cell to develop tension quickly (twitch).

The normal sequence of events during neuromuscular transmission

(1) Arrival of action potential in the nerve terminal.
(2) Release of ACh into the junctional cleft (width 20 nm).

(3) Diffusion of ACh down a concentration gradient towards the motor end plate.

(4) Association of ACh with the nicotinic cholinoceptors.

(5) Depolarization of the motor end plate to give an end plate potential (epp).

(6) When the epp crosses the threshold potential of excitability, an action potential is triggered and this travels out from the end plate to the muscle cell extremities.

(7) Passage of the action potential into the T-tubules and triggering of release of Ca^{2+} from intracellular sites causes shortening of myofibrils and the development of tension.

(8) Dissociation of ACh/receptor complex.

(9) Hydrolysis of ACh by AChE.

(10) Transport of choline back into the nerve terminal.

(11) Resynthesis of ACh.

(12) Storage of ACh in vesicles.

Under normal circumstances a single nerve action potential releases more than sufficient ACh to depolarize the end plate to threshold; that is, a safety factor exists for transmission. Normally only one muscle action potential is generated per nerve action potential since the transmitter is hydrolysed within the refractory period of the muscle cell (*Figure 2.13*).

The effects of agonists at nicotinic cholinoceptors on neuromuscular transmission

These agonists, which include ACh, *carbachol*, nicotine and **suxamethonium** (*Figure 2.14*), activate nicotinic cholinoceptors of the end plate and evoke depolarization. If this depolarization is large enough to cross the threshold of excitability, and does so rapidly enough, the muscle cell generates an action potential and contracts. Since these drugs are not readily hydrolysed by acetylcholinesterase (with the exception of ACh) the muscle cell often generates several action potentials and then enters a state where its end plate membrane remains depolarized at a level less inside-negative than the threshold of excitability. Under such circumstances, the muscle cell no longer responds to stimulation of its nerve supply by contraction. This is the state of depolarizing blockade of neuromuscular transmission (*Figure 2.15*). Blockade persists until such time as the end plate has repolarized to a level more inside-negative than the threshold of excitability. Depolarizing blockade of neuromuscular transmission can also be caused by inhibition of cholinesterases (ChEs, page 92).

The only agonist at nicotinic cholinoceptors shown in *Figure 2.14* that is useful for its action on skeletal muscle is **suxamethonium.** This drug is used in brief surgical or diagnostic procedures and in electroconvulsive therapy to produce brief (6 min) periods of paralysis. Iv injection causes asynchronous twitches of individual fibres in the bodies of muscles (fasciculation) due to the early phase of action potential firing. Then a phase of flaccid paralysis ensues due to depolarizing blockade of neuromuscular transmission.

Suxamethonium-induced paralysis is short lived due to rapid hydrolysis of the drug by cholinesterase. Patients genetically deficient in this enzyme (pages 30 and 90) suffer prolonged paralysis after **suxamethonium** injection.

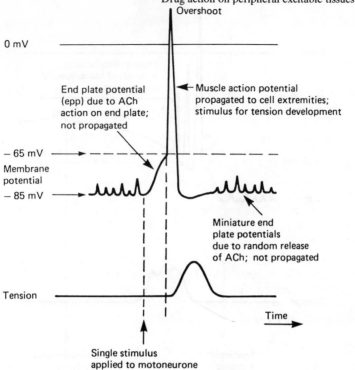

Figure 2.13 Twitch skeletal muscle: the motor end plate electrical activity and tension development of a single fibre evoked by stimulation of its nerve supply

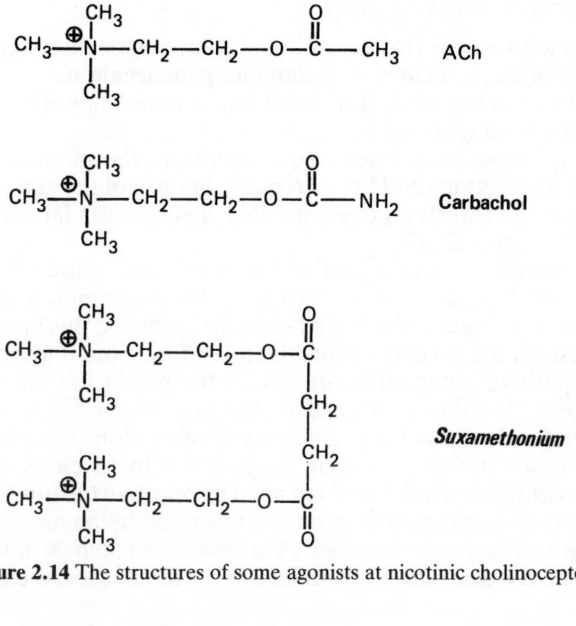

Figure 2.14 The structures of some agonists at nicotinic cholinoceptors

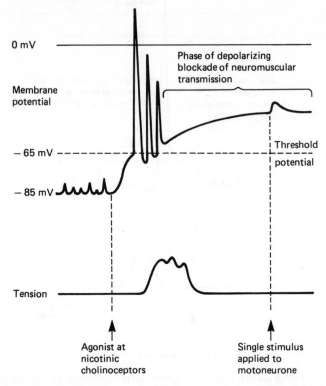

Figure 2.15 Twitch skeletal muscle: the effects of agonists at nicotinic cholinoceptors on the motor end plate electrical activity and tension development of a single fibre

Effects of antagonists at nicotinic cholinoceptors on neuromuscular transmission

Competitive antagonists (for definition of competitive antagonism, *see* page 14) – **tubocurarine,** *atracurium, gallamine,* **pancuronium.**
Noncompetitive antagonists (for definition of noncompetitive antagonism, *see* page 15) – α-bungarotoxin.

Any of the antagonists listed above decreases the number of transmitter/receptor interactions and hence reduces the size of the epp. If the epp no longer crosses the threshold of excitability, neuromuscular transmission to that cell fails (*Figure 2.16*).

When the effects of a competitive antagonist are followed *in vitro* or *in vivo*, a gradual depression of the twitch of the whole muscle is seen. Since transmission to a single cell is an 'all-or-none' process, this gradual onset of effect represents the successive inactivation of individual muscle cells.

The competitive antagonists are useful for producing muscle paralysis during surgery; they allow the anaesthetist to employ a relatively light level of anaesthesia and yet have adequate muscle relaxation. They are also useful in tetanus or strychnine poisoning (page 237). In all cases where tubocurarine-like drugs are used, there is a need to ventilate the lungs. The effects of the competitive antagonists can be terminated by an anticholinesterase drug, which increases the number of transmitter/receptor interactions by increasing the concentration of transmitter in the neuromuscular junction.

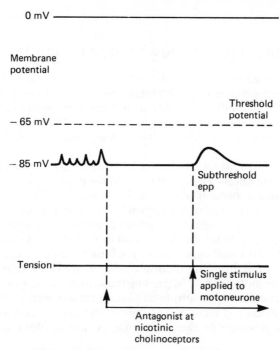

0 mV

Membrane
potential

Threshold
potential

– 65 mV

– 85 mV

Subthreshold
epp

Tension

Single stimulus
applied to
motoneurone

Antagonist at
nicotinic
cholinoceptors

Figure 2.16 Twitch skeletal muscle: the effects of antagonists at nicotinic cholinoceptors on the motor end plate electrical activity and tension development of a single twitch fibre

Tubocurarine causes histamine release (*see Table 4.13*) and ganglion blockade and hence lowers BP. These are not problems with **pancuronium**. *Atracurium* is particularly useful in patients with impaired liver or kidney function since its inactivation is largely brought about by spontaneous dissociation (nonenzymic Hofmann elimination – takes about 15 min).

α-Bungarotoxin is a component of the venom of a snake (the Taiwan banded krait, *Bungarus multicinctus*). It binds irreversibly and very selectively to the nicotinic cholinoceptors of skeletal muscle. It is not clinically useful but is a very valuable research tool, for example, in the localization and isolation of nicotinic cholinoceptors of muscle.

Clinically relevant interactions with neuromuscular blocking agents are shown in *Table 2.3*.

Table 2.3 Clinically relevant interactions with neuromuscular blocking agents

	Competitive (tubocurarine)	*Depolarizing* (suxamethonium)
General anaesthetics; **halothane**, *enflurane*, diethyl ether	+	0
Antibiotics; amino sugar **gentamicin**	+	0
Anticholinesterases; **neostigmine**	–	+
Hypothermia	–	+

+ = increases neuromuscular blocking activity; – = decreases neuromuscular blocking activity; 0 = no pronounced effect on neuromuscular blocking activity.

Multiply innervated (slow) skeletal muscle

In this kind of muscle each muscle cell has several neuromuscular junctions but there is no specialized muscle membrane (end plate) at these sites. This kind of muscle is relatively common in birds and amphibians but is uncommon in mammals. It should not be confused with the slow (red) focally innervated twitch fibres, which form a component of most mammalian muscles.

One site where multiply innervated muscle is found in mammals is in the intrafusal muscle fibres. These form part of the muscle spindles, the stretch receptors that are present within skeletal muscles. The muscle spindle consists of a central nuclear bag region, containing the sensory receptors. When stimulated these initiate the action potentials in afferent nerves that convey information about the degree and rate of stretch to the spinal cord and brain. The intrafusal muscle fibres are found at either end of the nuclear bag. The intrafusal fibres are themselves innervated by the small 'gamma-efferents' in the motor nerve. Increasing the activity of the gamma-efferents leads to contraction of the intrafusal fibres with consequent stretch of the nuclear bag region and increased activity of its sensory receptors, resulting in a reflex contraction of the contractile extrafusal fibres in the muscle concerned.

The fibres of multiply innervated slow muscles have nicotinic cholinoceptors, which respond to the same agonists, ACh, *carbachol* and **suxamethonium,** as the cholinoceptors of twitch muscle but the response evoked is a slow graded depolarization associated with a slow graded contraction of the muscle. Stimulation of the nerve supply during such a response has an additive effect on both the depolarization and the tension development (*Figure 2.17*). Note that the phenomenon of depolarizing blockade of transmission cannot occur in these muscle cells since they do not exhibit threshold behaviour. The soreness of muscles reported by patients after **suxamethonium** is probably due to excitation of the intrafusal fibres with consequent prolonged reflex activation of the skeletal muscle tone.

Antagonists at the nicotinic cholinoceptors of twitch fibres reduce the graded depolarization and graded contraction evoked in multiply innervated skeletal muscle by nerve stimulation or the administration of agonists at the nicotinic cholinoceptor (*Figure 2.18*).

The pharmacology of the cholinoceptors of ganglia

The sympathetic and parasympathetic ganglia are relay stations in autonomic efferent neural pathways. In most ganglia marked divergence occurs, i.e. the number of postganglionic fibres greatly exceeds the number of

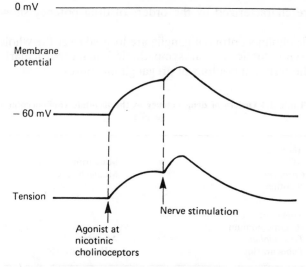

Figure 2.17 Slow skeletal muscle: the effects of agonists at nicotinic cholinoceptors on the electrical activity and tension development of a single fibre

preganglionic fibres. However, each preganglionic axon divides into many terminal branches so that each ganglion cell receives many synaptic contacts. In both the sympathetic and parasympathetic ganglia the transmitter released from the presynaptic terminals is acetylcholine.

The receptors were originally designated nicotinic since nicotine could readily mimic the action of ACh at these sites. Nicotinic cholinoceptors of

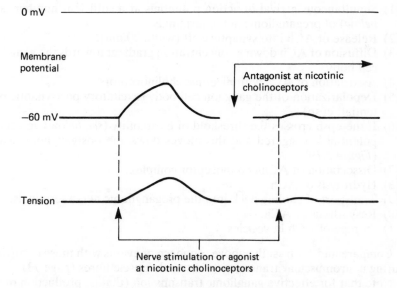

Figure 2.18 Slow skeletal muscle: the effects of antagonists at nicotinic cholinoceptors on the electrical activity and tension development of a single fibre

ganglia are characterized by the orders of drug potency shown in *Table 2.4.*

Nicotinic cholinoceptors of ganglia are located over the whole of the cell bodies of sympathetic and parasympathetic ganglia (particularly numerous beneath the terminal boutons of preganglionic fibres).

Table 2.4 Orders of drug potency at the nicotinic cholinoceptor of ganglia

Agonists		
ACh	> >	Muscarine
Carbachol		Methacholine
Nicotine		
Antagonists		
Hexamethonium		
Trimetaphan	> >	**Atropine**
Tubocurarine		α-Bungarotoxin

Note:

(1) Compounds to the left of the > > symbol are potent but not equally so; those to the right are so impotent that they may be regarded as inactive at this site.
(2) Nicotinic cholinoceptors of ganglia differ from those of skeletal muscle – particularly with regard to the order of antagonist potency (*Table 2.2*).

Normal sequence of events during ganglionic transmission

(1) Simultaneous arrival of action potentials at a sufficient number (*see below*) of preganglionic nerve terminals.
(2) Release of ACh into synaptic cleft (width 20 nm).
(3) Diffusion of ACh down a concentration gradient towards the ganglion cell body.
(4) Association of ACh with nicotinic cholinoceptors.
(5) Depolarization of the ganglion cell body (excitatory postsynaptic potential, epsp).
(6) If the epsp crosses the threshold of excitability (*see below*) an action potential is triggered and this moves down the postganglionic axon (*Figure 2.19*).
(7) Dissociation of ACh/cholinoceptor complex.
(8) Hydrolysis of ACh.
(9) Transport of choline back into the preganglionic nerve terminals.
(10) Resynthesis of ACh.
(11) Storage of ACh in vesicles.

Compare and contrast the above sequence of events with those occurring during neuromuscular transmission in twitch muscle fibres (page 73).

Note that for effective ganglionic transmission (that is, production of an epsp big enough to cross threshold) an appreciable number of preganglionic terminals must discharge transmitter in a synchronous fashion. Discharge of

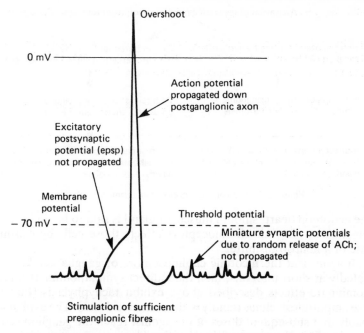

Figure 2.19 The electrical activity of an autonomic ganglion cell body

one terminal bouton would not normally evoke an action potential in the postganglionic cell body.

The effects of agonists at nicotinic cholinoceptors on ganglionic transmission

ACh, *carbachol*, nicotine

These activate nicotinic cholinoceptors of the ganglion cell body and evoke depolarization. If this depolarization is sufficiently large to cross the threshold of excitability, and does so sufficiently rapidly, the ganglion cell body generates an action potential. Since these drugs (even ACh, if in great excess) are not readily inactivated by acetylcholinesterase the ganglion cell body generally generates a burst of action potentials and then enters a state where its membrane potential is less inside-negative than the threshold of excitability. This is the stage of depolarizing blockade of ganglionic transmission (*Figure 2.20*). Under such circumstances the ganglion cell body becomes refractory (as regards action potential generation) to stimulation of the preganglionic neurones. Blockade of transmission persists until such time as the membrane of the ganglion cell body has repolarized to a level more inside-negative than the threshold of excitability.

Note the analogy with the actions of these drugs on neuromuscular transmission in twitch skeletal muscle fibres (page 74).

Agonists at the cholinoceptors of ganglia exert indirect sympathomimetic and parasympathomimetic effects on smooth muscle, cardiac muscle and exocrine glands because they trigger a burst of action potential discharge by the ganglion cell body (*Figure 2.21*).

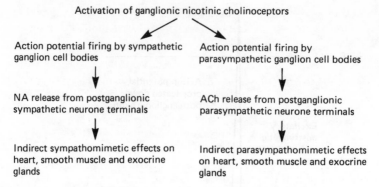

Activation of ganglionic nicotinic cholinoceptors

Action potential firing by sympathetic ganglion cell bodies

↓

NA release from postganglionic sympathetic neurone terminals

↓

Indirect sympathomimetic effects on heart, smooth muscle and exocrine glands

Action potential firing by parasympathetic ganglion cell bodies

↓

ACh release from postganglionic parasympathetic neurone terminals

↓

Indirect parasympathomimetic effects on heart, smooth muscle and exocrine glands

Figure 2.21 The consequences of ganglionic stimulation

The action on heart, smooth muscle or gland is said to be 'indirect' since the agonist at nicotinic cholinoceptors affects those cells by causing the release of a neurotransmitter.

If an agonist at the nicotinic cholinoceptors of ganglia is administered repeatedly at short intervals, then the indirect sympathomimetic/parasympathomimetic effects described above exhibit tachyphylaxis (that is, response amplitude declines rapidly with successive doses). The explanation is probably that subsequent doses of the agonist reach the ganglion cell body while it is still in the phase of depolarizing blockade.

Since these agents activate all sympathetic and parasympathetic ganglia,

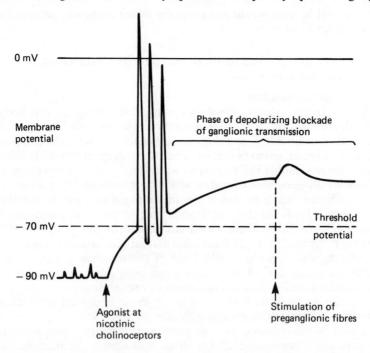

Figure 2.20 The effects of agonists at nicotinic cholinoceptors on the electrical activity of an autonomic ganglion cell body

their injection into the whole animal has very diverse effects. For this and other reasons, these agents are not used clinically for their action on ganglion cell bodies.

The effects of antagonists at the nicotinic cholinoceptors of ganglia

Hexamethonium, *trimetaphan*

These are competitive antagonists at the nicotinic cholinoceptors of ganglia. By reducing the number of transmitter/receptor interactions these agents reduce the epsp until it fails to cross the threshold of excitability. At this point ganglionic transmission fails (*Figure 2.22*).

These drugs block transmission through all ganglia (both parasympathetic and sympathetic) and at the adrenal medulla. They competitively antagonize ACh, nicotine or *carbachol* applied to these sites. *Table 2.5* shows their effects in the whole animal from which you can deduce whether an organ is normally dominated by parasympathetic or sympathetic tone.

Table 2.5 The important effects of ganglion blockade (for example, by hexamethonium, a competitive antagonist at nicotinic cholinoceptors of ganglia)

Sympathetic interruption	Organ	Parasympathetic interruption
	Eye	
	Ciliary smooth muscle	Relaxed
	Pupil	Dilated
Relaxed	Smooth muscle of nictitating membrane	
	Lacrimal and salivary glands	Reduced secretion
	Heart	
	SA node	Tachycardia, mild
	Gut, stomach to rectum	
	Propulsive smooth musculature	Reduced motility and constipation
	Alimentary and pancreatic exocrine glands	Reduced secretion
	Bladder	Retention of urine
	Genital apparatus	
Failure of ejaculation	Smooth muscle of seminal vesicles and vas deferens	
	Blood vessels of erectile tissue of external genitalia	Impotence
Dilated; postural hypotension	*All blood vessels*	
	Skin	
Relaxed	Pilomotor smooth muscles	
Reduced secretion	Eccrine sweat glands	

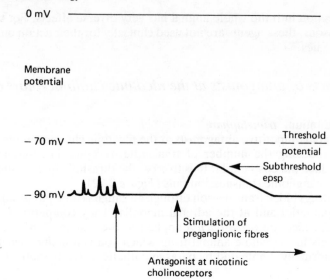

Figure 2.22 The effects of antagonists at nicotinic cholinoceptors on the electrical activity of an autonomic ganglion cell body

These agents have little therapeutic application because their effects in the whole body are so diverse. *Trimetaphan* is occasionally given by iv injection to lower BP and thereby minimize bleeding at the site of surgery ('bloodless' field). In addition to ganglion blockade, *trimetaphan* can lower BP by directly relaxing vascular smooth muscle and by evoking histamine release.

The pharmacology of the cholinoceptors of smooth muscle, cardiac muscle and exocrine glands

The receptors were originally designated muscarinic since muscarine could readily mimic the action of ACh at these sites. Muscarinic cholinoceptors of smooth muscle, cardiac muscle and exocrine glands are characterized by the orders of drug potency shown in *Table 2.6*.

Anatomy of parasympathetic neuroeffector junctions

Those smooth muscle, cardiac muscle and exocrine gland cells that receive a cholinergic innervation are supplied by postganglionic cholinergic neurones. Most neurones of this kind belong anatomically to the parasympathetic division of the autonomic nervous system. In the sympathetic division most postganglionic neurones are noradrenergic – but there are two kinds that are cholinergic:

(1) those supplying the eccrine sweat glands;
(2) those providing a vasodilator pathway to the arterioles of skeletal muscle.

Muscarinic cholinoceptors are probably located over the entire surface of effector cells. They are also found on cells that do not receive a cholinergic innervation, for example, the ventricular myocardium and the endothelial cells of blood vessels (*see* the footnote to *Table 2.7*).

Table 2.6 Orders of drug potency at the muscarinic cholinoceptor

Agonists		
ACh		
Methacholine		
Carbachol	> >	Nicotine
Pilocarpine		
Muscarine		
Antagonists		
Atropine	> >	**Tubocurarine**
Hyoscine		Hexamethonium
		α-Bungarotoxin

Note:
(1) Compounds to the left of the > > symbol are potent but not equally so. Those to the right are so impotent that they may be regarded as inactive at this site.
(2) The muscarinic cholinoceptors differ from nicotinic cholinoceptors both as regards the order of agonist potency and order of antagonist potency (*Tables 2.2 and 2.4*).

Normal sequence of events during cholinergic transmission to autonomic effector cells

(1) Arrival of action potential in the terminal branches of the postganglionic neurone.
(2) Release of ACh into the junctional cleft (width 20–1000 nm).
(3) Diffusion of ACh down a concentration gradient towards the effector cell.
(4) Association of ACh with muscarinic cholinoceptors on the effector cell.
(5) Induction of postjunctional events:
   (a) in effector cells where ACh has an excitatory action (*Table 2.7*), the transmitter/muscarinic cholinoceptor interaction may evoke an increase in membrane permeability to Cl^- and Ca^{2+} ions resulting in depolarization (excitatory postjunctional potential) and (in those cells that exhibit action potentials) an increase in

action potential frequency. Alternatively the transmitter/
muscarinic cholinoceptor interaction can stimulate the production
of the intracellular second messenger inositol trisphosphate, which
releases Ca^{2+} ions from stores in the endoplasmic reticulum.

(b) in effector cells where ACh has an inhibitory action, the transmit-
ter/muscarinic cholinoceptor interaction evokes a selective increase in membrane permeability to K^+ ions resulting in
hyperpolarization (inhibitory postjunctional potential) and (in
those cells that exhibit action potentials) a decrease in action
potential frequency.

Note that since many autonomic effector cells exhibit spontaneous electrical activity, the interaction of ACh with the muscarinic cholinoceptor tends not to initiate but rather to modify
ongoing electrical activity.

Table 2.7 The effects of ACh mediated by muscarinic cholinoceptors

Eye	
Ciliary smooth muscle	Contracted
Circular smooth muscle of iris	Contracted
Lacrimal and salivary glands	Secretion
Heart	
SA node	Reduced firing rate
AV node	Increased refractory period
Ventricular myocardium	Reduced contractile force*
Respiratory tract	
Airway smooth muscle	Constricted
Bronchial glands	Secretion
Gut, stomach to rectum	
Propulsive smooth musculature	Contracted
Alimentary and pancreatic exocrine glands	Secretion
Urinary system smooth muscle	
Detrusor	Contracted
Genital apparatus	
Blood vessels of erectile tissue	Dilated
Blood vessels	
All	Dilated*
Those in skeletal muscle involved in fainting and exercise	Dilated
Skin	
Eccrine sweat glands	Secretion

* Two effects of administered ACh that cannot be mimicked by autonomic nerve stimulation.
Muscarinic receptors are not restricted to cells receiving a cholinergic nerve supply. In blood
vessels muscarinic cholinoceptors lie on endothelial cells rather than smooth muscle cells and
modulate the release of an intermediate vasodilator substance, which is probably nitric oxide
(*see* page 138).

(6) Dissociation of the ACh/cholinoceptor complex.
(7) Hydrolysis of ACh by neural acetylcholinesterase and diffusion of ACh away from the site of action.
(8) Transport of choline back into the nerve terminal.
(9) Resynthesis of ACh.
(10) Storage of ACh in vesicles.

The effects of agonists at muscarinic cholinoceptors

ACh, methacholine, *carbachol* (*Figure 2.23*), *pilocarpine* and muscarine activate muscarinic cholinoceptors and cause changes (depolarization and/or inositol trisphosphate production; hyperpolarization) in effector cell activity analogous to the changes evoked by ACh released from cholinergic nerve terminals. Hence the agonists at muscarinic cholinoceptors can give rise to the excitatory and inhibitory effects listed in *Table 2.7*. Since many of the agonists at muscarinic cholinoceptors are less susceptible than ACh to hydrolysis by acetylcholinesterase, the cellular changes evoked by them are longer-lasting that those evoked by stimulation of cholinergic nerves.

The effects of agonists at muscarinic cholinoceptors are called (rather imprecisely) parasympathomimetic effects. Hence agonists at muscarinic cholinoceptors can also be called directly acting parasympathomimetic drugs. Contrast these agents with other drugs that can cause the same effects but by different mechanisms – the indirectly acting parasympathomimetic drugs. Examples include the agonists at the nicotinic cholinoceptors of ganglia (page 82) and anticholinesterase drugs (page 91).

ACh and muscarine are not used clinically.

Carbachol is used to stimulate the activity of the smooth muscle of the gut, bladder and ureters (for example, to expel gas from intestine prior to radiography, to reverse postoperative atony of the gut and bladder, to accelerate passage of ureteric stones).

Pilocarpine eye drops are useful for counteracting mydriatic drugs and also to lower intraocular pressure in acute attacks of narrow angle glaucoma (long-term relief from attacks may require surgery) and in long-term control of open angle glaucoma.

The effects of competitive antagonists at muscarinic cholinoceptors

Atropine, hyoscine [scopolamine], *tropicamide*
Quaternary ammonium derivatives – *ipratropium*

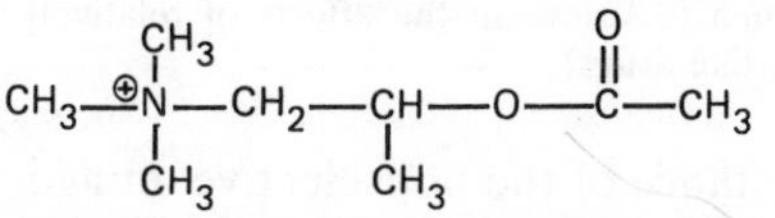

$$CH_3—\overset{\oplus}{\underset{\underset{CH_3}{|}}{\overset{\overset{CH_3}{|}}{N}}}—CH_2—\underset{\underset{CH_3}{|}}{CH}—O—\overset{\overset{O}{\|}}{C}—CH_3 \qquad \text{Methacholine}$$

Figure 2.23 Structures of some agonists at muscarinic cholinoceptors – *see Figure 2.14* for the structures of ACh and carbachol

Antimuscarinic drugs used in parkinsonism – *benzhexol*
Tricyclic antidepressive drugs – **imipramine**
Antidysrhythmic drugs – *quinidine*

These agents are all competitive antagonists of ACh at muscarinic cholinoceptors. Injection of these agents results in the effects shown in *Table 2.8*.

Measurements of the relative potencies of antagonists at muscarinic cholinoceptors suggest that such receptors can exist in the form of three distinct subtypes designated M_1, M_2 and M_3 cholinoceptors. *Pirenzepine* is a competitive antagonist exhibiting selectivity for the M_1 cholinoceptor. By blocking M_1 cholinoceptors on gastric parietal cells, *pirenzepine* can inhibit neurogenic gastric acid and pepsin secretion without exhibiting many of the other effects of **atropine**.

Table 2.8 The important effects of competitive antagonists at muscarinic cholinoceptors

Eye	
Ciliary smooth muscle	Relaxed (cycloplegia)
Circular smooth muscle of iris	Relaxed (mydriasis)
Lacrimal and salivary glands	Reduced secretion
Heart	
SA node	Tachycardia
AV node	Reduced refractory period
Respiratory tract	
Airway smooth muscle	Relaxed
Bronchial glands	Reduced secretion
Gut, stomach to rectum	
Propulsive smooth musculature	Reduced motility
Alimentary and pancreatic exocrine glands	Reduced secretion
Bladder	Difficulty of micturition
Skin	
Eccrine sweat glands	Reduced secretion

Note:
(1) *In vivo*, blockade of cholinergic autonomic neuroeffector transmission by **atropine** is more readily produced in some organs than in others. The order of susceptibility to blockade is: sweat, bronchial and salivary glands > heart and muscles of eye > smooth muscle of bladder and gastrointestinal tract > gastric glands.
(2) It is easier to prevent the effects of exogenous (injected) ACh than endogenous (released from nerve terminals) ACh. (The concentration of ACh in a narrow cleft during neuroeffector transmission can be high enough to surmount the effects of relatively large doses of atropine-like drugs).

Atropine is the type substance of the nonselective antagonists at muscarinic cholinoceptors. It has two actions that cannot be explained in terms of blockade of cholinergic transmission in the periphery:

(1) it causes histamine release, by virtue of its basicity (*see Table 4.13*), which results in dilatation of cutaneous vessels;
(2) it stimulates the CNS.

In therapeutic doses **atropine** stimulates the medullary vagal centre to evoke a transient bradycardia. This precedes the tachycardia due to occupation of myocardial muscarinic receptors by **atropine.** In toxic doses it causes restlessness, excitement, hallucinations, delirium, convulsions. Therapeutic uses are:

(1) anaesthetic premedication for effects on bronchial secretions and heart: **hyoscine** (sedative) is often preferred to **atropine** (CNS stimulant);
(2) routine mydriasis (diagnostic retinoscopy) carries a risk of precipitating glaucoma, particularly in the elderly, so choose a short-acting mydriatic – *tropicamide*;
(3) iritis and iridocyclitis are inflammatory conditions in which the iris tends to adhere to the anterior surface of the lens. A mydriatic with a long action is preferred – **hyoscine, atropine**;
(4) protection against undesired effects of anticholinesterase drugs during anticholinesterase drug therapy and poisoning (page 92);
(5) Parkinson's disease (page 219). Highly lipid soluble atropine-like drugs, for example, *benzhexol* are used to control tremor and excessive salivation;
(6) muscarinic (rapid-type mushroom) poisoning results from ingestion of toadstools that contain appreciable amounts of muscarine, for example, the red-staining inocybe (*Inocybe patouillardii*) – **atropine** is a specific antidote;
(7) travel sickness – **hyoscine** is useful (page 230);
(8) bronchoconstriction of chronic bronchitis – *ipratropium* is useful;
(9) gastric and duodenal ulceration – *pirenzepine* usefully reduces gastric acid and pepsin secretion and thereby promotes healing (page 370).

Cholinesterases and their inhibitors

Acetylcholinesterase

Acetylcholinesterase (AChE, EC 3.1.1.7) is found in and near the endings of all cholinergic axons and in erythrocytes. It is the activity of AChE that is primarily responsible for transmitter inactivation during cholinergic transmission (*Figure 2.11*).

AChE exhibits relatively high substrate specificity – it hydrolyses certain of the esters of choline (*Table 2.9*). Substrate attachment occurs both at the anionic and esteratic sites of the active centre of AChE (*Figure 2.24*).

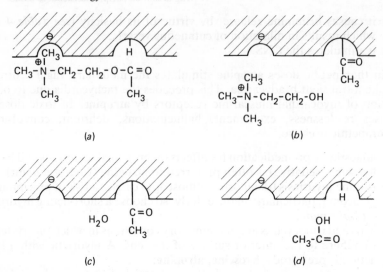

Figure 2.24 Hydrolysis of ACh by acetylcholinesterase: (a) attachment of ACh to anionic and esteratic sites; (b) acetylation of esteratic site with liberation of choline; (c) and (d) hydrolytic reactivation of esteratic site with liberation of acetic acid

Table 2.9 Hydrolysis of choline esters by AChE and ChE

Substrate	Rate of hydrolysis	
	AChE	ChE
ACh	+++	++
Methacholine	+	0
Carbamoyl esters of choline – *carbachol*	0	0
Suxamethonium	0	+

+ = hydrolysis; 0 = no hydrolysis.

Cholinesterase

Cholinesterase (pseudocholinesterase, butyrylcholinesterase, ChE, EC 3.1.1.8) is found in blood serum, in the liver and in certain effector cells.

The substrate specificity of ChE is low (*cf.* AChE). It not only hydrolyses certain choline esters (compare and contrast with AChE, *Table 2.9*) but will also hydrolyse esters unrelated to choline (for example, the ester kind of local anaesthetic agent, page 119).

Roughly 1 in every 3000 individuals is a homozygote with an abnormal gene pair that directs the synthesis of an atypical form of ChE. The atypical enzyme hydrolyses **suxamethonium** exceedingly slowly so that a homozygote producing the atypical enzyme stays paralysed for some hours when given this drug (page 30). Heterozygotes may hydrolyse **suxamethonium** slower than normal individuals but rapidly enough to present no clinical problem.

The atypical form of ChE is relatively resistant to inhibition by cinchocaine [dibucaine]. Measurement of the 'dibucaine number' (percentage inhibition of serum ChE activity produced by a standard concentration of dibucaine) gives an indication of whether the subject possesses abnormal genes for synthesizing ChE. A dibucaine number close to 80 indicates the absence of atypical ChE. A dibucaine number significantly lower than 80 indicates the presence of atypical enzyme.

Cholinesterase inhibitors

Competitive inhibitors

Neostigmine, *physostigmine* (eserine), *pyridostigmine, edrophonium, carbaryl*

The inhibition of AChE produced by these agents can be overcome by increasing the substrate (for example, ACh) concentration and the inhibited enzyme can readily be reactivated by subjecting it to dialysis – the inhibition is reversible. With the exceptions of *carbaryl* and *physostigmine*, all agents in this group have molecular structures that contain a quaternized N atom – and hence are fully ionized over a wide pH range. The positive charge on the quaternized N atom facilitates attachment of these agents to the anionic site of the active centre of AChE (*Figure 2.24*).

Since *physostigmine* is a tertiary amine its inhibition of AChE is pH-dependent. Attachment of *physostigmine* to the anionic site of AChE only occurs when the N atom of the amine group is positively charged.

Edrophonium is unique among the competitive inhibitors of AChE in that it is not an ester. *Edrophonium* cannot therefore combine with the esteratic site of AChE. This may explain the very brief duration of edrophonium's action *in vivo*.

AChE and ChE are equally sensitive to the actions of the competitive inhibitors.

Noncompetitive inhibitors

Malaoxon from *malathion*

The inhibition of AChE produced by these agents cannot be overcome by increasing the substrate (for example, ACh) concentration and the inhibited enzyme cannot be reactivated by dialysis – the inhibition is irreversible.

The noncompetitive inhibitors of AChE are organophosphorus esters and all can bind firmly to (phosphorylate) the esteratic site of AChE (*Figure 2.25*).

The noncompetitive inhibitors have higher affinities for ChE than for AChE.

Consequences of cholinesterase inhibition

Inhibition of AChE delays the biotransformation of ACh. The resulting accumulation of endogenous ACh evokes parasympathomimetic effects

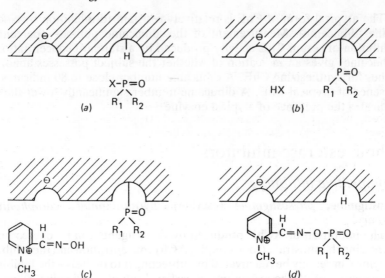

Figure 2.25 Organophosphorus inhibition of acetylcholinesterase: (a) and (b) phosphorylation of esteratic site with liberation of acid (HX); (c) and (d) reactivation of esteratic site by pralidoxime

(page 87 and *Table 2.1*) including excessive sweating, salivation and bronchial secretion, miosis, bradycardia and diarrhoea. These effects can be minimized by the administration of an antagonist at muscarinic cholinoceptors – **atropine**.

Inhibition of AChE can cause fasciculation of skeletal muscle and convulsions. However, when AChE is inhibited by about 80%, the accumulation of ACh at the skeletal neuromuscular junction evokes depolarizing blockade of neuromuscular transmission (page 74 and *Figure 2.15*). At this point death may ensue from respiratory paralysis – effectively due to ACh poisoning.

Uses of cholinesterase inhibitors

Competitive inhibitors of AChE are used in the diagnosis and treatment of myasthenia gravis (a disease in which cholinergic transmission at the skeletal neuromuscular junction is impaired and characterized by weakness and ready fatiguability of skeletal muscle). *Edrophonium* is a diagnostic agent – a positive result is indicated by a brief increase in muscular power following its injection.

Neostigmine and *pyridostigmine* are used in the symptomatic treatment of myasthenia usually in conjunction with **atropine,** which minimizes the effects of ACh at muscarinic cholinoceptors. Overdosage with **neostigmine** or *pyridostigmine* can itself precipitate muscle weakness due to excessive accumulation of ACh causing depolarizing blockade of neuromuscular transmission – a 'cholinergic crisis'. *Edrophonium* can be used to distinguish between a cholinergic crisis and the effects of under-treatment or increased disease severity. An injection of *edrophonium* will briefly exacerbate a cholinergic crisis but will briefly increase muscle power in the case of under-dosage with a ChE inhibitor.

Neostigmine is used to accelerate the offset of the neuromuscular blockade evoked by **tubocurarine** or **pancuronium** (*Table 2.3*). The injection of **neostigmine** is preceded by an injection of **atropine** in order to minimize the effects of ACh at muscarinic cholinoceptors.

Physostigmine is useful as a miotic, and for counteracting the actions of mydriatic drugs. It is useful for lowering intraocular pressure in congestive (narrow angle) glaucoma. Its use in the eye carries a risk of systemic toxicity since it is well absorbed from the conjunctival sac.

Malathion and *carbaryl* are used as insecticides in the treatment of pediculosis (page 269). Other organophosphorus anticholinesterases are agricultural insecticides or military nerve gases.

Reactivation of cholinesterases inhibited by organophosphorus compounds

The inhibition of esterases evoked by organophosphorus compounds is irreversible in the sense that the phosphorylated esteratic site cannot spontaneously hydrolyse. If, and only if, the phosphorylation is recent, the enzyme can be reactivated by agents that are more nucleophilic than water (for example, **pralidoxime**) (*Figure 2.25*).

Industrial, agricultural or military poisoning with organophosphorus anticholinesterases is treated by injection of both **atropine** and **pralidoxime.**

Noradrenergic neuroeffector transmission as a target of drug action

Revise

- The anatomy of the sympathetic nervous system (pages 56 and 60);
- The effects of stimulating sympathetic neurones (*Table 2.1*).

Noradrenergic neurones synthesize, store, and release NA as their transmitter. They include:

(1) most postganglionic sympathetic neurones (except those neurones supplying the eccrine sweat glands and those providing a vasodilator pathway to the arterioles of skeletal muscle – although anatomically sympathetic, these neurones are cholinergic);
(2) some neurones lying entirely within the CNS.

Anatomy of sympathetic neuroeffector junctions

The anatomy of sympathetic neuroeffector junctions is comparable with that of parasympathetic neuroeffector junctions (page 84). Those effector cells that receive a noradrenergic innervation (smooth muscle, cardiac muscle and exocrine gland cells) are supplied by postganglionic sympathetic neurones. The receptor sites for NA (α- and β-adrenoceptors, page 106) are located over the entire surface of the effector cells. They can also be found on cells that do not receive noradrenergic innervation (*Table 2.14*).

Drugs with noradrenergic prejunctional sites of action

Noradrenergic transmission

The process of noradrenergic neuroeffector transmission (*Figure 2.26*) is basically similar at all sites in the body.

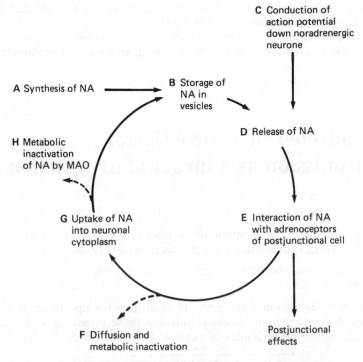

Figure 2.26 Noradrenergic neuroeffector transmission

Synthesis of NA

The biosynthesis of NA may arbitrarily be regarded as the first stage in the process of noradrenergic transmission. The starting material is dietary *l*-phenylalanine. This amino acid is actively absorbed from the gut and oxidized by hepatic phenylalanine hydroxylase to form *l*-tyrosine, which circulates in the bloodstream and is actively transported into the cytoplasm of noradrenergic neurones.

There (*Figure 2.27*) *l*-tyrosine is hydroxylated to form *l*-dihydroxyphenylalanine (*l*-dopa, **levodopa**). This reaction is catalysed by cytoplasmic tyrosine hydroxylase and is the rate limiting step in the biosynthesis of NA. The activity of tyrosine hydroxylase is governed by the cytoplasmic concentration of NA, a high NA concentration inhibiting enzyme activity. This is an example of feedback (product) inhibition.

Tyrosine hydroxylase exhibits some substrate specificity but is susceptible to inhibition by *metirosine* (α-methyltyrosine). This inhibits tyrosine hydroxylase and reduces catecholamine synthesis. It is useful in limiting the catecholamine output of a rare tumour of the adrenal medullary chromaffin cells (phaeochromocytoma) both preoperatively or as a long-term therapy in inoperable cases.

Aromatic *l*-amino acid decarboxylase is a cytoplasmic enzyme of low substrate specificity that converts *l*-dopa to dopamine. It can be inhibited by *benserazide* and by *carbidopa*. These agents are hydrophilic analogues of *l*-dopa and do not enter the brain (page 316). They can therefore provide a selective inhibition of peripherally located enzyme. This phenomenon is exploited in order to reduce the adverse peripheral effects (postural hypotension, tachydysrhythmias) and the dose of **levodopa** in the treatment of Parkinson's disease (page 220).

Dopamine, synthesized within the neuronal cytoplasm, is actively transported into the transmitter storage vesicles of the axon terminals. There, it is oxidized by dopamine β-hydroxylase (an enzyme of low substrate specificity) to form NA.

Storage of NA in vesicles

Endogenous NA is stored in membrane-limited vesicles, which are formed in the neuronal cell body and transported to the varicosities of the axon terminal by axoplasmic flow. Within the vesicles, storage of NA is aided by the presence of ATP (forms a weak complex), a sulphomucopolysaccharide and a soluble protein called chromogranin. The retention of NA inside vesicles results from the resistance to diffusion provided by the vesicular contents and of the continued operation of the amine uptake process in the vesicle membrane (a process requiring energy from the breakdown of ATP by Mg^{2+}-dependent ATPase).

Drugs that interfere with the vesicular retention of NA

Reserpine and *tetrabenazine* inhibit the amine uptake process in the vesicle membrane and thereby allow the leakage of NA into the cytoplasm where it is largely metabolized by neuronal monoamine oxidase (MAO, page 101). Furthermore, since vesicular dopamine uptake is inhibited, NA synthesis is

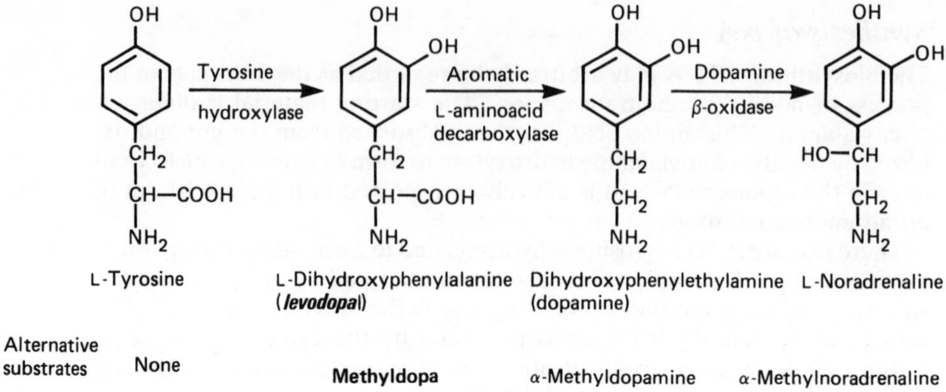

OH

Tyrosine
hydroxylase

OH
OH

Aromatic
L-aminoacid
decarboxylase

OH
OH

Dopamine
β-oxidase

OH
OH

CH_2
CH—COOH
NH_2

CH_2
CH—COOH
NH_2

CH_2
CH_2
NH_2

HO—CH
CH_2
NH_2

L-Tyrosine   L-Dihydroxyphenylalanine   Dihydroxyphenylethylamine   L-Noradrenaline
              (*levodopa*)   (dopamine)

Alternative
substrates   None

Methyldopa   α-Methyldopamine   α-Methylnoradrenaline

Figure 2.27 Synthesis of NA

impaired. For these two reasons the storage vesicles become depleted of NA (chromaffin cells of the adrenal medulla and noradrenergic, dopaminergic and tryptaminergic neurones within the CNS are also susceptible to this action of reserpine, page 221).

NA depletion is accelerated by action potential activity in the neurone. Noradrenergic neuroeffector transmission fails when NA content is reduced to about 25% of normal. When large doses of reserpine are used, recovery of neurone function depends upon the synthesis of new vesicles and their transport to the axon terminals (about 10 days).

Pretreatment with reserpine:

(1) abolishes the effects of sympathetic noradrenergic neurone activity;
(2) abolishes the effects of agents that cause the release of NA from axon terminals – the indirectly acting sympathomimetic agents (page 99);
(3) does not reduce responses of effector cells to exogenous NA or other directly acting sympathomimetic agents (page 104);
(4) has similar effects on noradrenergic, dopaminergic and serotoninergic neurotransmission in the CNS.

Reserpine was formerly useful in the treatment of severe hypertension. It is now rarely used because it can induce severe (suicidal) depression. Part of the hypotensive action of reserpine results from the impairment of aminergic transmission in blood pressure control centres of the CNS.

Tetrabenazine is of use in certain disorders of movement, for example, Huntington's chorea (page 221), presumably because *tetrabenazine* depletes the transmitter stores of central dopaminergic neurones. The usefulness of *tetrabenazine*, like reserpine, is limited by the development of severe depression.

Drugs that compete with NA for vesicular storage

Certain drugs, on gaining access to the neuronal cytoplasm, can compete with dopamine or NA for uptake into the vesicles. They may then stoichiometrically displace NA from its storage site. Drugs in this group include α-methyldopamine formed from *methyldopa* and certain indirectly acting sympathomimetic agents (tyramine, amphetamine).

As a consequence of NA displacement:

(1) less NA is available for release during neuroeffector transmission;
(2) the displacing drug may be released in the place of NA during neuroeffector transmission (false transmission);
(3) the response of the effector cell to the displacing drug may result from the pharmacological effects of displaced NA (*see* indirectly acting sympathomimetic agents, page 99).

Methyldopa (*cf.* triethylcholine acting on cholinergic transmission, page 72) is a substrate for aromatic *l*-amino acid decarboxylase and hence can be converted to α-methyldopamine. α-Methyldopamine is not a substrate for neuronal MAO (because it carries the α-methyl substituent, page 101) so it competes very successfully with dopamine for transport into the storage vesicles. Vesicular dopamine β-hydroxylase then oxidizes α-methyldopamine to yield α-methylnoradrenaline, which functions as a false transmitter since it can be stored in the vesicles and subsequently be released into the junctional cleft on arrival of the nerve action potential. α-Methylnoradrenaline is approximately equipotent with NA in evoking a response from effector cells in the periphery by agonist action at postjunctional α_1-adrenoceptors (page 106) but more potent than NA at presynaptic (release-inhibiting) α_2-adrenoceptors (page 107). It reduces neuroeffector transmission by reducing the amount of neurotransmitter released.

Pretreatment with *methyldopa*:

(1) reduces the effects of noradrenergic and dopaminergic neurone activity in the CNS;
(2) does not reduce the responses of effector cells to exogenous NA or other directly acting sympathomimetic agents, page 104.

Methyldopa is useful in the treatment of moderate to severe hypertension in patients in whom antagonists at β-adrenoceptors are contraindicated (page 115) and in pregnancy (page 383). Its main site of action in reducing cardiac output and peripheral resistance seems to be the central noradrenergic neurones involved in the control of BP. Adverse effects include drowsiness, depression and fluid retention.

Drugs that modify the release of noradrenaline

Neuronal action potential conduction

Action potential conduction in noradrenergic neurones is comparable with that in cholinergic neurones (page 70).

Action potential conduction down the noradrenergic axon can be prevented (and hence transmission will be prevented) by local anaesthetic agents (**lignocaine**) (page 117) and by tetrodotoxin (page 124). These agents prevent action potential conduction by membrane stabilization. They are not selective for noradrenergic neurones.

In contrast the noradrenergic neurone blocking agents (for example, *guanethidine*) selectively impair transmission at noradrenergic neuroeffector junctions. These agents are weak local anaesthetics but are selectively accumulated by noradrenergic neurones by the same mechanism that transports NA into the cell – the neuronal uptake pump (page 103). Thus, the noradrenergic neurone blocking agents are accumulated within noradrenergic neurones to local anaesthetic concentrations so that NA release is abolished by the prevention of nerve action potential conduction in terminal neuronal branches. In addition, these drugs may interfere with exocytosis. Large doses of *guanethidine* may cause structural damage in noradrenergic nerve terminals so that the axon partly and temporarily dies back towards the cell body.

The noradrenergic neurone blocking agents

(1) Prevent the effects of noradrenergic neurone activity;
(2) Prevent the effects of those indirectly acting sympathomimetic agents that initiate nerve action potential activity (nicotine, pages 81 and 99);
(3) Prevent the effects of those indirectly acting sympathomimetic agents that utilize the neuronal NA uptake mechanism to gain access to the neuronal cytoplasm (tyramine, amphetamine, page 99);
(4) Do not reduce the effects of exogenous NA or other directly acting sympathomimetic agents (page 104). Indeed, if the directly acting sympathomimetic agent is a substrate for the neuronal NA uptake process it is potentiated.

The selectivity of the noradrenergic neurone blocking agents and their ability to modify the actions of some indirectly or directly acting sympathomimetic agents all depend on their being substrates for the neuronal NA uptake process. The actions of noradrenergic neurone blocking agents are impaired by other drugs that compete with them for uptake into the neurone (tyramine) or that block the uptake process (*cocaine*, **imipramine,** page 104).

The noradrenergic neurone blocking agents are sometimes useful in the treatment of severe hypertension that is resistant to other drugs (page 380). Unwanted effects include postural and exercise hypotension, diarrhoea and failure of ejaculation.

Guanethidine eyedrops can lower intraocular pressure in chronic, simple, open-angle glaucoma and can reduce the exophthalmos and eyelid retraction of hyperthyroidism.

Release of NA from axon terminals

The release of NA from noradrenergic axons is comparable with the release of ACh from cholinergic axons (page 70).

In the absence of action potential traffic in noradrenergic nerves, the random migration of storage vesicles to the cell surface occasionally results in exocytosis. Although the amount of NA released is small, it can still influence the membrane of the postjunctional cell if the cleft is narrow, for example, spontaneous postjunctional potentials are seen in some noradrenergically innervated smooth muscles (*cf.* the miniature epp seen at the motor end plate of skeletal muscle, *Figure 2.13*).

Since spontaneous release does not require the arrival of nerve action potentials, it is unaffected by tetrodotoxin. Reserpine, by depleting the vesicles of stored NA (page 95), prevents both the spontaneous and action potential-evoked (*see below*) release of NA.

When an action potential invades the varicosities, membrane permeability changes occur. Na^+, Cl^- and Ca^{2+} enter the cell and K^+ emerges. The influx of Ca^{2+} triggers many storage vesicles to release NA, ATP, chromogranin and dopamine β-hydroxylase into the extracellular space (exocytosis) and this NA diffuses down its concentration gradient to stimulate adrenoceptors on the effector cell surface. The empty vesicles are probably retained within the cell and subsequently refilled with transmitter.

Since transmitter release by this mechanism requires the nerve action potential, it is prevented by local anaesthetic agents, tetrodotoxin and noradrenergic neurone blocking agents.

Since transmitter release by this mechanism requires the influx of Ca^{2+}, release is reduced if the extracellular environment is deficient in this ion or contains a high concentration of Mg^{2+}.

After treatment of tissues with *methyldopa*, action potentials release α-methylnoradrenaline (false transmission, page 97) rather than NA from the terminals of noradrenergic axons.

Indirectly acting sympathomimetic agents

The effects of activation of noradrenergic neurones are called (rather imprecisely) sympathomimetic effects. Hence an agonist at adrenoceptors can also be called a directly acting sympathomimetic agent. An indirectly acting sympathomimetic agent does not itself activate adrenoceptors. It evokes sympathomimetic effects either by promoting the release of neuronal NA (nicotine, tyramine) or by preventing the inactivation of NA (*cocaine*).

Agonists at the nicotinic cholinoceptors of ganglia

ACh, nicotine and *carbachol* cause action potentials to be generated in postganglionic sympathetic neurones and so evoke release of neural NA (*Figure 2.21*), thereby inducing sympathomimetic effects.

Tyramine-like indirectly acting sympathomimetic agents

Certain chemical modifications of the NA molecule (loss of catechol —OH groups; loss of the β-OH group; methylation of the α-C atom) yield agents that cannot themselves activate adrenoceptors. Examples include tyramine and amphetamine (*Figure 2.28*).

However, these drugs do act as substrates for the NA uptake process in the neuronal membrane (page 103) and gain access to the neuronal cytoplasm by that route. In addition, amphetamine is sufficiently lipid soluble to be able to gain access by diffusion across the neuronal membrane. From the cytoplasm they are then transported into the transmitter storage vesicles where they stoichiometrically displace NA. A high proportion of the displaced NA escapes from the neurone and subsequently activates postjunctional adrenoceptors because the MAO associated with the mitochondria (page 101), which would normally break down excess cytoplasmic NA, is occupied by a competing molecule. Tyramine is a substrate and amphetamine an inhibitor of MAO.

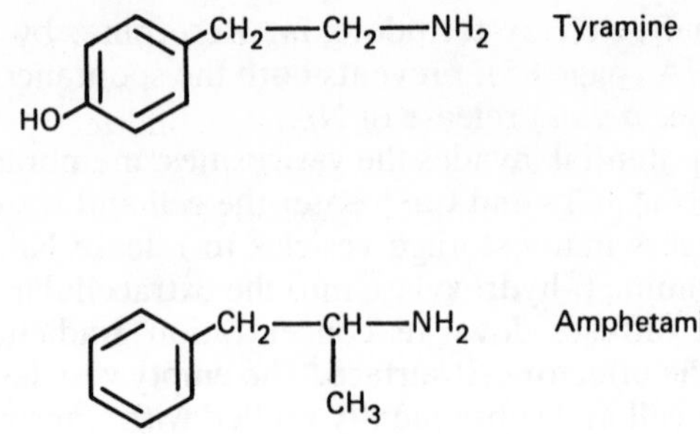

Figure 2.28 The structures of some indirectly acting sympathomimetic drugs

Table 2.10 Comparison of physiological directly acting and indirectly acting sympathomimetic agents

Directly acting, e.g. NA, adrenaline	Indirectly acting, e.g. tyramine, amphetamine	Explanation for property of indirectly acting drug
Chemically unstable	Chemically more stable	Drug molecule lacks catechol —OH groups
Pharmacological effects are brief	Pharmacological effects are more prolonged	Drug molecule relatively resistant to biotransformation
Poorly absorbed from gut	Better absorption from gut	Drug molecule lacks catechol —OH groups and is less polar
Poor penetration of CNS and thus CNS effects unremarkable	Better penetration of CNS and thus CNS effects more prominent	Drug molecule lacks catechol —OH groups and is less polar
Postganglionic sympathetic denervation potentiates	Postganglionic sympathetic denervation prevents action	Drug must enter neurone to be active; neurones degenerate
Cocaine and **imipramine** potentiate	*Cocaine* and **imipramine** prevent action	Drug must enter neurone to be active; entry into neurone prevented
Summates with NA	Potentiates NA	Drug competes with NA for neuronal uptake
Reserpine does not prevent action	Reserpine prevents action	Drug cannot displace neural NA; transmitter stores are depleted
Phenelzine does not modify action	**Phenelzine** potentiates	MAO inhibition delays biotransformation of drug or of NA released by drug
Repeated equal doses have equal effects	Tachyphylaxis occurs	Neuronal NA stores become depleted by repeated drug challenge

NA release evoked by tyramine-like agents does not require the discharge of neuronal action potentials.

The properties of the tyramine-like group of indirectly acting sympathomimetic agents are compared with those of NA and adrenaline, the physiological directly acting sympathomimetic agents, in *Table 2.10*.

Inhibitors of the neuronal uptake of NA

Cocaine and **imipramine** inhibit the neuronal uptake of NA (page 104). Endogenous NA (spontaneously released or released by neuronal action potentials) therefore accumulates in the junctional cleft and evokes sympathomimetic effects.

Drugs that modify the inactivation of noradrenaline

Enzymic degradation is not an important mechanism for the inactivation of NA released during neuroeffector transmission. The NA in the junctional cleft is largely inactivated by neuronal uptake (page 103).

Metabolic inactivation of NA

Sympathomimetic amines circulating in the bloodstream (amines from the diet, injected drugs, adrenaline released from the adrenal medulla) are inactivated by enzymic destruction to a variable extent. Metabolic inactivation assumes greatest importance if the circulating catecholamines are present in large amounts and are not substrates for neuronal uptake.

Circulating sympathomimetic amines may be metabolized by catechol-*O*-methyl transferase (COMT), by MAO, or by both enzymes (*Figure 2.29*).

COMT is found in the liver and certain effector cells but not in noradrenergic neurones. This enzyme can utilize any catechol as substrate. The *O*-methylated product may undergo conjugation (page 325) to form a sulphate or glucuronide, or may be oxidized by MAO to form the corresponding acid.

MAO is found in the intestine, in the liver and in mitochondria in the cytoplasm of noradrenergic neurones. MAO oxidatively deaminates its substrate. It can utilize many aryl- and alkyl-amines (NA, *adrenaline*, tyramine, 5-HT) as substrates but not those with a large N-substituent (*isoprenaline*, page 110) or those with an α-methyl substituent (amphetamine, α-methyldopamine). The product is the corresponding acid (in the periphery, *Figure 2.29*) or glycol (in the CNS).

The major product of biotransformation of both NA and adrenaline is 3-methoxy-4-hydroxymandelic acid (vanillylmandelic acid, VMA). The urinary excretion of VMA is raised in phaeochromocytoma and can be measured as a diagnostic test.

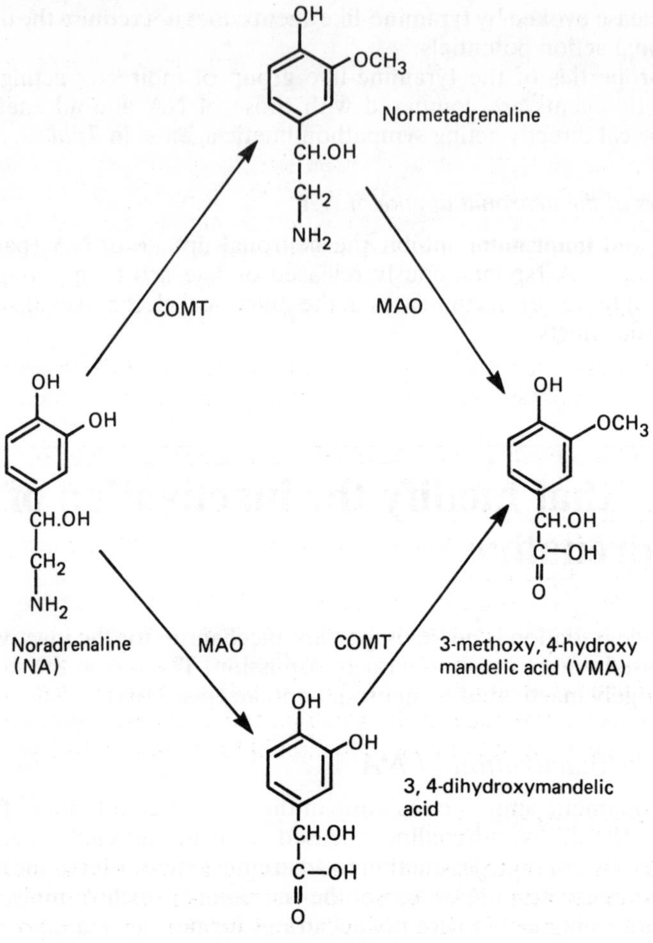

Figure 2.29 Metabolism of NA

Drugs that interfere with the biotransformation of NA

All catechols can act as competitive inhibitors of COMT but COMT inhibition is not therapeutically exploited.

MAO inhibitors are of two major kinds:

(1) competitive – *tranylcypromine*;
(2) noncompetitive (the hydrazine group) – **phenelzine**.

By inhibiting MAO, these agents potentiate dietary tyramine. Significant amounts of tyramine are found in cheese, beef extracts (Bovril), yeast extracts (Marmite), pickled herrings and some alcoholic drinks. Some sympathomimetic agents administered therapeutically (*adrenaline*, **levodopa** and indirectly acting sympathomimetic agent ingredients of proprietary cold remedies) are also potentiated and these, as well as tyramine in foodstuffs, can cause dangerous hypertensive crises.

MAO inhibition can potentiate sympathomimetic drugs by:

(1) delaying the biotransformation of the drug itself (*adrenaline*, tyramine);
(2) delaying the biotransformation of any NA released by the drug (tyramine).

The hydrazine MAO inhibitors lack selectivity for they can also inhibit the mixed function oxidase enzymes (page 324) of the liver. They can therefore delay the biotransformation of (and thus potentiate) many drugs that are not substrates for MAO (amphetamine, *pethidine* and **morphine**).

Tranylcypromine is a close structural and functional analogue of amphetamine; hence it has CNS stimulant properties (page 237) that further limit its usefulness.

MAO inhibitors have a place in the treatment of depression but are of limited usefulness because of the multiplicity of interactions with other drugs.

MAO is actually composed of several isoenzymes, the most abundant of which are called MAO-A and MAO-B. Both are found in most peripheral noradrenergic neurones but the liver and gut mucosa contain mainly MAO-A. More interestingly, parts of the brain contain mainly MAO-B – particularly the striatum.

Selegiline is a selective inhibitor of MAO-B (it forms an irreversible complex having been activated by the enzyme – a process known as 'suicide inhibition'). The 'cheese reaction' to dietary amine is not a problem during *selegiline* treatment because MAO-A is not inhibited. *Selegiline* is useful as an adjunct to **levodopa** in the treatment of Parkinson's disease (*cf. carbidopa*, page 95) as it allows a reduction in the dose of **levodopa**.

Neuronal uptake of NA

Uptake into the cytoplasm of noradrenergic neurones is the major mechanism for inactivating NA released during neuroeffector transmission or NA injected as a small iv dose. Blockade of uptake therefore potentiates exogenous NA or that released by a nerve impulse.

The uptake process is located in the axonal membrane and:

(1) operates against a concentration gradient;
(2) requires an energy supply;
(3) requires Na^+;
(4) is saturable;
(5) is moderately substrate specific.

Substrates for the neuronal NA uptake process

These include:

(1) the physiological directly acting sympathomimetic agents – NA and *adrenaline* (note that the synthetic drugs, *phenylephrine*, *isoprenaline* and **salbutamol** are not substrates);
(2) certain indirectly acting sympathomimetic agents – tyramine, amphetamine;
(3) the noradrenergic neurone blocking agents – *guanethidine*.

Drug interactions among the substrates for neuronal NA uptake

(1) The tyramine-like indirectly acting sympathomimetic agents and the noradrenergic neurone blocking agents potentiate NA and *adrenaline* by competing for neuronal uptake.
(2) The tyramine-like indirectly acting sympathomimetic agents and the noradrenergic neurone blocking agents are mutually antagonistic since they compete for the uptake process (and thus for access to their sites of action).

Nontransported inhibitors of neuronal NA uptake

Cocaine inhibits the NA uptake process at concentrations less than those required to produce local anaesthesia. *Cocaine* thus potentiates endogenous NA released either spontaneously or in response to an action potential from the axon terminal (for example, the mydriasis evoked by *cocaine* eyedrops). No other local anaesthetic drug has this property.

The antidepressive actions of the tricyclic agents **imipramine** and **amitriptyline** may be attributed to their blockade of amine uptake in the CNS (page 224).

Drug interactions with nontransported inhibitors of NA uptake

By blocking neuronal uptake, *cocaine* and tricyclic antidepressive drugs:

(1) potentiate NA and *adrenaline* (by delaying their inactivation);
(2) antagonize the tyramine-like indirectly acting sympathomimetic agents and the noradrenergic neurone blocking agents (by preventing their access to their sites of action).

Fate of NA transported into the neuronal cytoplasm

A small proportion of the NA entering the cytoplasm by way of the neuronal uptake process is metabolized by mitochondrial MAO. The majority is transported into the storage vesicles for subsequent transmitter use (*cf.* uptake of choline and its use in ACh synthesis, page 7).

Figure 2.30 summarizes the mechanisms of NA uptake and release from noradrenergic neurones.

Extraneuronal uptake of NA

Uptake of catecholamines (*isoprenaline* > *adrenaline* > NA), by a high capacity, low affinity active transport process, occurs at the effector cell membrane. This is their route of access to COMT. Inhibitors of extraneuronal uptake are not exploited therapeutically.

Agonists at adrenoceptors

The interaction of NA with postjunctional adrenoceptors

The NA/adrenoceptor interaction is comparable with the ACh/muscarinic cholinoceptor interaction (page 71).

Neurotransmitter NA that has been released into the extracellular space diffuses down its concentration gradient and forms reversible complexes with receptors (adrenoceptors) on the surface of the membrane of the effector cell. Some function of this interaction (page 13) determines the nature and size of the response. The response may comprise a change in ionic permeability of the effector cell membrane or a coupled change in enzyme activity, leading to a change in intracellular second messenger concentration.

(1) In effector cells where NA has an excitatory action (*Tables 2.12* and *2.14*), the NA/adrenoceptor interaction may evoke an increase in membrane permeability to Cl^- and Ca^{2+} resulting in depolarization (excitatory postjunctional potential) and (in those cells that exhibit action potentials) an increase in action potential frequency. Alternatively the

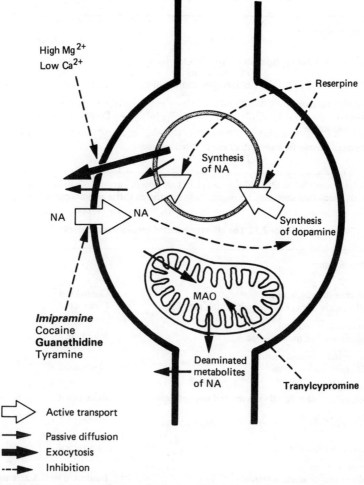

Figure 2.30 Summary of drugs influencing the fate of NA in a noradrenergic neurone

transmitter/adrenoceptor interaction may stimulate the production of the intracellular second messenger inositol trisphosphate, which releases Ca^{2+} from stores in the endoplasmic reticulum.

(2) In effector cells where NA has an inhibitory action, the NA/adrenoceptor interaction may evoke a selective increase in membrane permeability to K^+ resulting in hyperpolarization (inhibitory postjunctional potential) and (in those cells that exhibit action potentials) a decrease in action potential frequency. Alternatively, the transmitter/adrenoceptor interaction may stimulate the production of the intracellular second messenger cAMP, which enhances the uptake of Ca^{2+} into intracellular stores or the extrusion of Ca^{2+} from the cell.

Since many autonomic effector cells exhibit spontaneous electrical activity, the interaction of NA with the adrenoceptor tends not to initiate but rather to modify ongoing electrical activity.

Table 2.11 The α-adrenoceptor: relative orders of potency

Nonselective agonists		
NA	= *Adrenaline*	> > *Isoprenaline*
Agonists selective for subtypes of the α-adrenoceptor		
α_1	*Phenylephrine*	
α_2	α-Methylnoradrenaline	
Nonselective antagonists		
Phentolamine	> >	**Propranolol**
Phenoxybenzamine		
Antagonists selective for subtypes of the α-adrenoceptor		
α_1	*Prazosin*	

Note: Compounds to the left of the > > symbol are potent but not equally so; those to the right are so impotent that they may be regarded as inactive at the α-adrenoceptor.

Table 2.12 The effects mediated by α-adrenoceptors

α_1-*Adrenoceptors*	
Eye	
Radial smooth muscle of iris	Contracted
Smooth muscle of eyelids and nictitating membrane	Contracted
Gut, stomach to rectum	
Propulsive smooth musculature	Inhibited
Urinary system smooth muscle	
Bladder neck and trigone	Contracted
Genital apparatus	
Smooth muscle of seminal vesicles and vas deferens	Contracted
All blood vessels	Constricted
Skin	
Pilomotor smooth muscles	Contracted
α_2-*Adrenoceptors*	
Noradrenergic neurone terminals	Inhibition of NA release

There are two major kinds of adrenoceptor, which may be distinguished by characteristic relative orders of potencies for both agonists and antagonists: the α-adrenoceptor (*Table 2.11*) and the β-adrenoceptor (*Table 2.13*). Each of these receptors exists in the form of several subtypes.

Agonists at the α-adrenoceptor

The effects mediated by α-adrenoceptors are listed in *Table 2.12*.

Table 2.13 The β-adrenoceptor: relative orders of potency

Nonselective agonists		
Isoprenaline	> *Adrenaline*	> NA
Agonists selective for subtypes of the β-adrenoceptor		
β_1	Dobutamine	
β_2	**Salbutamol**	
Nonselective antagonists		
Propranolol	> >	**Phentolamine**
		Phenoxybenzamine
Antagonists selective for subtypes of the β-adrenoceptor		
β_1	**Atenolol**	

Note: Compounds to the left of the > > symbol are potent but not equally so; those to the right are so impotent that they may be regarded as inactive at the β-adrenoceptor.

Table 2.14 The effects mediated by β_1- and β_2-adrenoceptors

β_1-Adrenoceptors	
Heart	
SA node	Increased firing rate
AV node	Reduced refractory period
Conducting tissue	Reduced refractory period and increased automaticity
Ventricular myocardium	Increased contractile force
Gut, stomach to rectum	
Propulsive smooth musculature	Inhibited
Adipocytes+	Lipolysis
Liver cells+	Glycogenolysis
β_2-Adrenoceptors	
Respiratory tract	
Airway smooth muscle	Relaxed
Genital apparatus smooth muscle	
Uterus	Relaxed
All blood vessels*	Dilated
Skeletal muscle cells+	Tremor, glycolysis

* These vessels receive noradrenergic innervation but the NA released activates only α-adrenoceptors (*Table 2.12*). β-Adrenoceptors here are activated by circulating agonists – the resulting fall in BP is largely due to dilatation of arterioles in skeletal muscle because of the high proportion of body mass that muscles represent.

+ β-Adrenoceptors can be found on cells that do not receive a noradrenergic innervation (*cf.* muscarinic cholinoceptors, *Table 2.7*).

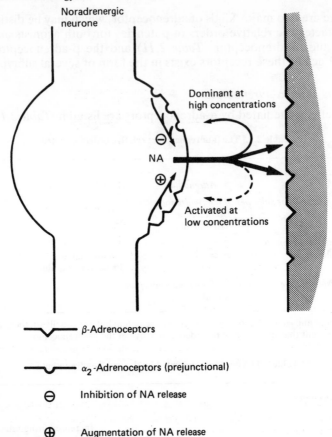

Figure 2.31 The physiological role of prejunctional α_2-adrenoceptors in the heart

The physiological role of prejunctional α_2-adrenoceptors is illustrated in *Figure 2.31* and is believed to be associated with conserving transmitter. α_2-Adrenoceptor activation results in a reduction in the amount of NA released at any given frequency of neuronal activity. This mechanism comes into play when the noradrenergic nerve terminal is exposed to high concentrations of NA.

Agonists at the β-adrenoceptor

The effects mediated by β-adrenoceptors are listed in *Table 2.14*.

In many effectors, the activation of β-adrenoceptors is accompanied by stimulation of adenylate cyclase and therefore an increase in cellular content of cAMP. The role of adenylate cyclase in lipolysis and glycogenolysis is illustrated in *Figure 2.32*.

The effects of agonists at adrenoceptors

Adrenaline, dopamine, dobutamine, isoprenaline, NA, phenylephrine, **salbutamol**

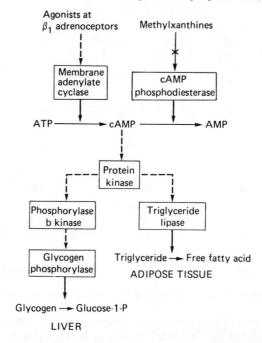

Figure 2.32 The second messenger function of cyclic nucleotide in mediating glycogenolysis and lipolysis. Note: in liver, protein kinase also phosphorylates and inhibits glycogen synthetase. --> = activation

These drugs activate one or both kinds of adrenoceptor and cause changes in effector cell activity analogous to the changes evoked by NA released from noradrenergic nerve terminals (depolarization and/or inositol trisphosphate production; hyperpolarization and/or cAMP production). Hence agonists at adrenoceptors can give rise to the excitatory and inhibitory effects listed in *Tables 2.11* and *2.13*. Since many agonists at adrenoceptors are less susceptible than NA to the uptake and biotransformation disposal mechanisms, the cellular changes evoked by them are longer-lasting than those evoked by stimulation of noradrenergic nerves.

Structure/activity relationships and selectivity of agonists at adrenoceptors

Most directly acting sympathomimetic agents are structural analogues of *adrenaline*. This agent is a potent agonist at both α- and β-adrenoceptors. Slight changes in the structure of the *adrenaline* molecule can yield compounds that selectively activate either α- or β-adrenoceptors. *Figure 2.33* shows a classification of agonists at the adrenoceptor according to their α:β selectivity.

Notes:

(1) An alternative name for 1,2-dihydroxybenzene is catechol, therefore 3,4- dihydroxyphenylethylamines are catecholamines.
(2) The β-carbon atom of phenylethanolamines is asymmetric; the

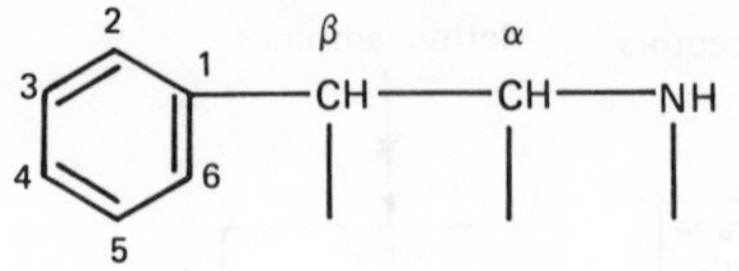

		β	α			Affinity for receptor type
3–OH		OH	H	CH$_3$	Phenylephrine	α
3–OH, 4–OH		OH	H	H	NA	α and β
3–OH, 4–OH		OH	H	CH$_3$	Adrenaline	α and β
3–OH, 4–OH		OH	H	CH(CH$_3$)$_2$	Isoprenaline	β
3–CH$_2$OH, 4–OH		OH	H	C(CH$_3$)$_3$	*Salbutamol*	β

Figure 2.33 Classification of directly acting sympathomimetic drugs

biosynthesis of the physiological compounds NA and adrenaline yields the *l*-isomer (in which much the greater biological activity resides).

(3) The physiological compounds, NA and adrenaline, have relatively low selectivity and therefore elicit effects mediated by both α- and β-adrenoceptors. The synthetic agonist drug *isoprenaline* elicits only the effects mediated by β-adrenoceptors (*Table 2.14*).

(4) In general, increasing the size of the substituent on the nitrogen atom of the 3,4-dihydroxyphenylethanolamine molecule increases selectivity for β-adrenoceptors.

(5) Provided that excessive drug concentrations are avoided, the synthetic agonist drug *phenylephrine* elicits only the effects mediated by α$_1$-adrenoceptors (*Table 2.12*) and the synthetic agonist drug **salbutamol** elicits only the effects mediated by β$_2$-adrenoceptors (*Table 2.14*).

Dopamine has a complex peripheral sympathomimetic pharmacology. It is a precursor in the synthesis of NA (page 95). Furthermore, when exogenously administered, it is an agonist at both β$_1$- and α$_1$-adrenoceptors. *Dopamine* is also an agonist at renal vascular dopamine receptors, mediating vasodilatation, and is an indirectly acting sympathomimetic agent.

Dobutamine is an analogue of *isoprenaline* that is an agonist at both β$_1$- and α$_1$-adrenoceptors. It has little chronotropic effect (contrast *isoprenaline*) because the vasoconstriction induces a rise in mean arterial BP and therefore a baroreceptor-mediated restraint on the heart rate.

Therapeutic uses

Eye drops containing *phenylephrine* or *adrenaline* produce brief periods of mydriasis during diagnostic retinoscopy. Such eyedrops are also effective in lowering intraocular pressure (possibly by reducing the production of aqueous humour) in primary open angle glaucoma.

Adrenaline is included in the formulation of some local anaesthetics for injection (see page 121). By causing vasoconstriction at the injection site it prolongs the local anaesthesia.

Adrenaline is given im in the control of anaphylactic shock (page 27) and other severe forms of urticaria. It usefully evokes vasoconstriction, bronchodilatation and a reduction in the permeability of capillaries to protein.

Salbutamol is useful for reducing airways resistance in bronchial asthma (page 393). It can relax bronchial smooth muscle at doses that have little or no cardiac stimulant activity. There is therefore less risk of tachycardia, ectopic beats and dangerous dysrhythmias than with the the the nonselective agent, *isoprenaline*. Most of the agonists selective at β_2-adrenoceptors that are used as bronchodilator drugs are neither substrates for uptake (page 103) nor for enzymic degradation by MAO or CQMT (page 101). Their resistance to COMT endows them with bronchodilator activity that outlasts that of *isoprenaline*.

Dopamine and *dobutamine* are useful, by iv infusion, to increase the force of contraction of the failing heart (page 379).

Antagonists at adrenoceptors

These drugs, to a certain extent, resemble NA structurally and are therefore able to combine with adrenoceptors but, unlike NA, are unable to activate adrenoceptors. Thus they do not evoke an active biological response from the effector cell.

Antagonists at the α-adrenoceptor

By combining with the α-adrenoceptor, these antagonists reduce the access of agonists. They thereby reduce those effects of sympathetic nerve activity or sympathomimetic drug (both directly and indirectly acting) action that are mediated by α-adrenoceptors (*Table 2.12*).

Nonselective

Phentolamine, phenoxybenzamine, chlorpromazine

These antagonists, while very selective for α- as opposed to β-adrenoceptors, have equal potency at (are nonselective between) the α_1- and α_2-subtypes.

Phentolamine and **chlorpromazine** are competitive (surmountable, reversible) antagonists (page 14) at α-adrenoceptors.

In contrast, **phenoxybenzamine** is a noncompetitive (nonequilibrium, insurmountable, irreversible) antagonist (page 15) at α-adrenoceptors. **Phenoxybenzamine** is a β-haloalkylamine. In neutral or alkaline solution it forms the highly reactive ethyleniminium ion. This ion either alkylates reactive groups of the cell membrane (for example, the α-adrenoceptor) or spontaneously condenses with water to form an inactive alcohol (*Figure 2.34*).

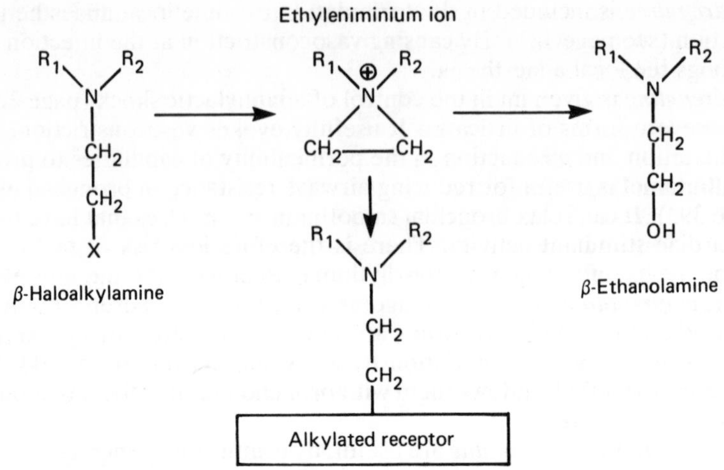

Ethyleniminium ion

β-Haloalkylamine

β-Ethanolamine

Alkylated receptor

Figure 2.34 Mechanism of alkylation by phenoxybenzamine

Note that a low concentration or short exposure time enables **phenoxybenzamine** to alkylate α-adrenoceptors selectively. A higher concentration or longer exposure time leads to the alkylation of other receptors – histamine H_1 receptors, $5\text{-}HT_2$ receptors and muscarinic cholinoceptors.

Selective

Prazosin is a competitive antagonist that is very selective for α- as opposed to β-adrenoceptors and also has a much higher affinity for α_1- than α_2-adrenoceptors.

Therapeutic uses

Phentolamine is occasionally a useful aid in the diagnosis of phaeochromocytoma. The diagnosis is supported when an iv injection of **phentolamine** produces a dramatic but brief fall in BP to near or below normal by antagonism of catecholamines (that are circulating in excessive amounts).

Phenoxybenzamine protects vascular smooth muscle from high circulating concentrations of catecholamines produced by phaeochromocytoma and is useful in providing this protection during surgical removal of such tumours or as symptomatic treatment in inoperable cases. In both circumstances it should be combined with an antagonist at β-adrenoceptors (page 115). Its irreversible action affords prolonged protection.

Phentolamine and **phenoxybenzamine** have not proved useful in the treatment of essential hypertension despite the fact that they produce a marked fall in peripheral resistance. This is because the resultant fall in blood pressure is accompanied by an unacceptable degree of reflex tachycardia.

Prazosin, however, produces much less tachycardia for the same fall in peripheral resistance and as a result has proved useful in treating hypertension. This difference arises because of the existence of prejunctional

α_2-adrenoceptors with structural requirements slightly different from the α_1-adrenoceptors on effector cells (page 106).

The explanation for the excessive reflex tachycardia in response to **phentolamine,** then, is that the normal feedback inhibition of NA release from cardiac sympathetic nerves that occurs during reflex tachycardia is abolished because **phentolamine** occupies prejunctional α_2-adrenoceptors (*Figure 2.35*). *Prazosin*, however, is selective for postjunctional α_1-adrenoceptors and the size of the reflex tachycardia can still be limited by the normal feedback inhibition via prejunctional α_2-adrenoceptors.

Other antagonists at α-adrenoceptors have useful properties unrelated to α-adrenoceptor blockade. **Chlorpromazine** (a phenothiazine) is an antipsychotic drug, which is valuable in the treatment of schizophrenia and can suppress vomiting. These actions of **chlorpromazine** on the CNS result from the drug's interaction with dopamine receptors (page 227). The antagonism

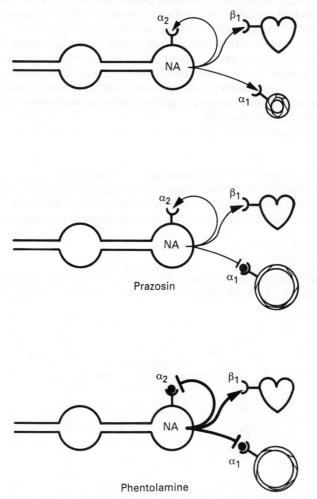

Figure 2.35 The propensity of phentolamine, when used as a hypotensive agent, to cause tachycardia is not shared by prazosin

at α-adrenoceptors evoked by **chlorpromazine** is responsible for some of the drug's unwanted effects (for example, hypotension).

Antagonists at the β-adrenoceptor

By combining with β-adrenoceptors, these antagonists reduce the access of agonists. They thereby reduce those effects of sympathetic nerve activity or sympathomimetic drug (both directly and indirectly acting) action that are mediated by β-adrenoceptors (*Table 2.14*).

Nonselective

Propranolol, while very selective for β- as opposed to α-adrenoceptors, has equal potency at (is nonselective between) the β_1- and β_2-subtypes. **Propranolol** is a competitive antagonist at β-adrenoceptors. In a concentration higher than that required for blockade of β-adrenoceptors, **propranolol** (but not **atenolol**) directly stabilizes the membranes of excitable cells (page 130).

Labetolol has a structure that confers affinity for both β- and α-adrenoceptors but is three times more potent as a competitive antagonist at β- than α-adrenoceptors. It is nonselective between the β_1- and β_2-subtypes but is selective for α_1-adrenoceptors, reducing the arteriolar response to NA without affecting the neuronal negative feedback mechanisms mediated by α_2-adrenoceptors (page 107).

Selective

Atenolol is a competitive antagonist that is very selective for β- as opposed to α-adrenoceptors and also has a higher affinity for β_1- than β_2-adrenoceptors. That is, it can antagonize NA on the heart at doses that have little or no effect on the relaxant action of NA on respiratory tract smooth muscle.

Therapeutic uses

Propranolol and **atenolol** lower the heart rate by occupying cardiac β-adrenoceptors. This prolongs diastole and reduces myocardial oxygen

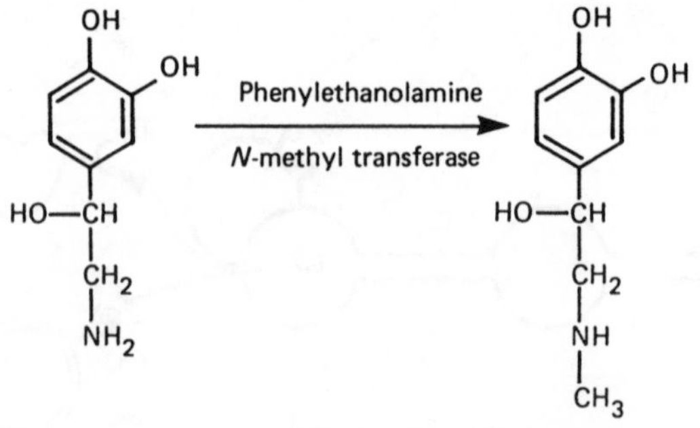

Figure 2.36 The synthesis of adrenaline by the adrenal medulla

demand, whereby increasing the exercise tolerance of patients with angina pectoris (page 388).

Propranolol and **atenolol** can be used to lower the BP of hypertensive patients (page 381). *Labetolol* is useful in both chronic hypertension and hypertensive emergencies (page 385).

Propranolol and **atenolol** are effective in the correction of certain cardiac dysrhythmias, especially those due to **digoxin** toxicity or thyrotoxicosis.

Propranolol and **atenolol** are useful in protecting cardiac β-adrenoceptors from high concentrations of circulating catecholamines prior to, or during, the surgical removal of a phaeochromocytoma.

Eyedrops containing an antagonist at β-adrenoceptors provide useful control of intraocular pressure in chronic simple glaucoma, probably by reducing the rate of production of aqueous humour. The drug can be absorbed from the conjunctival sac so that unwanted systemic effects can occur.

Unwanted effects of antagonists at β-adrenoceptors include the precipitation of cardiac failure in patients with a small cardiac reserve and aggravation of bronchoconstriction in asthmatic patients. The risk of precipitating bronchoconstriction is less with **atenolol** than with the nonselective antagonists at β-adrenoceptors but is nevertheless still significant. Unwanted effects of *labetolol* also include those mediated at α_1-adrenoceptors – postural hypotension and failure of ejaculation.

The adrenal medulla

The chromaffin cells that comprise the adrenal medulla arise embryologically from the same cells as those giving rise to postganglionic noradrenergic neurones. However, the embryonic adrenal medullary cells do not develop long axons or threshold electrical characteristics. Instead they develop a high capacity for the storage and release of catecholamines.

The medullary chromaffin cells synthesize NA (*Figure 2.27*) but also possess an additional enzyme for conversion of NA to adrenaline (*Figure 2.36*).

Adrenal medullary chromaffin cells bear nicotinic cholinoceptors (page 79) and are innervated by preganglionic cholinergic neurones. Receptor activation causes a small nonpropagated depolarization (analogous to an epsp, page 80 and *Figure 2.19*), Ca^{2+} influx and the subsequent Ca^{2+}-dependent exocytotic release of adrenaline into the bloodstream.

The released adrenaline can activate α- and β-adrenoceptors at all sites in the body. The effects of circulating adrenaline are thus all those of stimulating noradrenergic neurones together with:

(1) arteriolar dilatation in skeletal muscle;
(2) reduced capillary permeability;
(3) lipolysis (adipose tissue);

(4) glycogenolysis (liver);
(5) glycolysis (skeletal muscle);
(6) restlessness and anxiety (CNS).

Drug action on the adrenal medulla

Secretion of adrenaline is stimulated by agonists at nicotinic cholinoceptors (page 81) and inhibited by antagonists at nicotinic cholinoceptors (page 83).

The chromaffin cells are susceptible to the amine-depleting actions of reserpine and *guanethidine* (page 98).

3

Drug action on peripheral tissues – drugs acting on signalling and transduction mechanisms other than those directly related to receptors for neurotransmitters and hormones

Aims

The drugs described in this section are chosen by exclusion: they exert their effects on peripheral tissues by acting at peripheral sites (hence excluding them from Section 5) but their mechanism of action does not involve structural relationships with cholinergic or noradrenergic neurotransmitters (excluding them from Section 2) or with hormones (excluding them from Section 4).

For each drug you should seek to know:

- its mechanism of action and the direct and indirect consequences that stem from that fundamental process;
- its principal therapeutic applications and their rationale;
- its principal adverse effects.

Local anaesthesia

Local anaesthesia is the result of drug-induced reversible blockage of impulse generation and propagation in a restricted distribution of neurones. Sensation (and motor control of effectors) is impaired only in that part of the body subserved by the anaesthetized group of neurones. Drugs used to produce local anaesthesia include the amides **lignocaine,** *prilocaine* and *bupivacaine* and the ester *amethocaine* [tetracaine].

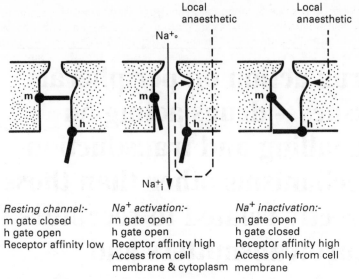

Figure 3.1 The sodium channel and the action of local anaesthetics (o = outside; i = inside)

Site and mechanism of action of local anaesthetic drugs

Most local anaesthetic drugs are relatively nonspecific in that they exert stabilizing effects on the plasma membranes of all kinds of excitable cells and even nonexcitable cells (for example, red blood cells).

The plasma membrane generally contains a bilayer of phospholipid molecules spanned by protein subunits arranged in a cylindrical structure with an internal pore. Such structures function as channels through which Na^+, K^+ or Ca^{2+} can cross the plasma membrane. In the case of electrically excitable cells, some of the protein subunits act as gates that control the passage of these ions. It is considered that the Na^+ channel has two such gates, the 'm' and 'h' gates (*Figure 3.1*). At the resting potential the 'm' gates are believed to be closed and the 'h' gates mainly open.

When the excitable cell is stimulated, the 'm' gates open rapidly allowing the influx of Na^+ (channel activation) and depolarization; this is observed as the upstroke of an action potential. On depolarization the voltage dependent 'h' gates close, although relatively slowly, terminating the influx of Na^+ (inactivation). Subsequently repolarization occurs aided by an efflux of K^+ through the voltage sensitive K^+ channels that open shortly after the upstroke of the action potential.

On repolarization the 'm' gates close quickly and the 'h' gates slowly reopen, the cell remaining refractory until the latter has occurred.

Local anaesthetic drugs act on the plasma membranes of excitable cells to inhibit the increase in Na^+ permeability that normally gives rise to an action potential. They are considered to produce this effect in two main ways. Partly, they may exert a nonspecific effect associated with their lipid soluble form (base). This, on dissolving in the phospholipid bilayer, increases its surface pressure thereby distorting the ion conducting proteinaceous channels thus reducing their ionic permeability.

Additionally some local anaesthetic drugs may act more specifically and block Na^+ channels by modifying gating. A receptor site is believed to be located toward the inner end of the Na^+ channel either at the membrane protein interface or within the channel pore or protein subunits of the channel. This receptor can be reached by local anaesthetic drug ingress either from the phospholipid bilayer or (provided the 'h' gate is open) from the cytoplasm.

Inhibition of Na^+ currents increases with repetitive depolarizations (use dependence; *see* also Calcium channel blockers, page 135) either because more channels become accessible during depolarization or because the channel conformations favoured by depolarization bind the drug with greater affinity; thus local anaesthetic drugs may bind more tightly to activated and inactivated channels than resting channels.

Attachment of the drug to the receptor inhibits Na^+ influx either by blocking the Na^+ channel and/or by increasing the probability of 'h' gate closure at any given level of membrane potential. This increases membrane stability but does not alter the resting membrane potential.

The nonspecific action resulting from dissolution of the drug in the phospholipid bilayer is important for some local anaesthetic drugs, especially *benzocaine*. However, most clinically useful agents exert their action predominantly through attachment to a receptor site in the Na^+ channel.

Active form of the local anaesthetic drug molecule

Local anaesthetic drugs are weak bases ($pK_a = 8-9$), which are combined with a strong acid (HCl) to provide a soluble salt for clinical use. They consist of a substituted amino group (hydrophilic) connected by an intermediate chain (usually a carbon chain) to an aromatic residue (lipophilic). The linkage between the intermediate and aromatic groups may be an amide (**lignocaine**, *prilocaine* and *bupivacaine*) or an ester (*amethocaine* and *benzocaine*) (*Figure 3.2*).

At tissue pH (7.4) local anaesthetic drugs exist in both ionized and unionized (base) forms, the relative percentage of each being dependent on the pK_a of the anaesthetic drug. Only the unionized (lipid soluble) form of the drug is able to cross membranous barriers (tissue, neural bundle) before

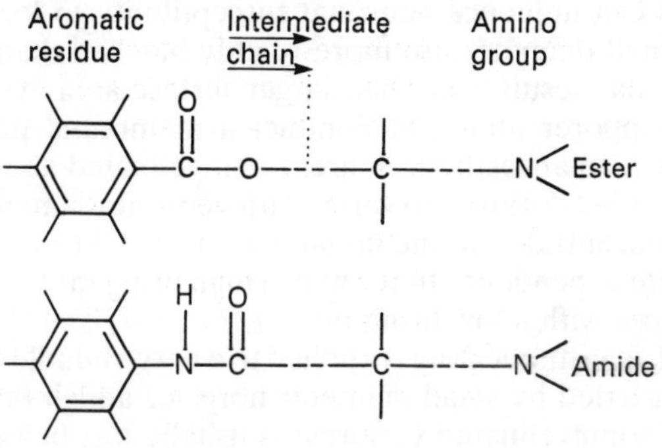

Figure 3.2 Ester and amide linkages between the aromatic part of the local anaesthetic molecule and the intermediate chain leading to the terminal amine

the site of action is reached and to dissolve in the neuronal plasma membrane. This form of the drug must therefore be responsible for local anaesthesia attributable to increased surface pressure in the phospholipid bilayer and for drug penetration to the neuronal cytoplasm or to the local anaesthetic drug receptor.

However, it is the cation, which forms about 75–95% (depending on the pK_a) of the drug in solution at pH 7.4, that binds to the local anaesthetic drug receptor.

Effects on the neuronal action potential

The action potential normally propagates because it acts as a suprathreshold stimulus (local circuit currents) for adjacent inactive regions of the neuronal membrane. For this reason and also because the drug effect against Na^+ influx is concentration dependent, local anaesthetic drugs can have graded effects on the action potential and its propagation.

A low concentration of a local anaesthetic drug increases the stimulus strength required to elicit an action potential (safety factor for conduction decreases). The rate of rise, amplitude and conduction velocity of that action potential are all reduced.

If sufficient local anaesthetic drug is applied the action potential becomes so reduced in amplitude that it ceases to act as a suprathreshold stimulus for adjacent inactive regions of the neuronal membrane and conduction ceases; hence action potentials can no longer be initiated or recorded irrespective of stimulus strength.

Preventing an increase in Na^+ permeability in a small part of an axon is however no guarantee of local anaesthesia. The local circuit currents responsible for action potential propagation can jump over a section of neurone in which permeability changes have been induced by a local anaesthetic drug. To prevent this action potential jumping about 5 mm of axon of a nonmyelinated neurone, or three successive nodes in a myelinated neurone, must be stabilized.

Differential blockage in mixed bundles of nerve fibres

Several factors can influence neuronal susceptibility to local anaesthesia. Neurones of small diameter are more readily blocked than those of large diameter. This may result from their larger surface area : volume ratio and therefore their poorer ability to conduct a membrane potential change passively through an anaesthetized area. In myelinated neurones the internodal distance (0.3–1.5 mm) also varies with neurone diameter; the Na^+ and K^+ gates are concentrated in the nodal region.

Because of use dependence fibres with a high firing rate are blocked more readily than those with a low firing rate.

When a local anaesthetic drug is applied to a nerve bundle the sensation of pain, which is carried by small diameter fibres of a high firing rate (myelinated A_δ and nonmyelinated C fibres) is usually lost before that of cold, warmth, touch or pressure (A_β fibres); motor fibres (large diameter fibres of low firing rate at rest) are blocked last.

Recovery from local anaesthesia

A local anaesthetic drug diffuses away from its site of administration down its concentration gradient in the interstitial fluid and is carried away by bulk flow of the interstitial fluid. Subsequently it enters local blood vessels. Most local anaesthetic drugs (for example, **lignocaine**) dilate blood vessels and by increasing local blood flow promote their systemic absorption and limit their duration of local anaesthesia. Some (*prilocaine*) do not. On reaching the systemic circulation esters are more rapidly destroyed (plasma and liver esterases including ChE) than are amides (liver microsomes).

Systemic effects of local anaesthetic drugs

Local anaesthetic drugs readily pass into the CNS where neurones are sensitive to plasma concentrations incapable of affecting peripheral nervous system activity. All nitrogenous local anaesthetic drugs cause stimulation of the CNS, resulting in restlessness, tremor, convulsions and respiratory stimulation. The stimulant effects may result from a selective depressant action on inhibitory neurones. Central stimulation is followed by depression; death following overdosage usually results from respiratory failure. Depressant effects (drowsiness, slurred speech) are prominent with **lignocaine.**

Local anaesthetic drugs also affect the cardiovascular system resulting mainly in myocardial depression and vasodilatation. The antidysrhythmic action of **lignocaine** is useful clinically (*see* page 128). Vasodilator effects are due partly to a direct effect on vascular smooth muscle and partly to an inhibition of sympathetic activity at arterioles. Combined myocardial depression and peripheral vasodilatation may result in life threatening hypotension.

Formulations of local anaesthetic drugs

Local anaesthetic drugs are available in a variety of formulations: eyedrops (beware corneal abrasion), lozenges, gels and ointments (beware contact dermatitis, page 436) and solutions for injection. The latter usually contain the hydrochloride salt buffered to pH 2.0–6.0.

Solutions for injection may also contain a catecholamine vasoconstrictor drug (*adrenaline*, noradrenaline). This prolongs the local anaesthesia by reducing the rate of systemic absorption. Formulations containing a catecholamine should not be used if the injection is intended for a digit or appendage. Patients receiving tricyclic antidepressive drugs (page 224) that potentiate catecholamines (page 104 may be at risk from cardiac dysrhythmias (especially *adrenaline*) and hypertension (especially NA). For such patients local anaesthetic drug formulations containing felypressin, an analogue of ADH, are available.

Other components of a local anaesthetic drug formulation for injection may include an antioxidant (to stabilize the vasoconstrictor if *adrenaline*), a buffering agent (to maintain pH), sodium chloride (to achieve isosmolality with interstitial fluids) and a preservative (to maintain sterility). The addition of preservatives (usually hydroxybenzoates) is now becoming an obsolete practice. Their exclusion further reduces the risk of allergic reactions.

Method of administration

Topical or surface anaesthesia

The drug is applied directly to mucous membranes, or the skin. To be effective for topical anaesthesia a drug must: (a) in its nonionized form, be relatively lipid soluble; (b) at pH 7.4, exist in appreciable amounts as its nonionized form (that is, have a pK_a of 8.5 or less, page 306).

Lignocaine, like most local anaesthetic drugs, penetrates mucosal surfaces readily. Only limited penetration of skin occurs, although a eutectic mixture of *prilocaine* and **lignocaine** applied under an occlusive dressing can provide surface anaesthesia for venepuncture.

Infiltration anaesthesia

The drug is injected sc or submucosally to anaesthetize fine sensory nerve branches.

Nerve block anaesthesia

The drug is injected alongside a nerve trunk. The transmission of both afferent and efferent impulses is prevented, which results in loss of sensation and muscle paralysis in the area supplied by the nerve trunk. The larger the nerve trunk bathed in drug the larger is the region anaesthetized. A special form of nerve block anaesthesia is termed epidural (or extradural) block. Here the drug is injected in relatively high concentration into the fatty material (*Figure 3.3*) outside the dura mater. The drug may have to diffuse into the subarachnoid space or outside the spinal canal before its effects can be mediated. However, the drug cannot penetrate to the brain because the epidural space terminates at the foramen magnum.

Spinal (or intrathecal) anaesthesia

The drug is injected to the subarachnoid space (*Figure 3.3*) usually in the lower spine where there is no danger of damage to the spinal cord. The dispersion of the injected fluid and hence the locus and extent of local anaesthesia depends on the:

(1) site of the injection;
(2) volume and speed of the injection;
(3) postinjection position of the patient;
(4) specific gravity (SG) of the injected solution.

The SG of the cerebrospinal fluid (CSF) varies from 1003 to 1009. A hypobaric solution (SG less than 1003) tends to rise through the CSF while a hyperbaric solution (SG more than 1009) tends to sink through the CSF. An isobaric solution tends to remain at the level of the injection site.

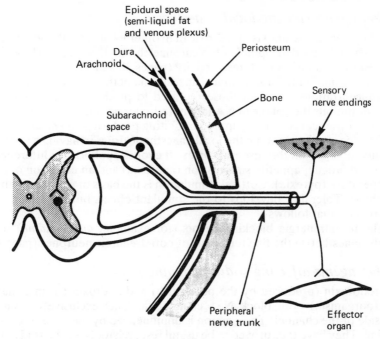

Figure 3.3 Sites for the production of local anaesthesia

Spinal anaesthesia produces analgesia (loss of pain sensation) and muscle relaxation without the patient losing consciousness. However, the level of anaesthesia within the spinal cord cannot be precisely controlled. Unwanted effects may include reduced cardiac output, hypotension and neurological complications.

Properties of individual local anaesthetic drugs

Lignocaine is widely used for all kinds of local anaesthesia. **Lignocaine** iv is effective in the control of cardiac dysrhythmias (page 128).

Prilocaine is suitable for all kinds of local anaesthesia. If large amounts enter the circulation methaemoglobin is formed. This can be reversed with methylene blue.

Bupivacaine has a slow onset of action. However, its long duration of action (up to 8 h) makes it particularly suitable for nerve block, epidural and spinal anaesthesia.

Amethocaine is an ester that is well and rapidly absorbed across mucous membranes. It provides useful topical anaesthesia of the skin, buccal mucous membranes and eye. Its toxicity and tendency to produce hypersensitivity reactions preclude its systemic use.

Benzocaine is an ester that is almost insoluble in water. It provides useful topical anaesthesia of mucous membranes of the mouth and the perianal area.

Other agents causing local anaesthesia

Cinchocaine [dibucaine] is more toxic than other local anaesthetic drugs but is occasionally used for spinal or topical anaesthesia. It is used in a biochemical test of pseudocholinesterase activity (pages 30 and 91).

Cocaine has limited use in topical anaesthesia of the eye, nose and throat. In concentrations less than those required to produce local anaesthesia, *cocaine* inhibits the uptake of NA into noradrenergic neurones (*see* page 104 for the consequences of the uptake-inhibiting properties of *cocaine*).

Cocaine is unique among the local anaesthetic drugs in having a powerful stimulant action on the cerebral cortex. It evokes euphoria, indifference to pain and fatigue, appetite suppression (anorexia) and an elevation of body temperature (pyrexia). Cortical stimulation is the basis of *cocaine*'s liability to abuse. Tolerance develops to the stimulant effects but not to the CNS depression that follows.

The noradrenergic blocking agents (for example, *guanethidine*) selectively anaesthetize the fine terminals of noradrenergic neurones (page 98).

Other agents affecting sodium channels

Tetrodotoxin (produced by the puffer fish) and saxitoxin (from a marine microorganism) both block Na^+ channels and act exclusively from the outside of the channel. Their action is uninfluenced by the state of channel gating. They have thus proved to be useful research tools for the study of the Na^+ channel. Whilst they selectively prevent action potential production mediated by increased membrane permeability to Na^+ (for example, action potentials of neurones and twitch skeletal muscle, or the early phase of the myocardial cell action potential), they do not influence the action potentials of smooth muscle cells since these are associated with the influx of Ca^{2+}. Hence tetrodotoxin can be used *in vitro* functionally to denervate smooth muscle leaving its contractility unaffected; this can be used to determine whether the action of a drug on smooth muscle is direct or whether it involves nerve action potentials.

Various highly lipid soluble substances (for example, the insecticides DDT and pyrethrins) and certain scorpion and sea anemone polypeptide toxins modify Na^+ channel gating to increase the probability of channel opening. This leads to cell hyperexcitability and spontaneous discharges although eventually cells become permanently depolarized and unexcitable (the ion channels remain inactivated). Such agents affect the heart causing dysrhythmia and may cause spontaneous discharges in nerve and muscle cells leading to twitching and convulsions.

Cardiac antidysrhythmic drugs

General features

Any disorder of cardiac rhythm is termed a dysrhythmia. This can result from disorders of impulse generation, impulse conduction or a combination of these.

Ionic basis of normal cardiac action potentials

In the normal heart the site (focus) for the generation of the heart beat is the SA node. From here electrical impulses are conducted through the atrial muscle to the AV node and thus, via the bundle of His and the Purkinje fibres to the ventricular muscle cells. The contractile cells of the atria and ventricles show a characteristic form of action potential associated with the movement of Na^+, Ca^{2+} and K^+ through specific ion channels. The opening and closing of these channels (their gating) is variously influenced by membrane potential, intracellular ionic concentrations and by intracellular metabolites. Gating processes are also usually time-dependent.

The cardiac action potential is conventionally divided into five phases (*Figure 3.4*), the most important of which for possible drug action are:

(1) depolarization (phase 0), which is caused by an increase in Na^+ permeability (fast inactivating);
(2) the plateau (phase 2), during which there are increased Na^+ (slowly inactivating) and Ca^{2+} permeabilities and reduced K^+ and Na^+ (fast inactivating) permeabilities;
(3) repolarization (phase 3) when there are declining Na^+ (slowly inactivating) and Ca^{2+} permeabilities and increasing K^+ permeability.

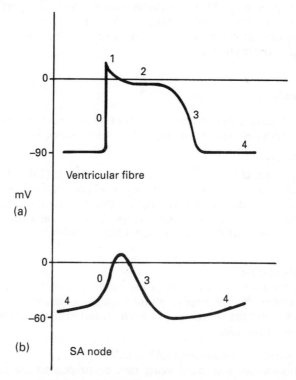

Figure 3.4 (a) Ventricular muscle cell action potential; (b) SA node cell action potential

In the normal SA nodal cells the action potential is characterized by the absence of a plateau and a diastolic transmembrane potential that is less negative than that of a ventricular cell. During diastole, the SA nodal membrane potential steadily becomes even less negative (the pacemaker potential, phase 4), until the threshold for firing a full action potential is reached. The pacemaker potential is caused by a steady rise in both Ca^{2+} and Na^+ permeabilities and a fall in K^+ permeability. In the SA and AV nodal cells the depolarizing phase of the action potential is carried almost entirely by Ca^{2+}, which enters through voltage-gated calcium channels. Na^+ influx plays only a minor role.

In the Purkinje fibres, the pacemaker tissue of the isolated ventricle, the pacemaker potential has an ionic basis that mainly involves a fall in K^+ permeability.

Types of dysrhythmia

Disorders of impulse generation

The most common problem is the development of an ectopic focus, a site of pacemaker activity additional to the SA node. Ectopic foci may be induced by damage to the cardiac muscle (myocardial infarction), drugs (general anaesthetic agents, page 246) or metabolic disturbances (hyperthyroidism, page 174). These dysrhythmias may be subdivided by the location of the focus into supraventricular (with the ectopic focus in the atria or AV node) and ventricular dysrhythmias.

Supraventricular dysrhythmias

The main problem for the patient arises from the increased ventricular rate, resulting in a reduced stroke volume and increased work load for the heart.

(1) Atrial flutter
This is characterized by a regular and very fast atrial rate (150–350/min). The AV nodal cells with their long refractory period cannot conduct impulses at this high rate; nevertheless, the ventricular rate becomes abnormally high, though regular. The cause is a single ectopic focus in the atrial muscle and the ECG shows several P waves for each QRS complex (in a 2:1, 3:1 or 4:1 ratio).

(2) Atrial fibrillation
The atrial action potential rate is in the range 200–600/min and the dysrhythmia is due to the presence of multiple atrial ectopic foci. There are no normal P waves and the ventricular rate is high and irregular, although much lower than the atrial rate.

(3) Supraventricular paroxysmal tachycardia
Sporadic episodes of increased heart rate occur due to the intermittent appearance of an atrial ectopic focus. Normal sinus rhythm can often be

induced by reflex vagal stimulation (by pressure applied to the eyeballs or to one carotid sinus).

Ventricular dysrhythmias

(1) Ventricular fibrillation
This is caused by the development of ventricular ectopic foci, leading to rapid uncoordinated ventricular contractions and a consequent severe reduction in cardiac output. Since it is rapidly fatal, DC electric shock (cardioversion) is indicated and pharmacological intervention has a limited role.

(2) Ventricular paroxysmal tachycardia
Sporadic episodes of increased heart rate due to the intermittent appearance of a ventricular ectopic focus. It is distinguished from the atrial type by an ECG record on which the QRS complexes outnumber the P waves.

Disorders of impulse conduction

Heart block

The most common sites of heart block occur in the AV node and the bundle of His. Different degrees of heart block are recognized.

In first degree block the PR interval is prolonged (longer than 0.2 s) but the ECG is otherwise normal. In second degree block some P waves do not initiate QRS complexes, indicating failure of AV conduction, but no additional beats arise from the ventricular pacemaker tissue. In third degree block AV conduction is blocked and ventricular contractions arise from the ventricular pacemakers. There is therefore a slower-than-normal ventricular rate and no coordination between P waves and QRS complexes.

In general, drug treatment is of limited value for heart block although agonists at β-adrenoceptors may be useful in the short term. In the long term the use of an artificial pacemaker is indicated.

Re-entry dysrhythmias

Since the whole heart muscle behaves like a complex syncytium, it might at first seem surprising that reverberatory circuits of excitation do not occur more frequently. This occurrence is avoided by the rapid conduction velocity and long refractory period that are characteristic of healthy cardiac muscle cells. However, if part of the heart muscle becomes damaged, as a consequence of myocardial infarction, or has had its excitability affected by drugs (agonists at β-adrenoceptors, **digoxin**, *quinidine*), abnormal conduction pathways may be set up. In damaged regions of the heart, the cardiac muscle cells tend to depolarize. Such an effect tends to inactivate (place in a nonconducting state) several kinds of cardiac ion channel with important consequences for antidysrhythmic drug action (*see below*).

One possible situation is illustrated in *Figure 3.5*. In the normal heart, shown in *Figure 3.5a*, the conduction wave passes down into the two bundle branches and is then conducted away on either side. The waves of conduction moving from the bundle branches towards the central portion of ventricular muscle extinguish each other. If, however, one of the bundle

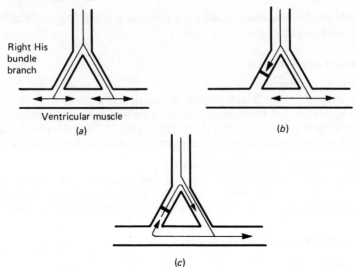

Figure 3.5 Establishment of a re-entry type of cardiac dysrhythmia: (a) normal conduction; (b) unidirectional block in right His bundle branch; (c) retrograde transmission through right His bundle branch

branches is damaged, so that anterograde but not retrograde conduction is blocked (*Figure 3.5b*), the wave of conduction from the normal branch may enter the damaged branch retrogradely (*Figure 3.5c*) and eventually reappear in the normal branch, thus completing a re-entry circuit. Similar re-entry circuits could occur anywhere in the cardiac muscle where damaged and normal muscle exist side by side.

A rare form of re-entry dysrhythmia occurs in the Wolff–Parkinson–White syndrome. Here an anatomically abnormal bundle of cardiac muscle joins the atria to the ventricles, bypassing the AV node. Thus the ventricles may be excited prematurely via this 'short-circuit' in addition to the normal AV node to Purkinje conduction. Following excitation via the latter pathway, the ventricular impulse may re-enter the atria through the bypass to set up a circus of excitation.

Some mild dysrhythmias (for example, occasional extrasystoles) require little treatment beyond reassurance of the patient. Others (for example, supraventricular paroxysmal tachycardia) may revert to normal rhythm spontaneously or can be induced to revert by reflex vagal stimulation. DC electroshock effectively induces the reversion of several types of tachycardia.

Antidysrhythmic drugs

Group 1: Inhibitors of Na⁺ influx

This group includes *quinidine, procainamide,* **lignocaine** and **phenytoin.** These drugs act mainly to inhibit the influx of Na^+ through both fast and slowly inactivating sodium channels (*cf*. local anaesthetic agents, page 118) although they may also have additional actions on both Ca^{2+} and K^+ channels of the cardiac cell membrane. Since action potentials in the SA node cells are much less dependent on Na^+ influx than those in atrial or ventricular cells, these drugs are more effective in suppressing ectopic than normal pacemaker activity.

Lignocaine and **phenytoin** are particularly effective in the suppression of the ventricular dysrhythmias observed after myocardial infarction, in which the damaged cells become depolarized. **Lignocaine** is able to block inactivated slow Na^+ channels resulting in selective suppression of excitation in the damaged regions. **Lignocaine** and **phenytoin** also reduce the action potential duration and shorten the effective refractory period, which may improve conduction in damaged cells in the bundle of His, reducing the likelihood of re-entry dysrhythmias.

Lignocaine has a rapid onset of action and a short $t_{\frac{1}{2}}$ (approximately 1 h), which means that it must be given by iv infusion. It is useful in emergency treatment during surgery. It is also an antagonist at muscarinic cholinoceptors and may therefore evoke mild tachycardia by removing the effect of vagal tone on the SA node. Adverse effects may be attributed to actions on the CNS and include confusion, fits, sweating and drowsiness.

Phenytoin is particularly effective in blocking ventricular dysrhythmias attributable to **digoxin** toxicity. Its general antidysrhythmic effectiveness is less than that of **lignocaine**. Unwanted effects include hypotension.

Quinidine and *procainamide* have very similar actions and are effective in blocking ectopic pacemaker activity both in atria and ventricles. Such ectopic foci cells are not abnormally depolarized and their Na^+ channels undergo normal cycles of activation and inactivation (*cf*. damaged cells in which Na^+ channels exist for a greater time in the inactivated state). Both *quinidine* and *procainamide* can block Na^+ channels in the activated state (*cf*. **lignocaine**). In addition they prolong the action potential and lengthen the effective refractory period. This may prevent the occurrence of re-entry dysrhythmias caused by retrograde transmission of the kind illustrated in *Figure 3.5c*.

Quinidine and *procainamide* each has a low therapeutic index and depresses the force of myocardial contraction at concentrations close to those required for the suppression of dysrhythmias. They may therefore precipitate cardiac failure in patients with low cardiac reserve. Their negative inotropic effects extend to skeletal muscle (aggravation of myasthenia gravis) and vascular smooth muscle (hypotension).

Quinidine is also an antagonist at muscarinic cholinoceptors (page 88). By removing the effect of vagal tone at the SA node it induces a mild tachycardia. This action at the AV node may precipitate a hazardous 'paradoxical' tachycardia in patients with atrial flutter or fibrillation. Cardiotoxic doses of *quinidine* directly depolarize Purkinje fibres and increase their automaticity (an effect opposite to that seen at therapeutic concentrations). Toxic doses may therefore induce hazardous ventricular dysrhythmias. Additional unwanted effects associated with *quinidine* include tinnitus (ringing in the ears), dizziness and other symptoms collectively known as 'cinchonism' (page 276).

Procainamide is a less effective antagonist at muscarinic cholinoceptors than *quinidine*.

Group 2: Antagonists at β-adrenoceptors

Since sympathetic stimulation produces a general increase in excitability of cardiac muscle, antagonists at β-adrenoceptors (**propranolol, atenolol**) can reduce the incidence of dysrhythmias by reducing automaticity, increasing the effective refractory period and decreasing conduction velocity. They reduce ventricular rate in atrial flutter and fibrillation by slowing AV conduction. In high doses they suppress the automaticity of ectopic foci and suppress re-entry dysrhythmias by mechanisms similar to those described for *quinidine*.

Propranolol and **atenolol** have a limited role in the management of dysrhythmias. They are effective in the treatment of dysrhythmias induced by catecholamines (phaeochromocytoma and thyrotoxicosis) and those attributed to **digoxin** toxicity. In concentrations close to those required for suppression of dysrhythmias, antagonists at β-adrenoceptors may depress the force of cardiac contraction and precipitate cardiac failure. The use of these drugs is particularly hazardous in patients with ventricular failure or low cardiac reserve who may depend on sympathetic drive to obtain an adequate cardiac output.

The use of the cardioselective antagonist at β_1-adrenoceptors, **atenolol,** may minimize the appearance of effects (bronchospasm, cold extremities) that follow from occupancy of β_2-adrenoceptors by the less selective **propranolol.**

Group 3: Drugs that prolong both the action potential and refractory period

K^+ channels play a crucial role in terminating the cardiac action potential and several K^+ channels with very different properties are involved. Blockade of cardiac K^+ channels delays repolarization and thus prolongs the refractory period with resultant antidysrhythmic effects. Very selective blockers of the delayed rectifier K^+ channel are currently on clinical trial.

Amiodarone prolongs the duration of the plateau (phase 2) of the cardiac action potential. Depolarization (phase 3) is delayed with a consequent lengthening of the effective refractory period. This effect is produced by blockade of K^+ channels, although *amiodarone* has several other actions (for example, Na^+ channel blockade) that may contribute to its antidysrhythmic effects. It is useful in the treatment of supraventricular tachycardias, particularly the Wolff–Parkinson–White syndrome.

Amiodarone must be administered in several doses daily for 2 weeks before therapeutic plasma concentrations are achieved. Its molecule contains iodine and released iodine may cause thyroid dysfunction during its long-term use. The high plasma concentrations of *amiodarone* encourage its deposition as microcrystals in the cornea, skin and other tissues, which act as reservoirs of the drug, so that its effects may persist for some time (weeks) after dosing is stopped.

Group 4: Inhibitors of calcium influx

Verapamil blocks the influx of Ca^{2+} through the slowly inactivating, voltage-dependent Ca^{2+} channels of the myocardial cell membrane, and predominantly affects the pacemaker tissue. **Verapamil** is therefore effective in blocking AV conduction and thus slows the ventricular rate in supraventricular tachycardias. The effect of **verapamil** is most marked when the frequency of action potentials is high – a phenomenon known as use-dependency. It is effective when the Ca^{2+} channels are either activated or inactivated.

Verapamil is effective in some types of re-entry tachycardia (in which the AV node is involved) but not in the Wolff–Parkinson–White syndrome (in which the accessory AV pathway is formed from ordinary cardiac muscle). **Verapamil** may indeed increase the frequency of conduction in the accessory tissue and is therefore contraindicated in the Wolff–Parkinson–White syndrome. **Verapamil** has a negative inotropic action and should therefore be used only with great care in patients receiving antagonists at β-adrenoceptors.

Not all calcium channel blockers (*see* page 135) show antidysrhythmic activity and **nifedipine** is an example of those that do not. It is only effective when the slow Ca^{2+} channels are in the activated state (*cf.* **verapamil**) and does not exhibit use-dependency.

Other antidysrhythmic drugs

Digoxin, by reducing conduction through the AV node, can reduce the rate at which the ventricles beat in response to atrial tachycardia, flutter or fibrillation (*see below*).

Cardiac glycosides

Digoxin is a glycoside extracted from the leaves of *Digitalis lanata* (foxglove family). It consists of an aglycone (a steroid nucleus, folded in a different way from the steroid hormones) that possesses the pharmacological activity, attached to three sugar (digitoxose) molecules that influence its pharmacokinetic behaviour (page 348). Other glycosides, which differ only in their pharmacokinetic properties, are available but little used.

Direct actions on cardiac cells

Membrane effects

Digoxin binds to and inhibits the Mg-dependent Na^+/K^+ activated ATPase that is located within the cardiac cell membrane and regulates the cellular

Na^+ and K^+ concentrations. Inhibition of this enzyme results in Na^+ accumulation within and K^+ loss from the cells and effectively lowers the membrane potential with two consequences:

(1) in some cells action potential propagation (and generation) is inhibited resulting in transmission block, especially in the AV node (useful in atrial fibrillation, *see above*);
(2) in other cells, especially in the bundle of His, automaticity is increased and ventricular dysrhythmias are produced (page 127). K^+ depletion (for example, associated with diuretic therapy and secondary hyperaldosteronism) enhances these actions and may lead to the development of fatal ventricular dysrhythmias.

Inotropic effects

The most important therapeutic action of **digoxin** is its ability to increase the force of myocardial contraction in the failing heart (page 378). Although it is not firmly established, this action may also result from inhibition of Na^+/K^+ ATPase. A build-up of Na^+ occurs within the cardiac muscle cells as a result of the inhibition of this enzyme and may allow more Ca^{2+} to enter the cell by a transmembrane exchange. This is sequestered into dynamic storage sites, from which more is released at each impulse producing a more powerful contraction. Tension development and relaxation occur faster and with relatively little increase in O_2 demand. This effect is best seen in patients with both heart failure and atrial fibrillation.

Indirect actions on cardiac cells

Digoxin augments vagal nerve activity by, in part, central vagal stimulation and also by increased cardiac effector sensitivity to ACh. These actions slow the heart and summate with the direct AV nodal blocking actions.

Toxicity

Digoxin has a very low therapeutic index. All its actions can be regarded as 'toxic' but in some instances (for example, the inotropic effect in congestive heart failure) these can be exploited to the benefit of the patient.

Nausea, anorexia and vomiting (due to stimulation of the CTZ) are all early features of **digoxin** toxicity, as are blurred vision and disturbances of colour vision, which may be due to inhibition of the Na^+/K^+ ATPase necessary for normal cone function. Later, cardiac dysrhythmias are common and almost any pathological dysrhythmia can be imitated by **digoxin** toxicity. Ectopic beats are common early signs and ventricular tachycardia and fibrillation terminate the sequence. The increased automaticity responsible for this arises in the Purkinje fibres where a high intracellular Ca^{2+} concentration causes membrane potential oscillations.

Treatment

In addition to terminating **digoxin** administration, increasing the plasma K^+ concentration stimulates the membrane Na^+/K^+ ATPase and hence aids Ca^{2+} extrusion. The antidysrhythmic drugs **phenytoin** (page 129) and **propranolol** are also useful. Digoxin-specific antibody fragments are also available for use in life-threatening situations.

Calcium channel blockers

These drugs are also known as inhibitors of calcium influx or calcium antagonists.

Role of calcium within the cell

In many effector cells (muscle, neuronal and secretory) an increase in free cytosolic Ca^{2+} concentration conveys to intracellular structures the information that the cell membrane is in an excited state. There are two sources of the extra cytosolic Ca^{2+}:

(1) it may be released from intracellular stores by membrane excitation;
(2) it may diffuse down the steep electrochemical gradient from ECF to cytosol through voltage-gated ion channels (*see below*) present in the cell membrane.

In all muscles Ca^{2+} is a necessary element of excitation contraction coupling. Contraction of skeletal muscle depends largely on Ca^{2+} release from intracellular stores. In cardiac and smooth muscle the influx of extracellular Ca^{2+} (see *Figure 3.6*) contributes to the contraction to a degree determined both by the cell and by the excitatory stimulus.

The dissipation of the Ca^{2+} signal, once excitation wanes, is by:

(1) active sequestration of Ca^{2+} into intracellular storage sites (prominent in skeletal muscle and other tissues that use an intracellular Ca^{2+} source);
(2) active extrusion from the cell (prominent in tissues that use an extracellular Ca^{2+} source).

Types of Ca^{2+} channel

Three types of voltage-gated Ca^{2+} channel are now recognized and some of their key properties are summarized in *Table 3.1*. L-channels (long-lasting) are activated for a long time on marked membrane depolarization. Such channels are the site of action of, and are blocked by, calcium channel blockers (*see below*). T-channels (transient) require little depolarization to become transiently activated. N-channels are found in neurones; relatively little is known about them and they require moderate depolarization to become activated.

Table 3.1 Properties of voltage-gated Ca^{2+} channels

	L	T	N
Ca^{2+} channel blocker sensitive	Yes	No	No
Duration of activation	Long	Transient	Intermediate
Channel conductance (Ca^{2+} flux per unit time)	Large	Small	Intermediate
Location	Cardiac, skeletal and smooth muscles	Widespread in excitable cells	Neurones

Types of Ca^{2+} channel blocker

Three types of Ca^{2+} channel blocker can be distinguished, largely on the basis of ligand binding and electrophysiological studies. Detailed studies have shown that the three types interact with distinct (but allosterically linked) sites within the L-type channel.

Blockade of channels by these inhibitors of Ca^{2+} entry reduces electromechanical coupling in cells dependent on extracellular Ca^{2+} and reduces contractile force. These drugs are thus calcium antagonists by virtue of their ability to reduce the access of Ca^{2+} to its site of action within the cell.

In addition to their effects in reducing excitation/contraction coupling, Ca^{2+} entry blockers can, in certain tissues and under certain circumstances, inhibit excitation. This occurs when Ca^{2+} entry forms a significant portion of the excitation process as in:

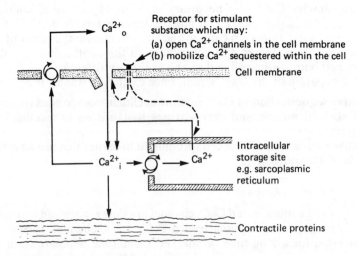

Figure 3.6 Mechanisms of modulation of the intracellular Ca^{2+} concentration that govern smooth muscle contraction (o = outside; i = inside)

(1) certain smooth muscle cells;
(2) cells of the SA node and AV node in the heart;
(3) other myocardial cells that are depolarized and where the Na^+ channel is therefore inactivated.

Nifedipine is the prototype dihydropyridine Ca^{2+} entry blocker. It interacts with a specific site within the L-channel, a process that is greatly enhanced the more depolarized the cell and if the channel is in an inactivated state. This interaction shows little dependency on the frequency with which the L-channel opens (lack of use-dependency).

Nifedipine has little action on the cardiac SA or AV nodes. The myocardium is affected and prominent peripheral vasodilatation occurs. **Nifedipine** is therefore useful in the management of essential hypertension (page 382) and angina pectoris (page 389). **Nifedipine** is well absorbed after oral (sublingual) administration and is strongly bound to plasma proteins. Its plasma $t_{\frac{1}{2}}$ is 4 h; sustained-release and iv formulations are available.

Verapamil is the prototype phenylalkylamine Ca^{2+} entry blocker. Its site of action within the L-channel is different from that of the dihydropyridines and the benzothiazepines (*see below*). Its interaction with the L-channel shows marked use-dependency and it binds preferentially to the channel in its inactivated state.

Verapamil inhibits Ca^{2+} entry in cardiac, vascular and gastrointestinal tissues.

In the myocardium it interferes with Ca^{2+} entry occurring during the plateau of the cardiac action potential and thereby reduces the contractility. Elsewhere in the heart it interferes with the Ca^{2+} entry that is important for excitation; this is exploited in the treatment of paroxysmal supraventricular tachycardia (page 131). It is also responsible for the very prolonged AV node transmission that can result from overdosage or combination of **verapamil** with an antagonist at β-adrenoceptors.

In arteriolar smooth muscle **verapamil** produces vasodilatation. This is exploited in the management of essential hypertension and angina pectoris but not in congestive heart failure (where further reduction in cardiac contractility is intolerable).

In gastrointestinal propulsive smooth musculature, similarly, contraction is weakened. This underlies the constipation that occurs as a side-effect of **verapamil.**

Verapamil is well absorbed orally and, like **nifedipine,** it is strongly bound to plasma proteins. Its $t_{\frac{1}{2}}$ is 6 h and iv formulations are available.

Diltiazem is the prototype benzothiazepine Ca^{2+} entry blocker. It interacts with a third site within the L-channel, a process that, like that of **verapamil,** is use-dependent. In profile, *diltiazem* is more like **verapamil** than **nifedipine** and it is capable of inhibiting cardiac tachycardias and producing bradycardia. Its main use is the treatment of angina pectoris.

Diltiazem is well absorbed on oral administration but little bound to plasma proteins. Its $t_{\frac{1}{2}}$ is 3–4 h.

Methylxanthines

Theophylline and *aminophylline* are the commonly prescribed methylxanthines. *Aminophylline* is the more water soluble and comprises a complex of *theophylline* with ethylenediamine. Coffee, tea, cocoa, chocolate and cola contain methylxanthines (caffeine, theobromine, theophylline).

Actions

Airways smooth muscle

Providing that plasma concentrations can be limited to the range 10–20 mg/l, *theophylline* and *aminophylline* evoke bronchodilatation with little effect on other smooth muscle-containing organs or on the heart. These agents are thus useful in the treatment of bronchial asthma (page 393).

The contribution of relaxation of airways smooth muscle to the therapeutic effect of the methylxanthines in bronchial asthma may depend on the treatment situation. When *aminophylline* is administered by iv infusion during the treatment of acute, severe asthma the rapidity of the therapeutic response suggests that relaxation of airways smooth muscle plays a more important role than resolution of inflammation. However, in the oral prophylaxis of asthma using sustained release formulations of *theophylline*, it is possible that anti-inflammatory actions of the drug (*see below*) assume greater importance.

Vascular smooth muscle

Methylxanthines dilate most blood vessels and thereby reduce peripheral resistance, though they may constrict cerebral vessels. Methylxanthine-induced venodilatation results in reduced central venous pressure and cardiac preload.

Other smooth muscles

Theophylline is capable, in high concentrations, of causing the relaxation of all kinds of smooth muscle.

Cells involved with inflammation in the lung

Mast cells, platelets, eosinophils and macrophages may all be involved with the process of inflammation in the lung. *Theophylline* can inhibit the release of mediators of tissue anaphylaxis from mast cells and can inhibit eosinophil accumulation within the lung. Actions of these kinds may allow *theophylline* to exert some anti-inflammatory activity in the asthmatic lung.

Kidney

Methylxanthines evoke a weak diuresis. This results mainly from inhibition of Na^+ reabsorption with a contribution from an increased GFR. The increased GFR is a consequence of the cardiac stimulant and vasodilator actions of the methylxanthines.

The heart

Theophylline and other methylxanthines stimulate the heart, producing an increase in force of contraction and rate. High concentrations of these drugs may induce dysrhythmias.

CNS

The methylxanthines stimulate the CNS. They increase alertness and reduce fatigue. Insomnia, restlessness, delirium and seizures are part of the acute toxic syndrome (see page 238) associated with overdosage.

Mechanism of action

Several mechanisms have been proposed for the pharmacodynamic actions of methylxanthines.

(1) Inhibition of cyclic nucleotide phosphodiesterase, thus raising cytosolic cAMP and cGMP concentrations (see *Figure 2.32*, page 109 and *Figure 3.8b*, page 139).

Theophylline inhibits cyclic nucleotide phosphodiesterase in tissue homogenates. However, significant increases in the tissue cAMP content are observed only at concentrations close to, or in excess of, those causing maximal relaxation of smooth muscle. This does not necessarily rule out phosphodiesterase inhibition as a mechanism for the smooth muscle relaxant action of *theophylline* because the changes in cAMP turnover crucial for relaxation may occur in a minor compartment not detectable by the assay of whole tissue cAMP content.

(2) Alteration of the Ca^{2+} handling of effector cells.

High concentrations of caffeine and *theophylline* can cause the release of Ca^{2+} from intracellular stores in smooth muscle. This action results in store depletion and does not depend on the intracellular accumulation of cAMP. In conditions (for example, low extracellular Ca^{2+} concentration) where store refilling is compromised, methylxanthines can therefore prevent the actions of spasmogenic agents that are dependent on a functional intracellular Ca^{2+} store. There is evidence to suggest that high concentrations of methylxanthines can directly inhibit cellular influx of Ca^{2+} through voltage dependent channels in the plasmalemma.

(3) Antagonism of adenosine (and related nucleotides) at cell surface adenosine receptors.

Adenosine acts on neuronal terminals to inhibit neurotransmitter release. This action may be prevented by methylxanthines. Antagonism of adenosine may explain the ability of the methylxanthines to stimulate the CNS and to cause gastric irritation.

Nitrates

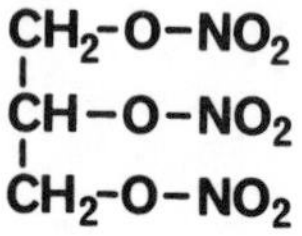

$$CH_2-O-NO_2$$
$$CH-O-NO_2$$
$$CH_2-O-NO_2$$

Figure 3.7 Structure of **glyceryl trinitrate**

Glyceryl trinitrate (*Figure 3.7*) and *isosorbide mononitrate* are organic esters of nitric acid and are sufficiently lipid soluble to penetrate smooth muscle cell membranes. The molecules can be regarded as carriers of the nitrite ion (NO_2^-) that is the precursor of the active species nitric oxide (*see below* and *Figure 3.8a*).

Mechanism of action

Within the smooth muscle cells, organic nitrates are reduced by sulphydryl groups to release nitric oxide (NO) via a nitrite intermediate. The pool of sulphydryl groups available for this step can become exhausted resulting in tolerance to the relaxant actions of the organic nitrate. (Dithiothreitol, a source of sulphydryl groups, has been used experimentally to reverse the tolerance.) Nitric oxide activates soluble guanylate cyclase, a process that also requires —SH groups, although the pool of these seems different from that involved in the formation of NO. The resulting increase in cGMP concentration produces smooth muscle relaxation, probably by activating protein kinase. This initiates a series of biochemical changes that effectively reduce intracellular free Ca^{2+} concentration (*see Figure 3.8a*).

The actions of organic nitrates can be inhibited experimentally by methylene blue, an inhibitor of soluble guanylate cyclase, and potentiated by phosphodiesterase inhibitors that slow the breakdown of cGMP (*Figure 3.8b*).

Actions

Smooth muscle

Blood vessels

There is generalized relaxation of vascular smooth muscle leading to vasodilatation. The effect on veins and venules is greater than that on the

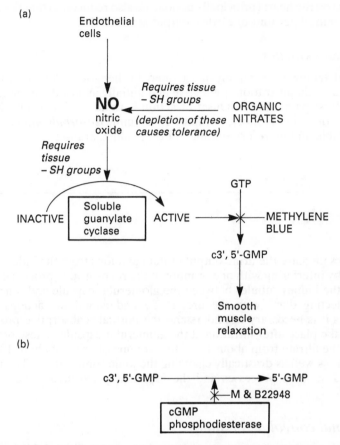

Figure 3.8 (a) Mechanism of action of the organic nitrates. These synthetic agents mimic the action of the body's endogenous vasodilator, nitric oxide, which is liberated from the vascular endothelium; (b) breakdown of cyclic 3'5' GMP

arteriolar tree resulting in skin flushing. The filling pressure at the heart (preload) is reduced to a greater extent than total peripheral resistance (after load).

Adverse effects that follow from the vasodilatation include skin warmth and sweating, throbbing headache (stretching of cranial vessels) and fainting. Therapeutic exploitation of the reduced preload occurs in angina of effort (page 388) and in congestive heart failure (page 378).

Other smooth muscle

Organic nitrates are capable of relaxing all kinds of smooth muscle including that of the bronchi, biliary tract, gut and genitourinary tract.

The heart

Tachycardia arises reflexly from nitrate-induced vasodilatation (*see above*).

The load on the heart (principally preload) is also reduced so that the cardiac work required per unit of cardiac output is reduced.

Pharmacokinetics

Glyceryl trinitrate is rapidly inactivated by hepatic reductase enzymes. Sublingual administration is effective and initially avoids the hepatic circulation ('first pass effect'). Onset of action is rapid, within 1 min, but the duration of action is short, normally 15–30 min. *Isosorbide mononitrate* is more stable and therefore suitable for oral administration.

Diuretics

Diuretics increase the urine output of fluid and ions from the kidney. They do this by interfering with one or more of the reabsorptive processes occurring in the kidney tubules between the glomerular capsule and junction of the collecting ducts with the ureter. To understand the actions of the diuretics it is necessary to understand the normal reabsorptive processes, which take place after filtration at the glomerular capsule. These processes reduce the filtrate from about 12.5 l to a volume of urine of about 100 ml in 100 min, as well as drastically changing the ionic composition. The regions involved in these processes and the functions performed in each are as follows.

Proximal convoluted tubule

(1) Reabsorption of a substantial portion of the filtered Na^+, accompanied by Cl^- and water to maintain electrochemical and osmotic balance.
(2) Reabsorption of most of the filtered K^+ accompanied by Cl^- and water.
(3) Reabsorption of filtered HCO_3^-. This involves the production of HCO_3^- and H^+ within the tubular epithelial cells under the influence of cytoplasmic carbonic anhydrase, the transfer of the HCO_3^- to the peritubular vessels and the exchange of the H^+ with Na^+ in the filtrate. This Na^+ is transferred to the peritubular fluid, the H^+ interacts with HCO_3^- in the filtrate, catalysed by carbonic anhydrase on the brush border membrane, producing water and CO_2 (which may diffuse into the epithelial cells and be used in the production of more HCO_3^-). This HCO_3^- reabsorption can take place throughout the nephron but the major site appears to be the proximal tubule.

Descending limb of the loop of Henle

The tubular membranes are relatively impermeable to anything other than water, which is removed by osmotic forces.

Ascending limb of the loop of Henle

Reabsorption of Na^+ and Cl^- by a cotransport mechanism. The tubule cell membranes are relatively impermeable to water, thus the rate of absorption of the ions exceeds that of water, leaving a tubule fluid that is hypotonic as it enters the distal tubule. Ca^{2+} and Mg^{2+} are also reabsorbed in this region.

Distal convoluted tubule

Reabsorption of Na^+, accompanied by Cl^-, and further reabsorption of Ca^{2+}.

Collecting duct

(1) Active reabsorption of Na^+ in connection with secretion of K^+, this 'exchange' is increased by aldosterone (page 178) and by increased delivery of Na^+ to the region.
(2) Reabsorption of water unaccompanied by ions, which is regulated by ADH released from the posterior pituitary gland (page 188). ADH increases the permeability of the tubule cells and normally results in a tubule fluid that is hypertonic to the general ECF when it leaves the collecting duct. Changes in plasma tonicity influence the release of ADH such that more, or less, water is reabsorbed to restore the tonicity to normal.

Compounds reducing or blocking these reabsorptive processes for solutes result in the production of an increased volume of urine with increased concentration of one or more ions.

Benzothiadiazides and related diuretics

A large group of diuretics comprising the benzothiadiazides ('thiazides'), having a basic structure in common (**bendrofluazide** [bendroflumethiazide]) and related compounds (*chlorthalidone, metolazone*), that do not have the basic structure of the thiazides but produce essentially the same effects. Members of the group appear to have the same mechanism of action, produce the same maximum effect on urine production and have the same potential for side-effects. The drugs are concentrated in the kidney partly by glomerular filtration and partly by active secretion into the proximal tubule by the organic acid secretory mechanism located there. These diuretics differ from each other mainly in their onset and duration of action. This latter appears to depend on the degree of plasma protein binding, the longer acting compounds being more extensively bound, and lipid solubility.

The major action of the drugs is to reduce the reabsorption of Na^+ (and Cl^-) in the distal tubule. The mechanism is not clear but may involve a decreased permeability to Na^+ (and Cl^-) at the luminal membrane. The increased delivery of Na^+ to the collecting ducts results in increased K^+ secretion in association with increased Na^+ reabsorption at this site. Some members of the group are able to inhibit carbonic anhydrase and potentially increase HCO_3^- loss in the urine; this is not the explanation for their main diuretic activity. The net effect is an increased urine volume with an increased loss of Na^+ and Cl^- and possible accompanying K^+ and HCO_3^- loss. The thiazides are classed as being of moderate efficacy and can result in 5–10% of the filtered Na^+ being excreted (cf. 1% excreted in the absence of diuretic administration).

Other renal effects are a reduction in uric acid secretion (due in part to competition for proximal secretory processes), enhanced excretion of Mg^{2+}, a decreased excretion of Ca^{2+} (due to increased reabsorption in the distal tubule) and a decreased GFR possibly due to a direct action on the renal vasculature.

The increased K^+ secretion may result in hypokalaemia and present problems, particularly in patients receiving **digoxin** (page 132). This problem may be reduced by the use of K^+ supplements (effervescent potassium tablets), or of K^+-sparing diuretics (see below). In susceptible patients the hyperuricaemia may induce gout.

Adverse effects that are not of renal origin include the induction of hyperglycaemia and aggravation of pre-existing diabetes mellitus.

In patients with diabetes insipidus (due either to lack of ADH or lack of responsiveness of the kidney to ADH) the thiazides produce a reduction in the urine volume. The Na^+ depleting effect appears to be essential for this action. It is suggested that the loss of Na^+ causes a reduction in ECF volume and GFR and an increased reabsorption of Na^+ and water in the proximal tubule. A reduced Na^+ and water load is delivered to the distal tubule and a smaller volume of less dilute urine is produced.

The thiazide and related diuretics also produce a sustained antihypertensive effect, which may be due, initially, to the diuretic action but subsequently is independent of this effect, may be obtained with lower doses and is probably due to a direct relaxation of arteriolar smooth muscle. *Diazoxide* (a thiazide analogue) causes profound relaxation of arterioles whilst causing salt and water retention and antagonizing **bendrofluazide,** thus lending support to the suggestion that the antihypertensive effect of the thiazides is distinct from their diuretic action. *Diazoxide* is useful in the treatment of hypoglycaemia (page 188).

High ceiling or loop diuretics

Like the thiazides, **frusemide** and *bumetanide* are absorbed after oral administration, are protein bound in the plasma and enter the kidney partly by filtration and partly by active secretion into the proximal tubule by the organic acid secretory mechanism. Unlike that of the thiazides, the diuretic action is rapid in onset, short in duration and dose related. As the group name suggests, the response is more marked than with other diuretics.

The major action is to reduce the Na^+ and Cl^- cotransport from the lumen to the cell in the ascending limb of the loop of Henle, although there may be minor actions on Na^+ reabsorption in the proximal tubule. Na^+/K^+ ATPase is involved in the movement of Na^+ from the tubule lumen to the peritubular fluid but although loop diuretics can be shown to inhibit the enzyme *in vivo* it is not clear if inhibition plays any role in their diuretic effect. K^+ secretion (associated with Na^+ reabsorption) is increased because of the higher Na^+ load delivered to the collecting duct. There is thus an increased urine volume with loss of Na^+ (15–30% of the filtered Na^+ may be lost), Cl^- and K^+. The Cl^- loss may induce alkalosis and the K^+ loss provoke **digoxin** intoxication. In contrast to the thiazides, loop diuretics cause the loss of both Ca^{2+} and Mg^{2+}. Loop diuretics also cause increased renal blood flow, an action that may be mediated via the prostaglandins, PGE_2 and $PGF_{2\alpha}$. Uric acid secretion may be reduced, resulting in gout in susceptible patients. The very rapid, marked reduction in ECF volume has resulted in cardiovascular collapse and may cause urinary retention in patients with an enlarged prostate gland.

Potassium sparing diuretics

Amiloride and triamterene

The major action of **amiloride** and *triamterene* is to reduce K^+ secretion in the collecting duct by a primary effect on Na^+ reabsorption (which normally provides a potential to aid K^+ secretion). The mechanism of action of these drugs is not clear but does not involve antagonism of aldosterone (*see below*).

Amiloride binds to a receptor on the luminal membrane, blocking the Na^+ channels and limiting the entry of Na^+ to the tubular cells. As a result, K^+ secretion and the Na^+/H^+ exchange are reduced. *Triamterene* may have a similar action. This gives a mild diuresis with loss of Na^+ (up to 5% of that filtered) and a reduced loss of K^+. The main problem associated with the use of these compounds is the danger of hyperkalaemia. Diuretics of this kind are generally used in combination with thiazide diuretics to reduce the loss of K^+ normally associated with the use of this group.

Aldosterone antagonists

Spironolactone inhibits the Na^+ reabsorption and associated K^+ secretion in the distal tubule promoted by aldosterone by competing with it for intracellular receptors. The magnitude of the effect depends on the involvement of aldosterone in the reabsorption. **Spironolactone** is useful in combination with the thiazides to reduce the K^+ loss normally associated with their diuretic effect. Again the main adverse effect is the likelihood of raised plasma K^+ concentrations but disturbances of endocrine function (gynaecomastia) may also occur, presumably due to the ability of **spironolactone** to interact with steroid receptors.

Other diuretics of limited use

Carbonic anhydrase inhibitors

Acetazolamide produces a noncompetitive inhibition of carbonic anhydrase and therefore reduces the formation of H^+ and HCO_3^- within the epithelial cells of the tubule; this reduces the reabsorption of HCO_3^-. The loss of HCO_3^- may result in metabolic acidosis as the plasma buffer concentration falls; this limits the diuresis as sufficient H^+ is generated from metabolism to exchange with Na^+ in the tubule and thus re-establish HCO_3^- reabsorption from the tubule fluid.

Adverse effects include paraesthesiae (tingling and similar sensations), hypokalaemia, anorexia, drowsiness and depression. These problems and the self-limiting nature of the diuresis restrict the use of this group of diuretics.

Acetazolamide is useful in the treatment of open angle glaucoma (inhibition of carbonic anhydrase reduces the formation of HCO_3^- and the secretion of aqueous humour causing intraocular pressure to fall) and epilepsy (page 417).

Osmotic diuretics

Osmotic diuretics (*mannitol*) are compounds that are filtered at the glomerulus and are not significantly reabsorbed from the tubules. The presence in the filtrate of the osmotically active solute limits the reabsorption of water and therefore increases urine output. Osmotic diuretics, by this mechanism, are able to maintain urine volume even when GFR is reduced; they are thus used in the prophylaxis of acute renal failure. Other uses, dependent on the same mechanism, are to reduce the volume and pressure of CSF and intraocular fluid (in acute closed angle glaucoma).

Anticoagulant, antithrombotic and fibrinolytic compounds

These are used:

(1) to prevent the clotting of blood in extravascular situations (blood samples, heart-lung machines, artificial kidneys);
(2) in an attempt to prevent the formation or enlargement of thrombi (intravascular clots) in the venous circulation and on prosthetic heart valves (anticoagulants) or in the arterial circulation (antiplatelet drugs);
(3) to break down pre-existing thrombi.

The normal clotting process is activated by tissue damage or contact of the blood with a foreign surface. These result in the conversion of the inactive precursor prothrombin, normally present in the plasma, to the enzyme thrombin. This catalyses the conversion of the soluble protein fibrinogen (also normally present in the plasma) to the insoluble fibrin (*Figure 3.9*), activates fibrin stabilizing factor (Factor XIII), which causes the formation of covalent bonds between the monomers of fibrin, thus stabilizing it, and acts on platelets to promote aggregation and the release of thromboxane A_2 (*see below* and page 200).

Prothrombin is activated by either the intrinsic pathway, involving conversion of Factor XII (Hageman factor) to its active form, which results in a 'cascade' of factors (XI, IX, X, V) being successively converted to their active forms, or the extrinsic pathway involving tissue damage, the production of thromboplastins, and Factors VII, X and V. The later stages of the two

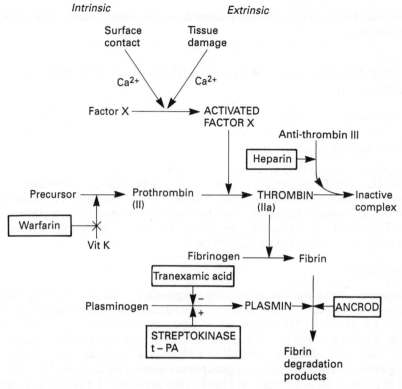

Figure 3.9 The blood clotting and clot dissolution processes and the sites of drug action. Words in CAPITALS represent active proteasers. Boxes enclose names of drugs acting at the sites indicated

pathways are common and in addition to the involvement of various factors require the presence of Ca^{2+} and the aggregation of platelets. Thromboxane A_2, synthesized in platelets from arachidonic acid, promotes platelet aggregation and vasoconstriction whilst prostacyclin, synthesized by the vessel wall from arachidonic acid (page 200), inhibits platelet aggregation and exerts vasodilator actions.

Thrombus formation

Thrombi occur most commonly in the deep veins of the calf following surgery and bed rest when blood flow is sluggish and there may be changes in the blood (elevated platelet count, increased stickiness of platelets and raised concentration of fibrinogen). Thrombus formation starts with the aggregation of platelets at the vessel endothelium, the activation of coagulation resulting in the formation of fibrin and the entanglement of passing red cells. The resulting mass of platelets, fibrin and red cells is the thrombus. In arterial thrombus formation, which typically occurs in a fast flowing circulation, platelet aggregation plays a more important role than does coagulation. For this reason compounds with anticoagulant activity are less successful than those inhibiting platelet function in the prevention of arterial thrombosis.

Drug interference with coagulation or thrombus formation

There are several means by which compounds can affect coagulation.

Removal of calcium ions

In practice this method is restricted to *in vitro* application. Removal of Ca^{2+} inhibits several stages of the process. Ca^{2+} can be removed by precipitation (as the insoluble fluoride, sulphate, oxalate) or by chelation (with sodium edetate). Blood for transfusion is often prevented from clotting by the use of citrate, which forms a soluble complex with Ca^{2+}. Citrate has the advantage that it is metabolized in the Krebs' cycle.

Heparin

Heparin occurs naturally in the body at a number of sites including the liver, lungs and mast cells. Heparin is a sulphated mucopolysaccharide of varying MW (4000–30 000 Da), built up of repeating units of glucosamine and glucuronic acid, and glucosamine and iduronic acid. The anionic sulphate and carboxylic acid groups result in a highly acid molecule with a high net negative charge, these negative groups are essential for activity. The activity of **heparin** as an anticoagulant requires the presence of a cofactor, plasma antithrombin III. This cofactor inhibits the activity of thrombin (and the factors in the cascade) by forming inactive complexes. **Heparin** greatly increases the rate at which these inactive complexes are formed by binding to antithrombin and causing a conformational change that aids thrombin's access to the active site. High MW **heparin** shows higher activity because it contains more of the necessary binding sites but low MW **heparin** is claimed to show selective activity at different points in the cascade (Factor X) and to be free of effects on platelet behaviour (*see below*). The anticoagulant effects of **heparin** are exerted both *in vivo* and *in vitro*. Despite the presence of **heparin** in the body and the mechanism of its anticoagulant activity there is no evidence that it plays any role in the physiological control of blood clotting.

Platelet aggregation may be decreased by **heparin**, because of the decrease in thrombin activity. Some 25–30% of patients experience a mild fall in platelet numbers (thrombocytopenia) because of aggregation and destruction, and a smaller number experience a severe fall, which may be due to the formation of antiplatelet antibodies against the **heparin**/antithrombin III complex. By releasing or activating lipoprotein lipase ('clearing factor') from tissues **heparin** increases the removal of lipids from the plasma.

As a fully ionized molecule **heparin** is not absorbed after oral administration and it is therefore given by iv injection, iv infusion or sc injection. It should not be given by im injection because of possible haematoma formation at the site of injection. **Heparin** may be used *in vivo*, in extracorporeal circulations and to preserve blood samples.

The main problem associated with the use of **heparin** is haemorrhage, especially if the patient has a hidden potential source of bleeding (peptic ulcer). Transient alopecia may occur several months after use. **Heparin** is of animal origin and thus hypersensitivity and anaphylactic reactions may occur but these are not frequent.

Antagonists to heparin

Excessive anticoagulant activity or minor haemorrhage is controlled by ceasing administration of **heparin.** For major haemorrhage resulting from **heparin** use of an antagonist is required. **Protamine sulphate** is a simple, low MW protein that is strongly basic and combines with heparin forming a stable complex with no anticoagulant properties. It is given by slow iv injection, usually 1 mg to 100 units of **heparin** but the dose required declines with the time after **heparin** administration. Because **protamine sulphate** has some anticoagulant properties (inhibits thrombin/fibrinogen interaction), care must be taken not to exceed the amount required to neutralize **heparin.**

The injection of **protamine sulphate** may cause bradycardia, dyspnoea, flushing and a feeling of warmth by releasing histamine (page 193) – it is usually not antigenic.

Ancrod

Ancrod is a glycoprotein extracted from the venom of the Malayan pit viper. It converts fibrinogen to an unstable fibrin, which is removed by the reticuloendothelial system. It is usually given to dissolve deep vein thrombi by slow iv infusion and its effect monitored by plasma fibrinogen concentration or by measuring the size of the clot that can be formed in blood samples. The major problem associated with its use is haemorrhage (as fibrinogen is consumed), which is treated with antivenom (which may cause anaphylaxis) or fibrinogen.

Oral anticoagulants

There are two groups of compounds each with essentially the same mechanisms of action and drawbacks. They are the coumarin **warfarin** and the indanedione *phenindione*. These compounds act as competitive antagonists of vitamin K (similar chemical structure), which is essential for the formation in the liver of prothrombin and Factors VII, IX and X. During the carboxylation of precursors of these factors, vitamin K is converted to its inactive oxide and then metabolized back to its active form. The oral anticoagulants prevent this reconversion and thus reduce the formation of prothrombin and other factors. There is a delay in the onset of the anticoagulant effect as the preformed factors (prothrombin, VII, IX and X) must first be depleted. The varying plasma $t_{\frac{1}{2}}$ of the factors (prothrombin 60 h, Factor VII 6 h) complicates control. The action is exerted only *in vivo* and is influenced by the vitamin K intake and the fat content of the diet (affects absorption of vitamin K). Concurrent use of broad spectrum antibiotics that alter gut bacterial flora and thus vitamin K production, may affect the action of the oral anticoagulants.

Warfarin, a racemic mixture of *dextro R-* and *laevo S*-isomers, is completely absorbed after oral administration, is almost totally protein bound in the plasma and is metabolized by nonspecific MFO in the liver. The peak anticoagulant effect is exerted from 36–72 h, the *S*-isomer being four times more potent than the *R*-isomer. The duration of this effect after withdrawing the drug is 4–5 days. Adverse effects other than haemorrhage or interaction with other drugs (*see below*) rarely occur. **Warfarin** crosses the placenta and should be avoided in pregnancy (page 36).

The less widely used *phenindione* is also completely absorbed after oral administration, is protein bound in the plasma and metabolized in the liver. Its peak effect is exerted for 24–48 h and its duration is 1–4 days. The commonest problem is haemorrhage. Adverse effects are more numerous and common including hypersensitivity reactions, renal damage, hepatitis and agranulocytosis. A product of the metabolism colours the urine red-orange, which may alarm the patient.

Drug interactions

Warfarin is subject to several clinically important pharmacokinetic interactions by the mechanisms of induction of MFO (page 41), competition for plasma protein binding sites (page 40) and inhibition of metabolism (page 43). *Sulphinpyrazone* selectively inhibits the metabolism of the more active *S*-isomer and so potentiates **warfarin.**

Aspirin causes a reduction in prothrombin concentration in the blood and may add to the effects of the oral anticoagulants. Gastric haemorrhage commonly produced by **aspirin** may cause greater problems in the presence of oral anticoagulants.

Drugs affecting platelet function (by influencing thromboxane A_2 and prostacyclin formation) may also interact with oral anticoagulants.

Antagonists to the oral anticoagulants

Minor haemorrhages and excessively reduced prothrombin concentration respond to withdrawal of the drug. Some situations may need more rapid action, whole blood (containing the missing factors) or vitamin K_1 (**phytomenadione** [phytonadione]) may be given.

Drugs affecting platelet function

Aggregation of platelets and their adhesion to the vessel wall is essential for clotting and thrombus formation. This is decreased by prostacyclin (derived from vessel walls) through a mechanism involving elevated concentration of cAMP within the platelets.

Epoprostenol

Epoprostenol (prostacyclin, PGI_2) is available for use in extracorporeal circulations (cardiopulmonary by pass, renal dialysis, charcoal haemoperfusion) with or without **heparin**. It cannot be used in other situations because of its extremely short $t_{\frac{1}{2}}$ (30 s–3 min) and marked vasodilator action giving hypotension, headache and flushing.

Dipyridamole

By inhibiting the enzyme phosphodiesterase *dipyridamole* reduces the metabolism of cAMP and results in elevated concentration within the platelet. This decreases platelet adhesiveness and may reduce thrombus formation. For best effect it is used in combination with **aspirin** or **warfarin.**

Aspirin, other NSAIDS and sulphinpyrazone

These drugs inhibit cyclo-oxygenase and reduce the synthesis of the products of the arachidonic acid pathway. It is claimed that it is possible to inhibit thromboxane A_2 formation without inhibiting that of prostacyclin (because of the inability of the platelet to synthesize more cyclo-oxygenase and possibly greater sensitivity of the platelet enzyme to inhibition) and thus reduce thrombus formation. Dose appears to be critical and results from clinical trials for prophylaxis against coronary thrombosis are equivocal.

Dissolution of thrombus

In the normal clotting process *in vivo* the clot is finally broken down to soluble fibrin degradation products (*Figure 3.9*) by the action of plasmin (fibrinolysin). This is formed from an inactive precursor plasminogen (fibrinolysinogen) by a Factor XII dependent activator formed during the clotting process. Activators of this mechanism may be used in an attempt to breakdown pre-existing thrombi. **Streptokinase** (from haemolytic streptococci) and urinary-type plasminogen activator (*urokinase* from urine) are both able to activate this mechanism and show most success in dissolving fresh clots. Additionally **streptokinase** and tissue-type plasminogen activator (*alteplase*, produced by recombinant DNA technique) are useful in acute myocardial infarction. **Streptokinase** may cause allergic reactions and anaphylaxis.

One danger associated with such attempts to dissolve clots is that fibrinogen and other factors may be used up in maintaining the clot with the resultant risk of haemorrhage. Should this occur an inhibitor of plasminogen activation, *tranexamic acid*, or *aprotinin*, which primarily inhibits plasmin, may be used. Another danger associated with attempts at dissolution is the loosening of the clot from its site of attachment and subsequent movement through the circulation as an embolus.

Lipid-lowering drugs

Hyperlipidaemia, in particular cholesterol and triglyceride in combination with low density lipoprotein, is associated with atherosclerosis. Lipids are transported in the blood within chylomicrons, which are broken down at the interface of adipose tissue and capillaries. Most of the lipid is absorbed into the tissue but the remnants of the chylomicron are metabolized by the liver to give rise to the low density lipoproteins.

Hyperlipidaemia is difficult to define quantitatively and the pathology is often obscure. Lipid concentrations fluctuate widely within an individual, however it is generally thought that plasma cholesterol concentrations above 6 mmol/l require treatment.

Dietary modification is always the first treatment.

Severe hyperlipidaemia may be alleviated by *cholestyramine*, an ion exchange resin that promotes cholesterol excretion by preventing the enterohepatic circulation of the cholesterol contained within the bile salts. Fat soluble vitamins may be lost from the body.

Bezafibrate and related drugs alter the pattern of hepatic lipid metabolism and the beneficial effects arise from the lowered production of low density lipoproteins and cholesterol at the expense of raised high density lipoproteins.

4

Endocrine pharmacology

Aims

- To provide a framework of physiology of the important endocrine systems.
- To explain the site and mechanism of action of endogenous hormones, their structural analogues and other compounds that interact with endocrine systems.
- To produce a scientific basis for the therapeutic use of compounds that interact with endocrine systems.

Introduction

In the mammalian body chemical messengers are often employed to transmit information from one cell to itself (autocrine), within the tissue (paracrine) and to distant organs (endocrine). The peripheral (page 55) and CNS (page 211) sections deal with the theme of drugs that interact with one class of chemical messengers – the neurotransmitters. The theme of this section is interaction with chemical messengers other than neurotransmitters (*Table 4.1*).

Table 4.1 Classification of chemical messengers

	Cell type of origin	Transport medium
Neurotransmitter (paracrine)	Nerve	Interstitial fluid
Local hormone (paracrine)	Non-nerve	Interstitial fluid
Neurohumour (endocrine)	Nerve	Blood
Hormone (endocrine)	Non-nerve	Blood

Hierarchy of endocrine hormones

Several endocrine systems consist of a hierarchy of endocrine glands and hormones in which the secretion of one hormone influences the secretion of a second hormone and that in turn affects the production of a third hormone. This third hormone may act on a peripheral target tissue. *Example: Figure 4.1.*

Usually homeostasis is maintained by a negative feedback whereby a change in the plasma concentration of the peripherally produced hormone alters the secretion of the centrally produced hormone in the opposite direction. A similar but simpler link occurs between plasma glucose concentration and insulin secretion. Consequently pharmacological manipulation at one point in an endocrine system tends to influence the whole system because of this hierarchy and feedback.

Table 4.2 Mechanisms of hormone action

	Membrane-mediated	*Nucleus-mediated*
Mechanism of action	Hormone action mediated extracellularly Interaction with a cell membrane receptor Change in intracellular activities of second messengers (Ca^{2+}, cAMP, protein kinase) Increase in cellular metabolic activities	Hormone action mediated intracellularly (*see Figure 4.2*) Interaction with an intracellular receptor Binding of receptor complex to DNA in the nucleus Synthesis of mRNA, proteins and enzymes
Examples	*Hormone – target* Insulin – liver Adrenaline – adipose cells Protirelin – anterior pituitary Thyroxine – most tissues	*Hormone – target* Glucocorticoids – liver Oestrogens – uterus Androgens – prostate Thyroxine – most tissues
Onset of action	Rapid (min)	Slow (h), often with a delay
Offset of action	Rapid	Persistent due to slow turnover of enzymes/proteins
Correlation between plasma concentration of hormone and time course of action	Good	Poor as action slow and delayed

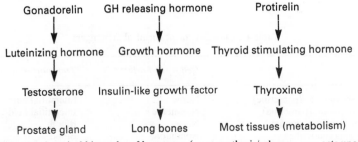

Figure 4.1 A typical hierarchy of hormones ($\rightarrow$ = synthesis/release; $\rightarrow$ = acts upon)

Mechanisms of hormone action

Hormones act by regulating pre-existing processes. The actions of hormones can be divided into those that are cell membrane-mediated and those that are cell nucleus-mediated (*Table 4.2*).

Most reproductive and nonreproductive steroid hormones have a similar molecular mechanism of action. Tissue selectivity is achieved by the presence of one of a family of specific soluble protein receptors which are occasionally found in the cytoplasm (may be an artefact) but are mainly in the nucleus of the target cell (for example, oestrogen-specific in the uterus, androgen-specific in the prostate). Steroids pass from the blood into the cell, combine with the receptor which allows the complex to bind to the DNA of the nucleus (*Figure 4.2*). Here an interaction with the tissue specific chromatin sites produces the metabolic events unique to that target tissue.

The time course of onset and offset of a drug modifying an endocrine system is influenced by whether the actions are membrane-mediated or nuclear-mediated. For example, *soluble insulin* given iv has a very rapid onset and offset of action due in part to the membrane-mediated nature of the action of insulin and in part to its rapid metabolism. Therefore, many formulations of insulin have been developed to produce a slower onset and more prolonged duration of action (page 184). Conversely, the benefits of glucocorticoids given in the relief of chronic asthma take several hours rather than a few minutes to appear, due to the genomically mediated action of these drugs.

Therapeutic uses of drugs affecting endocrine systems

Most therapeutic uses can be divided into four categories.

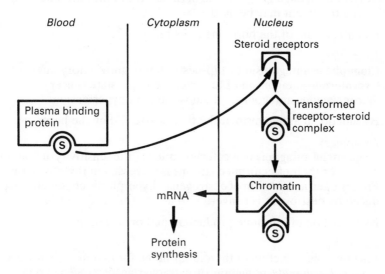

Figure 4.2 The interaction of steroids with target cells

Replacement therapy

Where there is hyposecretion of an endogenous hormone this can be replaced by the administration of the hormone or a structural analogue.

Examples:
Insulin for diabetes mellitus
Thyroxine sodium for hypothyroidism
   Many hormones, unlike neurotransmitters, are proteins or polypeptides and, therefore, it is more difficult to produce structural analogues and such analogues are unlikely to be orally active.
   Alternatively, residual endogenous hormone secretion can be stimulated by drugs either directly at the site of endocrine deficiency or by an action higher in the endocrine hierarchy.

Examples:
Tolbutamide to stimulate insulin secretion
Gonadorelin to treat female infertility
   The dosage used is such that the endocrine system is functioning within the normal physiological range and, therefore, unwanted effects are usually few. Treatment is particularly easy when a constant action is required (for example, treatment of hypothyroidism).
   However, when a varying magnitude of effect is required (for example, diabetes mellitus, page 186) replacement therapy may present more problems.

Decrease of hormone action

Endocrine diseases due to hypersecretion of a hormone or excess response of a peripheral target tissue to a hormone can be treated by surgical (for example, adrenal origin of Cushing's disease) or radiological (for example, hyperthyroidism, page 176) removal of the source of the hormone. Alternatively drug treatment may be used.

(1) By antagonism of the hormone at its receptor.

   Examples:
   Clomiphene antagonism of 17β-oestradiol in anovulatory infertility
   Cyproterone antagonism of testosterone in prostate cancer
   Spironolactone antagonism of aldosterone in hypertension

(2) By functional antagonism at the tissues affected by the hormone.

   Examples:
   Propranolol antagonism of catecholamines – the sensitivity of β-adrenoceptors or their effector mechanisms is increased in thyrotoxicosis
   Progestogen antagonism of oestrogens – hyperplastic endometrium produced by oestrogens is converted to a secretory endometrium

(3) By reduction of hormone production and/or secretion.

   Examples:
   Carbimazole reduction of thyroid hormone formation in thyrotoxicosis
   Aminoglutethimide reduction of extraovarian oestrogen formation in postmenopausal breast cancer

Captopril prevention of conversion of angiotensin I to angiotensin II in hypertension
Combined contraceptive steroid inhibition of gonadotrophin secretion and prevention of ovulation

Functional tests of endocrine systems

An endogenous hormone, structural analogue or synthesis inhibitor is given to determine the site of under or excess secretion of a hormone.

Examples:
Hypothalamic-pituitary-adrenal system (page 181)
Hypothalamic-pituitary-thyroid system (page 176)

Drugs affecting endocrine systems for nonendocrine diseases

The commonest uses of such drugs fall in this category:

Examples:
Glucocorticoids (**prednisolone**) for inflammatory reactions and immune responses in suppression of rheumatoid arthritis and asthma
Mineralocorticoid antagonists (**spironolactone**) for hypertension
    As the dosage required by agonists is greater than in the replacement dose situation so the unwanted effects tend to be greater.

Hypothalamo-pituitary axis

The pituitary gland is situated at the base of the brain and is connected by the pituitary stalk to the hypothalamus. The posterior pituitary gland secretes antidiuretic hormone (ADH, vasopressin, page 188) and oxytocin (page 190) from nerve endings. These nerves have their cell bodies in the hypothalamus. The anterior pituitary gland comprises noninnervated endocrine gland cells that synthesize, store and secrete the proteinaceous pituitary trophins which include:

(1) follicle-stimulating hormone (FSH);
(2) luteinizing hormone (LH);
(3) prolactin (PRL);
(4) thyroid-stimulating hormone (thyrotrophin, TSH, page 173);
(5) lipotrophin (LPH, page 216);
(6) adrenocorticotrophic hormone (corticotrophin, ACTH, page 177);
(7) growth hormone (GH) – biosynthetic human *somatropin* is expensive but effective in the treatment of short stature in children due to a deficiency of growth hormone secretion.

    The secretion of pituitary trophins is controlled by neurohumours synthesized in neurones in the hypothalamus. The neurohumours are released into the blood of capillaries which unite to form the sole blood supply of the anterior pituitary gland (a portal system).

Hypothalamo-pituitary neurohumours

These are substances that promote or inhibit the synthesis and secretion of an anterior pituitary hormone. They are also called hypothalamic releasing or release inhibiting hormones.

Generally there is one neurohumour for each anterior pituitary hormone. Supraphysiological doses of the neurohumours may affect the secretion of other anterior pituitary hormones.

(1) There is only one neurohumour controlling FSH and LH secretion, FSH/LH releasing hormone or *gonadorelin*, which is a decapeptide. The mechanism of differential release of FSH and LH is poorly understood. In both men and women gonadotrophin secretion is episodic.

Gonadorelin or analogues given in short iv pulses stimulate ovarian and testicular development and can be used to treat infertility. Sustained activity at the receptor causes down regulation and inhibition of gonadal activity, an observation that has led to the introduction of potent analogues (*goserelin*) for the treatment of hormone dependent breast and prostate cancer.

(2) Prolactin secretion is inhibited by prolactin release inhibiting hormone, the major component of which is dopamine, acting upon dopamine receptors in the pituitary.

(3) TSH secretion is promoted by TSH releasing hormone which is a tripeptide, *protirelin*. This is not entirely specific as it can also release prolactin.

(4) Somatostatin or GH release inhibiting hormone is a tetradecapeptide that inhibits GH secretion, whereas the release factors are larger polypeptides of between 37 and 44 amino acids.

(5) Corticotrophin releasing hormone, which controls lipotrophin, ACTH (page 177) and β-endorphin (page 216) secretion, is also a large molecule and consists of 41 amino acids.

These neurohumours are not exclusively localized in the hypothalamus and may possess other actions both centrally and peripherally, for example, somatostatin is found in the pancreas and may inhibit both insulin and glucagon secretion (page 182). The plasma $t_{\frac{1}{2}}$ of each neurohumour is very short (less than 5 min) therefore clinical applications are mainly limited to diagnostic procedures that require tests of pituitary integrity.

Feedback mechanisms

Feedback in the control of anterior pituitary hormone secretions involves the central (hypothalamus and/or pituitary) monitoring of the plasma concentration of a peripherally produced hormone and the consequent alteration of anterior pituitary hormone secretions to maintain a predetermined concentration. Feedbacks may be overridden by higher physiological processes, for example, stress will increase ACTH and hence adrenal steroid secretion so that normal physiological plasma concentrations are exceeded. A unique transient positive feedback operates to promote gonadotrophin secretion above the set point in pubertal and adult females and is usually seen where high plasma concentrations of oestrogen follow low priming concentrations – as occur preceding ovulation.

Drug interactions

Various drugs that disturb hypothalamic neurotransmitter processes also produce disturbances in anterior pituitary secretion (barbiturates, phenothiazines and **morphine** inhibit gonadotrophin secretion, leading to decreased libido and infertility).

Phenytoin increases GH secretion, so producing hyperplasia of the gums. *Bromocriptine* suppresses GH release in acromegalic patients (and so is useful to prevent excessive growth in stature) whereas in normal subjects GH release is paradoxically increased.

High serum prolactin concentrations associated with gynaecomastia (increased breast size), galactorrhoea (inappropriate breast secretion), impotence and infertility can result from the use of drugs modulating dopamine storage, release and action. **Chlorpromazine** reduces the neuronal drive from higher centres to the hypothalamic dopaminergic nerve endings. *Metoclopramide* (and perhaps **chlorpromazine**) antagonizes prolactin release inhibiting hormone at its pituitary (dopamine) receptor. An agonist at dopamine receptors, *bromocriptine* is useful therapeutically to decrease prolactin secretion. *Bromocriptine* is the drug of choice to suppress lactation. It also promotes fertility in both sexes where raised prolactin plasma concentrations, possibly as a result of a pituitary adenoma, are associated with disturbances of gonadal activity and/or impotence. Oestrogens promote the synthesis and subsequently the secretion of prolactin. This accounts for the increased plasma concentrations of prolactin seen late in pregnancy and after the combined contraceptive pill and *stilboestrol* for prostatic carcinoma.

The feedback mechanisms are also exploited for therapeutic purposes. The combined type of oral contraceptive inhibits gonadotrophin release and therefore ovulation does not occur. Oestrogens and progestogens are administered to men to reduce LH and hence androgen secretion in an attempt to influence androgen-dependent prostatic cancer. **Clomiphene** (an oestrogen antagonist) prevents the negative feedback action of oestrogens, so generating a surge of gonadotrophin secretion and ovulation. Therefore it is useful in infertility associated with high plasma oestrogen concentration (Stein–Leventhal syndrome characterized by polycystic ovaries, infertility and oligomenorrhoea – decreased menstrual blood loss).

Gonadotrophins

A gonadotrophin is a substance producing growth and development of the gonads. The gonadotrophins, except prolactin, are high MW (25 000 to

70 000 Da) glycoproteins. Prolactin is a protein (MW about 25 000 Da). FSH, LH, *chorionic gonadotrophin* (and TSH too) consist of a common α-chain and different β-chains. The β-chain provides specificity of action. *Follicle-stimulating hormone* is a mixture of gonadotrophins, mainly FSH, extracted from the urine of postmenopausal women. *Chorionic gonadotrophin* is similarly obtained from pregnant women.

Gonadotrophic actions in the female

It is cyclical changes in the pituitary gonadotrophin secretions that produce corresponding ovarian changes and hence the changes characteristic of the human menstrual cycle.

At birth each human ovary contains about 200 000 oocytes, each enclosed in follicular cells to form primordial follicles. Oocytes have partially undergone first meiotic division. FSH (cooperating with a small concentration of LH as during the follicular phase of the menstrual cycle) promotes growth of a few oocytes and their follicular cells. It also promotes 17-β-oestradiol secretion by the thecal cells of these follicles (*Figure 4.3*) which leads to a surge of LH secretion (positive feedback, page 156).

The LH induces final maturation of one (usually) oocyte and completion of first meiotic division. Ovulation and conversion of the remaining follicle to a corpus luteum occurs about 10 h later. This corpus luteum secretes 17-β-oestradiol and progesterone under the influence of LH.

If the oocyte is fertilized the resulting blastocyst implants onto the endometrium of the uterus about 7 days after ovulation. The trophoblast soon secretes HCG, which maintains the steroidogenic activity of the corpus luteum. Immunoassay of HCG may be used for the diagnosis of pregnancy. In a menstrual cycle in which the ovum is not fertilized, the corpus luteum regresses, due to lack of gonadotrophins, and steroid secretion declines. This withdrawal of steroid hormones produces loss of endometrium (menstruation).

Steroid synthesis

Steroid synthesis to the progesterone stage is common for the adrenal cortex, testis and ovary (*Figure 4.4*).

FSH, LH (and ACTH) increase steroid synthesis, probably by increasing conversion of cholesterol to pregnenolone. FSH and LH selectively stimulate synthesis in the gonads. This selective synthesis of testosterone and 17-β-oestradiol derives from the presence of receptors and enzymes in the gonads and the relative absence of enzymes capable of forming corticosteroids. Similarly, only thecal cells of the ovary possess large amounts of enzymes converting precursors to 17-β-oestradiol. In the testis, LH stimulates synthesis and secretion of mainly testosterone (plus some androstenedione and 17-β-oestradiol). Note, testosterone secretion in the female derives mainly from the adrenal cortices.

Prostaglandin $F_{2\alpha}$ (*dinoprost*) reduces progesterone synthesis by causing the atrophy of the corpus luteum. This may be the basis of menstrual cycling.

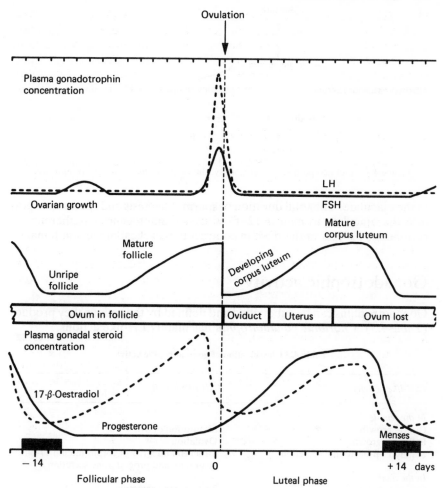

Figure 4.3 Events occurring during the human menstrual cycle

Gonadotrophic action in the male

In the pubertal male gametogenesis is mainly controlled by FSH and steroid-ogenesis by LH. In the adult spermatogenesis is mainly dependent upon LH-stimulated androgen. Sites of sperm production are the seminiferous tubules of the testes. Between the tubules are Leydig cells, which are the major site of testosterone synthesis and secretion.

Before puberty, the seminiferous tubules are lined by diploid spermato-gonia. FSH stimulates continued cell divisions so that there are increased numbers of diploid spermatogonia and spermatocytes (*Figure 4.5*). Also, FSH induces the Sertoli cells to secrete an androgen binding protein, which maintains a high androgen concentration in the tubule lumen. Meiosis is stimulated by FSH and testosterone. Spermatozoa pass to the epididymides where final maturation occurs and it can be 1–3 weeks before sperm appear

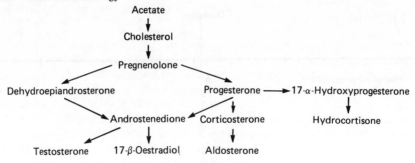

Figure 4.4 Simplified pathways of steroid synthesis in adrenal cortex, testis and ovary

in the ejaculate. The total duration of spermatogenesis and sperm transport into the ejaculate in man is 12–15 weeks. Gametogenesis is therefore a continuous process in the male in contrast to a cyclical process in female.

Gonadotrophic activity

Gonadotrophins can be subdivided and defined by the actions they produce (*Table 4.3*). *Chorionic gonadotrophin* has mainly LH-like actions.

Table 4.3 Classification of gonadotrophic activity

FSH-like activity	LH-like activity
In the female	
Oocyte growth	Maturation of ova
Follicular growth	Ovulation
Mainly 17-β-oestradiol secretion	Structural integrity of corpus luteum 17-β-oestradiol and progesterone secretion
In the male	
Spermatogenesis	Testosterone secretion

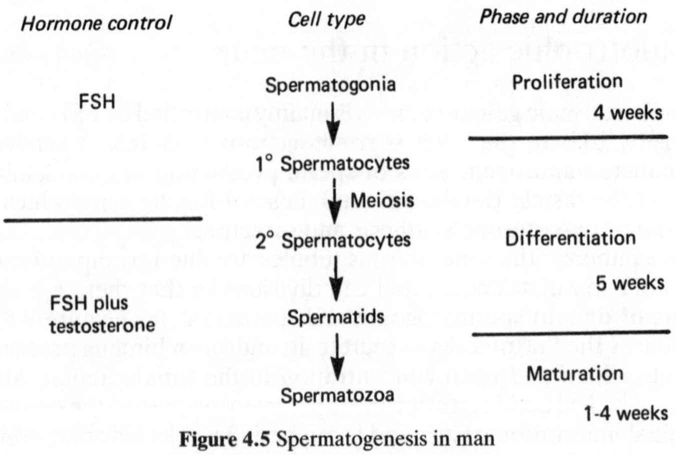

Hormone control	Cell type	Phase and duration
FSH	Spermatogonia	Proliferation
	↓	4 weeks
	1° Spermatocytes	
	↓ Meiosis	
	2° Spermatocytes	Differentiation
	↓	5 weeks
FSH plus testosterone	Spermatids	
	↓	
		Maturation
	Spermatozoa	1-4 weeks

Figure 4.5 Spermatogenesis in man

Therapeutic use

One cause of female infertility is irregular and insufficient endogenous gonadotrophin secretion and therefore absence of ovulation. Replacement therapy with *follicle-stimulating hormone* followed by *chorionic gonadotrophin* mimicking the physiological sequence can lead to ovulation and pregnancy if the ovaries are capable of responding. Ovarian stimulation is easier to manage if endogenous gonadotrophin secretion is inhibited by a gonadorelin agonist. Excessive response leads to ovarian enlargement and haemorrhage, multiple ovulations and multiple pregnancy. This can be avoided by monitoring the rise in plasma oestrogens as a measure of the number of follicles developing in response to *follicle-stimulating hormone*. If this is excessive then *chorionic gonadotrophin* is not given. Multiple ovulations are deliberately induced for subsequent collection of ova for *in vitro* fertilization of the ovum in the treatment of infertility.

Exogenous gonadotrophins have proved of little value in the treatment of male infertility that is due to reduced secretion of endogenous gonadotrophins. In part this may be due to the long time (10–13 weeks) between the first spermatogonial division and final maturation.

Replacement therapy for steroid hormone deficiencies usually involves the use of steroids rather than pituitary trophins.

Oestrogens, progestogens and androgens

An oestrogen, progestogen or androgen is a compound that produces a similar range of effects to those produced by 17-β-oestradiol, progesterone or testosterone respectively. Most such compounds show specificity of action but some possess properties of the other types of steroid at higher doses (for example, an androgen could possess progestogenic activity due to an inherent property of the compound or due to the production of a metabolite possessing progestogenic activity). Some nonendocrine drugs combine with steroid receptors and this accounts for some of their adverse effects. **Spironolactone** and **digoxin** can produce gynaecomastia by acting as agonists at the oestrogen receptor. **Cimetidine,** an antagonist at H_2 histamine receptors, also displaces testosterone from its receptor so that the background oestrogens can be expressed (removal of functional antagonism).

All naturally occurring steroid hormones have a short plasma $t_\frac{1}{2}$ (less than 4 h) and are inactive orally due to high first-pass metabolism. Simple structural alterations of the steroid molecule produce dramatic changes in biological activity (*Figure 4.6*). Modification of the basic structure by conjugation, esterification or alkylation (at positions 1 or 17) extends the $t_\frac{1}{2}$ into the therapeutically useful range. The esters exhibit significant first pass metabolism but a sustained effect (days) occurs after parenteral administration by slow de-esterification. Steric hindrance by alkylation at position 17 (by an ethinyl group —C≡CH) greatly reduces first pass metabolism so these derivatives are orally active with $t_\frac{1}{2}$ of about 1 day.

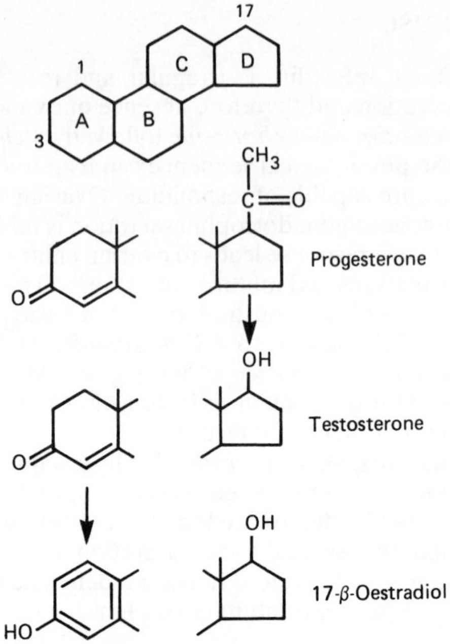

Figure 4.6 The steroid nucleus, position numbering and substituents of some physiological steroids

Steroids are extensively bound to albumin or specific binding globulins. Free steroids are metabolized by the liver and conjugated to form the sulphate and glucuronide. Excretion of the metabolite is mainly in the urine but some is excreted in the bile. Once in the gut bacteria act upon some of the conjugates to release free steroid which is then reabsorbed – a process referred to as enterohepatic circulation. The remainder is excreted in the faeces.

Oestrogens

The major secretory product of the ovarian follicles is 17-β-oestradiol which is rapidly metabolized to less potent oestrogens – oestriol and oestrone. *Figure 4.3* shows the steroid secretion pattern during the menstrual cycle.

Preparations

Steroidal

Oestradiol is available as trans- and subdermal preparations, thus the first pass effect is avoided.

Ethinyloestradiol is active orally because its 17-ethinyl group sterically hinders first pass metabolism by MFO. Mestranol is the 3-methyl ether of ethinyloestradiol and is an active prodrug converted by the liver and the gut wall to the more potent ethinyloestradiol.

Table 4.4 Effects of oestrogens

System affected	Consequence
Female reproductive organs	
Fallopian tubes, uterus, vagina	Growth and development
Mammary glands	Growth and development of ducts
Uterine endometrium	Proliferation (irregular menstruation)
Cervical epithelium	Thin and copious mucus (good sperm penetration)
CNS	
FSH and LH secretion	Positive and negative feedback
Prolactin secretion	Increases
Libido	Indispensable in nonprimate mammals; role in humans not clear
Chemosensitive trigger zone	Nausea and vomiting
Metabolic actions	
Coagulation factors	Predisposition to thromboembolic phenomena
Hormone binding globulins	Increases plasma concentration
Carbohydrate metabolism	Weak diabetogenic action
Fluid mobilization	Salt and water retention
High density lipoproteins increased	Protection against atherosclerosis
Other actions	
Long bones	Growth early; reduces bone reabsorption
Epiphyses	Closure
Axillary and pubic hair	Growth in female pattern
Oestrogen-dependent cancers	Growth after low doses
Carcinogenesis	Endometrial carcinoma may be induced in postmenopausal women by chronic treatment with high doses

Nonsteroidal

These are orally and topically active preparations; *stilboestrol* [diethylstilbestrol] and dienoestrol. This group of oestrogens is suspected of carcinogenic activity, therefore their use is restricted to topical applications or postmenopausal breast cancer or prostate cancer.

All are agonists at oestrogen receptors producing the effects in *Table 4.4*.

Therapeutic use

Oestrogens are used for either their direct actions or indirect hypothalamus-pituitary negative feedback actions. Oestrogen therapy alone is not recommended due to the high incidence of side-effects, for example thromboembolic phenomena or uterine endometrial hyperplasia which in postmenopausal women is associated with progression to carcinoma. Progestogens are usually administered concurrently in the form of the combined contraceptive tablet to obtain the desired effect (page 167).

Replacement therapy

These effects occur with small doses and result from direct actions on target tissue receptors.

Primary ovarian failure. Oestrogens initiate pubertal changes, which are maintained with combination therapy.

Relief of menopausal symptoms (natural or premature), which include vasomotor instability, anxiety, depression and atrophy of secondary sexual organs. Oestrogens do not relieve osteoporosis but may prevent its development. Oestrogen should only be used alone as replacement therapy if the patient has had a hysterectomy (see page 163).

Note: atrophic vaginitis or vulvitis is the only indication for topical (pessary or cream) application to produce a local effect.

Neoplastic disease

These palliative effects occur only with large doses and result from a combination of direct actions on target tissues receptors and nonreceptor-mediated effects. Examples are:

(1) androgen-dependent carcinoma of the prostate;
(2) advanced breast cancer (page 303).

Oestrogen antagonists

These compete with 17-β-oestradiol for the cytoplasmic receptors (*Figure 4.2*). **Clomiphene** and **tamoxifen** are nonsteroidal orally active compounds which antagonize oestrogens at all their specific target organ receptors. They are partial agonists with very long $t_{\frac{1}{2}}$.

Therapeutic use

Induction of ovulation

Oestrogen antagonists can induce ovulation in an infertile patient with an intact hypothalamus-pituitary-ovarian axis and raised plasma oestrogen concentration, for example, Stein–Leventhal syndrome (page 157), or in amenorrhoea on discontinuing contraceptive tablets. In combination with *chorionic gonadotrophin* they produce multiple ovulations for ovum collection for *in vitro* fertilization. A short period of administration induces ovulation and initiates menstrual cycles by preventing oestrogen's inhibitory (negative feedback) action at the hypothalamus, allowing gonadotrophin secretion and therefore follicular development.

Advanced breast cancer

Thirty per cent of breast tumours respond by regression to hormone manipulations, that is, empirical treatment which may involve the removal of the hormone-producing gland, ovary or adrenal (premenopause), or the administration of large doses of androgens, oestrogens or antioestrogens. Breast tumours containing detectable oestrogen receptors respond more favourably. **Tamoxifen** has replaced all other endocrine manipulations as the treatment of choice. Regression can only be obtained during continuous therapy, which is relatively free of adverse effects.

Progestogens

Physiologically the major progestogen is progesterone which is secreted by the corpus luteum of the ovary as well as by the placenta during pregnancy. Most progestational effects are only seen after previous priming of the target organs with oestrogens.

Table 4.5 Effects of progestogens

System affected	Consequence
Female reproductive organs	
Fallopian tubes, uterus, vagina	Growth and development
Mammary glands	Growth and development of the lobular-alveolar system
Uterine endometrium	Increased secretion. Withdrawal leads to tissue necrosis and menstruation
Cervical epithelium	Viscous and scanty mucus (poor sperm penetration)
CNS	
FSH and LH secretion	Negative feedback
Libido	Synergistic with oestrogens in lower mammals
Consciousness	Sedative (large doses)
Body temperature	Thermogenic
Pregnancy	
Uterus, placenta, fetus	Necessary for normal course of pregnancy
Metabolic actions	
Fluid mobilization	Salt and water loss (aldosterone antagonism)
High density lipoproteins	Adversely lowered

Preparations

Progesterone derivatives

Medroxyprogesterone acetate is an ester and only weakly active after oral administration, due to high first-pass metabolism; it is given by deep im injection.

Desogestrel is an orally active, potent and selective agonist at progesterone receptors, used only as the progestogen component in the combined contraceptive tablet.

19-Nortestosterone derivatives

Norethisterone is one of a group of steroids having an ethinyl substitution at the 17-α-position, which makes them orally active and extends the $t_{\frac{1}{2}}$. Ethynodiol is a prodrug that is converted to norethisterone. Levonorgestrel is the commonest progestogen in combined contraceptive tablets.

These compounds are all agonists at progestogen receptors and produce the same effects as progesterone (*Table 4.5*). In addition members of this group may possess androgenic, oestrogenic or antioestrogenic activity because of either intrinsic efficacy of the parent molecule or metabolism to active compounds. Relative to the peripheral progestational effects they more strongly inhibit gonadotrophin secretion than the progesterone derivatives.

Testosterone derivatives

Danazol is a mixed androgen and progestogen that inhibits pituitary gonadotrophin secretion but shows less peripheral progestogenic and androgenic effects.

Therapeutic use

Progestogens are usually used in combination with oestrogens. However, the following list indicates where a progestogen has been found useful alone.

Contraception

(1) Continuous oral administration of 19-nortestosterone derivatives in doses lower than those contained in the combined oral contraceptive tablets has a contraceptive effect. The action is a combination of the effects (see *Table 4.5*) upon the CNS, pituitary, ovary, Fallopian tube, endometrium and cervical mucus. Ovulation is suppressed in about 50% of women and breakthrough menstrual bleeding is common. Ectopic pregnancy is not prevented.

(2) Three-monthly im depot injections of the esters *medroxyprogesterone acetate* or *norethisterone enanthate* have a contraceptive effect. Gonadotrophin secretion is suppressed so ovulation does not occur. Menstruation is irregular and amenorrhoea may occur after 12 months. Continued patient compliance is not required therefore it is useful when pregnancy is contraindicated, for example, following rubella vaccination.

Both approaches are useful during lactation and in women who suffer from oestrogen-related adverse effects of the combined oral contraceptive tablets.

Endometriosis

Endometriosis is the growth of endometrial tissue in inappropriate (ectopic) positions, such as in the peritoneal cavity. Continuous long-term use of progestogens is aimed at producing regression of the tissue mass by the withdrawal of endogenous oestrogen support.

Neoplastic disease

Large doses of progestogens produce remission in inoperable endometrial carcinoma and breast cancer, which is maintained for about 15 months.

Progestogen antagonist

Mifepristone is a progestogen antagonist. As progesterone is necessary for the maintenance of pregnancy, mifepristone can be useful for the termination of early pregnancy.

Oestrogen plus progestogen

Oral combined therapy (one oestrogen [**ethinyloestradiol** or mestranol] plus one progestogen [a 19-nortestosterone derivative] or desogestrel) is used at lower doses than single drug therapy as the constituents are synergistic.

The synthetic steroidal oestrogens are combined with the orally active progestogens. The combination is usually administered as a 21-day course followed by a 7-day tablet-free interval during which withdrawal bleeding from the endometrium occurs (not true menstruation). Practically any cycle length can be produced by continuing administration of these drugs. The oestrogen plus progestogen exert a negative feedback action at the hypothalamus-anterior pituitary resulting in decreased FSH and LH secretion and preventing the midcycle surge of secretion of these gonadotrophins. Consequently, ovulation is prevented and endogenous 17-β-oestradiol and progesterone secretion markedly reduced. However, the peripheral action of the steroid hormones is replaced by that of the synthetic hormones. The pattern of administration of these synthetic compounds is in a different sequence from that of the endogenous hormones, so disrupting the finely tuned processes necessary for ovulation, fertilization and pregnancy. Reduction of the daily dose of oestrogen below 30 μg is likely to lead to breakthrough bleeding and lower contraceptive efficacy due to failure to inhibit gonadotrophin secretion and suppress the endogenous cycle.

Drug interactions

Drugs that increase the mixed function oxidase activity of the liver, for example, **rifampicin** [rifampin], **phenytoin** or the barbiturates decrease the plasma concentrations of the steroids and hence the efficacy of the contraceptive tablet – recognized by breakthrough bleeding or later by pregnancy. Oral antibiotics that reduce the gut content of bacteria may also produce these effects by decreasing the enterohepatic circulation of the steroids especially.

Therapeutic uses

Replacement therapy

In the treatment of menopausal symptoms and primary ovarian failure where there is deficient endogenous hormone secretion, the combination provides better cycle control than oestrogens alone and avoids continuous therapy.

Menstrual irregularities

In the treatment of dysmenorrhoea (painful menses) and dysfunctional uterine bleeding (abnormal menstrual pattern) the therapeutic aim is to impose regular drug-induced cycles by inhibiting the endogenous ovarian hormonal rhythm.

Contraception

The combined type of oral contraceptive tablet produces almost complete suppression of gonadal activity and therefore no ovulation. Other progestational effects contribute to the contraceptive action (page 166). Triphasic and biphasic formulations seek to mimic the pattern of hormone secretion during the menstrual cycle. Adverse effects can be alleviated by changing the oestrogen/progestogen content.

Postcoital contraception

The contraceptive action can occur up to 72 h after intercourse. Possible mechanisms are interference with sperm migration, increases in tubal transport of the ovum or prevention of implantation by asynchronous development of the endometrium. The incidence of acute side-effects is increased compared to that seen with conventional oral contraception as a larger dose is necessary for effectiveness postcoitally.

Adverse effects

Adverse effects that show tolerance

Some adverse effects tend to disappear after the first month of administration.

(1) Oestrogenic – nausea, vomiting, headache, weight gain, enlarged and tender breasts, decreased libido.
(2) Progestogenic – increased appetite, weight gain, decreased libido, depression, cramps, acne.

Less transient adverse effects

Most of these effects arise because the dose of the administered steroids is greater than the replacement dose, and are similar to the changes that can occur in early pregnancy. The overall risk is less than that of pregnancy.

(1) Thromboembolic disorders. The mortality due to deep vein thrombosis is increased two times and that due to cerebral thrombosis is increased four times. These mortality increases are greater above 35 years of age and with longer medication and higher dose of the oestrogenic and possibly progestogenic component. Combined contraceptive tablets contain 50 μg or less of **ethinyloestradiol** or mestranol to reduce the incidence of thromboembolic disorders.

(2) Arterial diseases. Cerebrovascular and ischaemic heart disease is associated with the progestogenic component, which raises cholesterol and lowers high density lipoprotein concentrations in the serum. Their incidence is increased 2–6 times while that of hypertension is reversibly increased about three times. The risk of dying from a vascular disease is greater with age, cigarette smoking, obesity and family history of hypertension.

(3) Genitourinary tract infections. The incidence is increased about 1.5 times, probably by increasing vaginal pH.

(4) Glucose tolerance is decreased but the incidence of diabetes mellitus is not increased.

(5) Thyroid function tests are impaired.

(6) Amenorrhoea may follow cessation of use; however, fertility is not significantly different from that in nonusers 18 months after ceasing treatment.

(7) There is no association between usage and cancer, except cancer of the cervix which is increased. This may be due to changes in pregnancy rate and sexual practices and not to the drugs.

Advantageous effects

Beneficial health effects can be demonstrated for dysmenorrhoea, menorrhagia, iron deficiency anaemia, pelvic inflammatory disease, fibroids, endometrial and ovarian cancer as well as benign breast disease.

Contraindications

Breast feeding, diabetes mellitus and migraine (not absolute), cardiovascular disease including hypertension and thromboembolism, liver disease, pregnancy, young oligomenorrhoeic girls, abnormal vaginal bleeding, hormone dependent cancer, elective surgery and immobilization.

Androgens

Androgens are substances that cause masculinization. Testosterone is the most important androgen and is secreted by the Leydig cells of the testis and to a smaller extent by the adrenal cortex of both sexes. Testosterone is converted to the more potent derivative 5-α-dihydrotestosterone in the target tissues of the body.

Table 4.6 Effects of androgens

System affected	Consequence
Reproductive organs	
Internal and external genitalia	Sexual differentiation in the fetus
	Growth and development
Spermatogenesis	Low concentrations stimulate
	High concentrations inhibit via negative feedback on gonadotrophin secretion
CNS	
LH secretion	Negative feedback
FSH secretion	Negative feedback in combination with the testicular factor inhibin
Fetal hypothalamus	Imprinting of male behavioural and acyclic control of gonadotrophin secretory patterns
Libido and aggression	Augments in both sexes
Metabolic actions	
General	Marked net anabolic action (nitrogen retention)
Fluid mobilization	Salt and water retention
Other actions	
Long bone	Growth
Epiphyses	Closure
Muscle	Growth
Hair	Growth in male pattern. Paradoxically responsible for male pattern baldness
Skin	Thickening. Increased secretion from sebaceous glands (acne)
Vocal cords	Growth
Blood	Increased erythropoiesis
Liver	17-α-alkylated derivatives cause cholestatic jaundice

Preparations

Testosterone

A *testosterone ester* is given by injection in oil im weekly. It is hydrolysed to the active drug testosterone. The dosage interval can be extended by administering a mixture of *testosterone esters* that are hydrolysed at different rates.

Mesterolone

Alkylation in position 1 results in oral activity and the lack of 17-α-alkylation in a low incidence of hepatotoxicity. *Mesterolone* is a weak androgen that has primarily peripheral actions.

Anabolic steroids

Nandrolone is alkylated at the 17-α-position, which reduces the rate of metabolism. This results in oral activity but also some hepatotoxicity (cholestatic jaundice). Androgens have useful anabolic actions and nandrolone shows some separation between the anabolic and androgenic actions but its ratio of anabolic to androgenic potency is only 2–3 times that of testosterone, which militates against its use particularly in women and children. Abuse of these drugs is common among athletes.

Therapeutic use

Replacement therapy

Androgens initiate or maintain the growth of the male secondary sexual characteristics, for example, after castration or gonadal failure with delayed puberty. *Mesterolone* is useful as it acts peripherally and does not decrease gonadotrophin secretion. Premature fusion of the epiphyses may occur in boys.

Treatment of infertility

Male infertility of endocrine cause is usually resistant to treatment. Spermatogenesis requires gonadotrophins plus androgens while the latter usually suppress gonadotrophin secretion by negative feedback. In hypopituitarism fertility can be restored with *chorionic gonadotrophin* and *follicle-stimulating hormone* which stimulate both androgen production and spermatogenesis.

Advanced breast cancer

Androgens are sometimes used after recurrence of metastatic breast cancer. The action may be exerted via the negative feedback at the pituitary or directly upon the tissue. The adverse effects are virilization (growth of facial hair), hoarseness of voice and an increase in libido (*see* page 170).

Stimulation of erythropoiesis

Large doses of the anabolic steroids are administered for at least 2 months in aplastic anaemia, leukaemia and refractory anaemia. The response is variable and said to be mediated by increased production of erythropoietin by the kidney, which then acts upon the stem cells of the bone marrow.

Androgen antagonists

Cyproterone competes with testosterone for the androgen receptor (page 161) and antagonizes androgens at all their specific target organs. It is also a very potent progestogen, so activating the negative feedback upon gonadotrophin secretion.

Therapeutic use

It decreases sexual drive in sexual offenders but does not alter the direction of the desire. Severe hirsutism in women, due to excess adrenal androgen secretion, can be treated with **cyproterone**. Severe acne in women may be treated with an oral preparation of **ethinyloestradiol** and **cyproterone**. Prostate cancer also responds to this androgen antagonist.

Antispermatogenic effects of drugs

A number of drugs and chemicals modify spermatogenesis although none are currently suitable for use as male contraceptives. Such compounds either inhibit spermatogenesis or modify the sperm such that fertilization does not ensue. There are two major mechanisms of drug action as follows.

Direct action on sperm cells

Many alkylating agents and antimetabolites when used in cancer chemotherapy (page 300) inhibit spermatogenesis at specific stages leading to infertility. The time from commencement of drug administration to sterility is dependent on the stage of spermatogenesis affected. For example, *busulphan* selectively kills spermatogonia. The stages from spermatocytes onward continue at the normal rate and therefore sterility does not occur for upwards of 14 weeks. Irreversible ablation of spermatogenesis often occurs after **cyclophosphamide** or *mustine* and *procarbazine*. The ovary is also affected. Infertility is a particular problem after the successful treatment of young people for Hodgkin's disease or children for acute lymphoblastic leukaemia. The effects of these drugs are related to widespread inhibition of cell proliferation. The mechanism producing reversible infertility during treatment of inflammatory bowel disease with *sulphasalazine* is unknown.

Indirect action via suppression of secretion of gonadotrophins

As the gonadotrophins are necessary for spermatogenesis, any drug that suppresses their secretion sufficiently and for a prolonged period eventually produces sterility. Therefore oestrogens, progestogens and androgens can all produce sterility via their negative feedback actions at the hypothalamus or anterior pituitary gland. The time to the onset of sterility is usually at least 14 weeks. Most endocrine drugs do not affect the stem cells within the seminiferous tubules, so that fertility usually returns after cessation of drug treatment. This may take several months.

The thyroid gland and drugs used in thyroid abnormalities

The function of the thyroid gland is the synthesis, storage and release of the thyroid hormones l-thyroxine (T_4) and l-tri-iodothyronine (T_3).

Synthesis and release

Dietary iodine is converted to I^- and absorbed from the alimentary canal. The thyroid concentrates I^- 20–200 times with respect to the plasma concentration by active transport (the I^- pump) involving a cAMP-dependent Na^+/I^- cotransport system, from the blood to the thyroid follicular cells and ultimately, by diffusion, to the colloid-containing lumen of the follicle. At the apical surface of the follicular cell the I^- is converted to an active iodinating species by the action of a haem-containing thyroid peroxidase that requires H_2O_2. The iodinating species appears not to be iodine itself but an intermediary, which may be a sulphenyl iodide. Whatever the nature of this species it reacts with tyrosine molecules within the thyroglobulin (a complex glycoprotein present in the luminal colloid of the thyroid follicle) to yield monoiodotyrosine (MIT) and di-iodotyrosine (DIT). These compounds have respectively one or two molecules of iodine attached to the benzene ring of tyrosine. Two molecules of DIT undergo condensation, with the elimination of alanine, to form T_4. Some T_3 is similarly formed from the condensation of MIT and DIT. The condensation reactions are oxidative and utilize thyroid peroxidase as a catalyst. In normal circumstances more T_4 than T_3 is produced but when iodine is deficient the ratio may be reduced. At this stage MIT, DIT, T_3 and T_4 are in peptide linkage to the thyroglobulin. Release involves the proteolytic breakdown of the peptide bonds between iodinated compounds and thyroglobulin. T_4 and T_3 pass out of the thyroid cells into the circulation. MIT and DIT are deiodinated by microsomal iodotyrosine deiodinase to I^- and tyrosine, which are reused in synthesis. Ninety-nine per cent of the plasma thyroid hormones are protein bound, particularly to an α-globulin called thyroxine binding globulin; 90% of the circulating hormone is T_4, the remainder is T_3. T_4 is slowly eliminated from the body ($t_\frac{1}{2}$ 6–7 days) whereas the $t_\frac{1}{2}$ of T_3 is 2 days. Both compounds are conjugated in the liver with glucuronic and sulphuric acids. There is an enterohepatic circulation of the hormones.

In peripheral tissues, T_4 is converted to T_3, which is about four times as active as T_4. The rate of this conversion in each tissue is therefore a determinant of its biological response to thyroid hormone.

Control of synthesis and release

This involves the hypothalamus and anterior pituitary gland (see page 155). TSH stimulates all stages of synthesis (but especially I^- uptake) and release of the thyroid hormones. Most of the actions of TSH are dependent upon cAMP as an intracellular second messenger. A negative feedback system exists such that increased concentration of free thyroid hormone in the blood reduces the output of TSH from the anterior pituitary.

Effects of thyroid hormone

In general, thyroid hormones increase the O_2 consumption of most metabolically active tissues (exceptions: brain, testes, uterus, spleen and anterior pituitary). They stimulate lipid catabolism, protein synthesis and intestinal carbohydrate absorption. These actions are believed to be exerted through interaction with both membrane and nuclear receptors (page 152). The effect on body systems can best be illustrated by comparison between the hypothyroid and hyperthyroid states (*Table 4.7*).

Table 4.7 Comparison of hypothyroid and hyperthyroid states

Effect	Hypothyroid state	Hyperthyroid state (thyrotoxicosis)
Body weight	Gain	Loss
Oxygen consumption	Decreased	Increased
Heat production	Decreased	Increased
Basal metabolic rate	Decreased	Increased
CNS	Impaired mentality Poor memory and concentration Drowsiness	Excitability, restlessness apprehension, insomnia
Somatic motor nervous system	Decreased activity	Increased activity
Sympathetic nervous system	Decreased activity	Increased activity
Cardiovascular system	Bradycardia, fall in cardiac output and BP	Tachycardia, increase in cardiac output and BP
Gastrointestinal tract	Activity diminished, constipation	Activity increased, diarrhoea
Sensitivity to catecholamines	Decreased	Increased

Use of thyroid hormone

Thyroxine sodium and *liothyronine sodium* are only used as replacement therapy to treat hypothyroid states (adult myxoedema, childhood cretinism). *Thyroxine sodium* is normally the drug of choice for maintenance therapy but *liothyronine sodium* may be preferred when a rapid onset of action (hypothyroid coma) or shorter duration of action (hypothyroidism with ischaemic heart disease) is required.

Thyroid hormones may enhance the effects of the oral anticoagulants although the mechanism of the interaction is not clear. The hormones can be shown to inhibit the metabolism of anticoagulants and to displace them from protein binding sites but this is probably not the case with therapeutic plasma concentrations and other mechanisms are likely to be involved.

Thyrotoxicosis

In thyrotoxicosis there is an excess of circulating thyroid hormones. This may be due to:

(1) a diffusely enlarged gland producing excess hormone – this is Graves'

disease, which is associated with autoantibodies directed against TSH receptors on the thyroid follicular cells. Unlike TSH, the synthesis of these thyroid-stimulating antibodies is not subject to feedback control by thyroid hormones.

(2) a multinodular goitre;

(3) stimulation of the thyroid by excess TSH from a pituitary thyrotroph tumour (not subject to feedback control);

(4) an autonomously functioning nodule (toxic adenoma).

Drugs used in thyrotoxicosis

Thioamide derivatives

Carbimazole and *propylthiouracil*. These compounds prevent both the iodination of the tyrosine residues and also the condensation reaction between the mono- and di-iodotyrosines; this latter occurs at a concentration lower than that needed to inhibit the iodination. As both stages of the synthesis involve tyrosine peroxidase and a reactive oxidation derivative of iodine it seems likely that the thioamide compounds interfere with the action of the peroxidase enzyme or interact with the intermediate, possibly sulphenyl iodide, itself.

Propylthiouracil also prevents the peripheral metabolism of T_4 to the more active T_3. The drugs are well absorbed from the intestine and widely distributed in tissues. Response to treatment takes several weeks with the euthyroid state produced in 1–2 months. To avoid relapse treatment should be prolonged (1.5–2 years), even then relapse is common: up to 50%, many within 3 months of stopping treatment. Thioamides may also be used before thyroid surgery and to hasten euthyroidism after radiation therapy. Side-effects include skin rashes, lymphadenopathy and fever (3–5% of patients treated) and agranulocytosis (0.5%). If the dosage is too high and a hypothyroid state is produced enlargement of the gland (goitre) may result, TSH being released from the anterior pituitary in response to the low circulating concentrations of thyroid hormones and stimulating the gland causing hyperplasia.

Propylthiouracil is useful when rashes develop to **carbimazole** as there is not usually cross sensitivity. When used during pregnancy or lactation there is a danger of neonatal goitre and hypothyroidism as the drugs can enter the fetus from the placenta and the newborn from the milk.

Monovalent ions

Iodide. The daily intake of I^-, in amounts considerably above the normal requirement of 100–200 μg, is able to control hyperthyroidism. The mechanism of action is unclear but I^- promotes involution of the hypertrophied tissue with an increased colloid storage and a decreased release of thyroid hormones. A possible explanation for this action (autoregulation) is that I^- reduces the stimulation by TSH on cAMP synthesis in thyroid cells. The effects are rapid in onset (10–15 days for maximal effect) but not sustained. I^- is useful before surgery to prepare the gland for subtotal thyroidectomy, but only after prior treatment with antithyroid drugs, and together with other antithyroid drugs and supportive measures in thyrotoxic crisis. It is prescribed as *iodine aqueous solution*. Adverse effects include hypersensitivity reactions and painful salivary glands.

Radioactive iodide

Radioactive I⁻ (given as sodium iodide) is treated exactly as unlabelled iodide by the body and is rapidly and efficiently trapped by the thyroid gland, incorporated into the iodoamino acids and deposited into the colloid of the follicles. Several isotopes of iodine are available (*Table 4.8*). ^{131}I is the one normally used in the treatment of hyperthyroidism. The dose needed is large compared with that used in diagnostic tests. The radioactive iodine is deposited in the colloid of the follicles from where the destructive β-particles originate. The average depth of penetration of the particles is 0.5 mm, which means that radiation damage occurs to the parenchymal cells lining the follicles of the thyroid gland with little or no damage to surrounding tissue. The response is slow (this is overcome by administering antithyroid drugs postdosing) and there is a high incidence of myxoedema (up to 50% of cases in 8 years after dosing) due to the difficulty in estimating the effective dose. There is a late increase in the incidence of thyroid cancer. Radioactive isotopes are also used in the testing of thyroid function (*see below*).

Table 4.8 Medically useful isotopes of iodine

Isotope	$t\frac{1}{2}$	Radiation emitted	Application
^{125}I	57 days	Gamma rays	Diagnostic aid
^{131}I	8 days	β particles Gamma rays	Diagnostic aid and treatment of hyperthyroidism
^{132}I	2.3 h	β particles Gamma rays	Diagnostic aid

Antagonists at β-adrenoceptors

Propranolol (page 114) and other antagonists at β-adrenoceptors reduce many of the signs and symptoms of thyrotoxicosis, including nervousness, atrial fibrillation and increased myocardial contractility and cardiac output. There is no effect on basal metabolic rate or I⁻ utilization. **Propranolol** is valuable before thyroidectomy, after irradiation and in thyrotoxic crisis (in conjunction with antithyroid drugs and supportive measures). As sole treatment for thyrotoxicosis the success rate differs little from the spontaneous remission rate and the patient remains biochemically hyperthyroid throughout the treatment.

Testing of the hypothalamic-pituitary-thyroid system

TRH stimulation test

Protirelin (TRH) is used as a diagnostic aid because of its ability to stimulate the anterior pituitary gland and influence the output of TSH (page 156.)

A patient with normal thyroid function will respond to an iv injection of *protirelin* with an increased output of TSH (and consequential increased plasma concentrations of T_3 and T_4). In thyrotoxicosis this increased output is prevented by the negative feedback exerted by the elevated concentrations of thyroid hormones. TSH concentrations may also fail to rise in hypothyroidism due to pituitary failure.

Radioactive iodide uptake test

The percentage of an administered dose (as NaI solution) absorbed by the thyroid at set time intervals is determined. The pattern of uptake distinguishes hypo-, hyper- and euthyroid patients. ^{131}I (in small doses) can be used but the ultrashort $t_{\frac{1}{2}}$ of ^{132}I has the advantage of delivering much lower radiation doses and this isotope may be preferred for diagnostic tests in infants and young children, during pregnancy or whenever sequential tests of thyroid function are planned.

T_3 suppression test

The uptake of ^{131}I or ^{132}I is determined before and after administration (several days) of T_3. The second uptake should be reduced through the feedback activity of T_3 at the anterior pituitary (reduced TSH output). A failure to suppress indicates the presence of ectopic TSH or an autonomously functioning gland.

The adrenal cortex and the corticosteroids

The function of the adrenal cortex is the synthesis and release of the adrenal steroids hydrocortisone [cortisol], corticosterone and aldosterone (minor amounts of 11-deoxycorticosterone and androgens are also produced).

Synthesis is from cholesterol (*Figure 4.4*).

Control of synthesis and release

The rate of release of adrenocortical hormones is virtually identical to the rate of synthesis as the hormones are not stored. The role of the hypothalamus and anterior pituitary gland in synthesis and release of adrenocortical hormones is discussed on page 155. ACTH stimulates the production of hydrocortisone by increasing activity of the enzyme, cholesterol esterase, that regulates the conversion of cholesterol to pregnenolone. ACTH release is under hypothalamic control mediated by corticotrophin releasing factor (CRF), which is secreted into the hypophyseal portal venous circulation.

A negative feedback system operates with increased plasma concentration of free hydrocortisone reducing release of CRF and ACTH. A circadian rhythm exists in hydrocortisone production, output being maximum shortly after awakening. In the plasma, hydrocortisone is largely protein bound to a high affinity α_2-globulin (transcortin). Metabolism occurs in the liver giving water soluble metabolites with little or no activity that are excreted by the kidney. Approximately 0.5% of hydrocortisone is excreted unchanged in the urine. This is of clinical significance as 'urinary free hydrocortisone' reflects plasma free hydrocortisone and can be used to assess adrenal cortical hyperactivity.

Aldosterone synthesis and release is under the control of the renin-angiotensin mechanism (page 190). Renin is released from the juxtaglomerular apparatus in the kidney in response to a fall in blood volume, renal perfusion pressure or plasma Na^+ concentration. Both the action of the released aldosterone in the promotion of Na^+ retention and of the angiotensin II in constricting blood vessels reduce the stimulus for further renin release.

Effects of the adrenal steroids

The adrenal cortex functions as an organ of homeostasis enabling the body to maintain a constant internal environment in response to changing environmental demands. The adrenal steroids exert a number of actions on all aspects of metabolism resulting in effects classed as mineralocorticoid and glucocorticoid.

Mineralocorticoid effects are: electrolyte balance – increased Na^+ retention and K^+ loss by the kidney.

Glucocorticoid effects are:

(1) peripheral amino acid mobilization;
(2) decreased glucose uptake and increased gluconeogenesis;
(3) mobilization of fatty acids from adipose tissue.

These effects are believed to be exerted by interaction of the steroids with specific steroid receptors (see page 152).

Supraphysiological doses of steroids with glucocorticoid activity reduce immune and inflammatory responses. The effect on the immune response is the result of decreased release of interleukin 2 (IL-2) by T-cells in response to antigenic stimuli. The anti-inflammatory action reduces manifestations of the inflammatory response, both macroscopic (warmth, redness, swelling, pain) and microscopic (leucocyte accumulation and activation of mononuclear cells), regardless of the cause. This involves the stimulation of synthesis and release by leucocytes of a protein, lipocortin, that inhibits phospholipase A_2 thus preventing the formation of products of the arachidonic acid pathway (PGs and LTs) involved in inflammatory responses (page 198). Associated with these functions is a reduction in lymphoid tissue mass. These actions on immune and inflammatory responses are classed as glucocorticoid.

Aldosterone exerts exclusively mineralocorticoid effects, hydrocortisone exerts mainly glucocorticoid activity but large doses also influence electrolyte balance.

The use of ACTH

Preparations

ACTH (*corticotrophin*) is a 39-amino acid polypeptide chain in which the first 24 amino acids are common to all species and are essential for the physiological activity. The remaining 15 amino acids are species specific, not essential for activity and confer specific antigenicity.

Tetracosactrin is a synthetic analogue consisting of the adrenocortico-trophic component of ACTH, that is, the first 24 amino acids. Both structures have a short plasma $t_{\frac{1}{2}}$. To reduce frequency of administration they are formulated with gelatin (*corticotrophin*) or zinc (*tetracosatrin*) to give depot preparations.

Uses

(1) Diagnostically – to determine if adrenal insufficiency is due to pituitary or adrenal failure. This test assesses adrenal cortex reserve. Blood for hydrocortisone assay is collected at standard times in relation to an injection of a standard dose of short acting soluble ACTH. In the normal individual a significant increment and peak value is seen. In adrenal insufficiency both increment and peak value are smaller.

(2) Treatment of anterior pituitary failure, although replacement therapy with glucocorticoids is usually preferred, ACTH may have a role in children where growth retardation by corticotrophin is less than that produced by glucocorticoids.

The main problem with the use of ACTH is the necessity for parenteral administration to avoid proteolytic destruction of the polypeptide structure. Hypersensitivity reactions occur only infrequently with *tetracosatrin*.

The use of adrenal steroids

Preparations

Modification of the structures of the natural adrenal steroids has produced compounds that have the following properties:

(1) mainly glucocorticoid activity but with some significant mineralocorti-coid activity, **prednisolone;**

(2) glucocorticoid activity with no significant mineralocorticoid activity, *betamethasone, beclomethasone, dexamethasone, fluocinolone;*

(3) mineralocorticoid activity with no significant glucocorticoid activity, **fludrocortisone.**

It has not yet proved possible to produce compounds showing anti-inflammatory activity without the other glucocorticoid actions.

Alteration in structure also changes plasma $t_{\frac{1}{2}}$ by influencing protein binding and metabolism. Hydrocortisone has a very short $t_{\frac{1}{2}}$ of about 2 h; synthetic steroids can be classified as short acting, ($t_{\frac{1}{2}}$ less than 36 h **prednisolone**) or longer acting ($t_{\frac{1}{2}}$ greater than 48 h *dexamethasone*).

Uses

Corticosteroids are useful for replacement therapy or in nonendocrinological diseases for their other (particularly anti-inflammatory) actions.

Replacement therapy

There is little risk of side-effects when adrenal steroids are used for replacement therapy as plasma concentrations are in the physiological range. The type of analogue (mineralocorticoid or glucocorticoid) chosen will depend on the condition treated. Acute adrenal failure usually requires only a glucocorticoid (*hydrocortisone sodium succinate* given iv) together with measures to correct fluid and electrolyte imbalance. Chronic adrenal insufficiency requires both glucocorticoid (*hydrocortisone*) and mineralocorticoid (**fludrocortisone**) replacement. In anterior pituitary failure a glucocorticoid alone is sufficient as ACTH does not regulate aldosterone secretion. In congenital adrenal hyperplasia abnormalities in the steroid synthetic pathway lead to deficient glucocorticoid secretion, elevated ACTH secretion and androgen production as the precursors are diverted from the nonfunctioning to the functioning pathways. Potent and longer acting compounds (*dexamethasone*) are preferred in this instance as they have to replace deficient steroids and suppress ACTH secretion in order to reduce androgen production. Mineralocorticoid replacement may be necessary depending on the nature of the defect in the synthetic pathway.

Treatment of nonendocrinological disorders

The steroids are used for their effects on immune and inflammatory responses. Compounds with high glucocorticoid and low mineralocorticoid activity (for example, **prednisolone**) are used.

Among conditions treated with glucocorticoids are those in which tissue inflammation and autoimmunity play a part (asthma, page 395), allergic rhinitis and conjunctivits, eczema, systemic lupus erythematosus). Topical application of glucocorticoids can be useful in reducing inflammation in skin (page 439) and eye diseases. However care should be taken to avoid their use in infective situations as in herpes simplex. Glucocorticoids can be used for their ability to cause involution of lymphoid tissue in achieving temporary remission in leukaemia (page 302) and prevent transplant rejection. In all these situations glucocorticoids themselves are not curative.

Treatment with glucocorticoids presents two main risks:

(1) Abrupt withdrawal after prolonged high dosage may result in life threatening acute adrenal insufficiency due to suppression of ACTH and atrophy of the gland. When treatment is discontinued the dose should be reduced gradually over several weeks or months. However a corticosteroid given for periods less than 7 days as in acute severe asthma can be withdrawn rapidly with little danger. Alternate day therapy and the

use of minimal effective doses can be used to prevent suppression of the hypothalamo-pituitary-adrenal axis. High doses especially those larger than 7.5 mg daily can cause hypothalamo-pituitary-adrenal axis suppression. Attempts to reduce the dose often results in disease relapse.

(2) Prolonged treatment in supraphysiological doses always carries risks, which must be weighed against benefits in serious disabling illness. Many of these adverse effects are clearly extensions of the physiological actions and include hyperglycaemia, salt and water retention, increased susceptibility to infection, muscle wasting, osteoporosis and a state resembling Cushing's syndrome. Disruption of the local gastric defence against the acid environment may predispose to peptic ulceration. Other adverse reactions include cataract, euphoria, psychosis, and increased intraocular pressure. This latter is genetically determined in patients with a predisposition to open angle glaucoma and occurs more readily to topical treatment.

Nonsystemic application or administration of glucocorticoids does not necessarily protect against these two risks – liberal application of the older, more potent compounds in the treatment of various skin problems was associated with suppression of the hypothalamo-pituitary-adrenal axis (sparing application of less potent compounds is now employed). More recently asthma therapy with inhaled glucocorticoids has been implicated in the development of cataracts. In both these situations there is sufficient absorption from the site of application to produce a significant systemic drug concentration.

Interference with synthesis or action of the adrenal steroids

Metyrapone decreases the synthesis of hydrocortisone, corticosterone and aldosterone by inhibiting the enzyme that converts 11-deoxyhydrocortisone to hydrocortisone and 11-deoxycorticosterone to corticosterone. It can be used to test pituitary function and in the treatment of ectopic ACTH secretion and malignant adrenal tumours to reduce steroid output. *Aminoglutethimide*, which inhibits conversion of cholesterol to pregnenolone, can also be used to treat such tumours. The ability of *aminoglutethimide* to inhibit the conversion of androgens to oestrogens in peripheral tissues leads to its use in the treatment of breast cancer in postmenopausal women. Concurrent steroid replacement therapy (*dexamethasone*) is required.

Spironolactone acts as an antagonist to aldosterone and is a potassium-sparing diuretic (page 143).

Testing of the hypothalamic-pituitary-adrenal system

(1) *Corticotrophin* or *tetracosactrin*: a test of adrenal reserve that helps in the diagnosis of adrenal insufficiency and the distinction between pituitary and adrenal failure.

(2) *Metyrapone*: the fall in plasma hydrocortisone concentration results in

an increase in ACTH release. This stimulates the adrenal cortex causing an increase in urinary metabolites of adrenocorticoid steroids. Such a rise indicates that both the anterior pituitary and adrenal glands are functioning. Absence of a rise may be due to failure of either.

(3) *Dexamethasone* suppression test: this is used in the diagnosis of Cushing's syndrome. Decreased urinary steroid metabolite or plasma hydrocortisone concentration following *dexamethasone* demonstrates suppression of ACTH output by negative feedback and indicates pituitary-dependent steroid production. Failure to suppress indicates production of steroids by adrenal neoplasms or under control of ectopically produced ACTH.

Tests 2 and 3 are used less often today as it is possible to assay plasma ACTH concentration.

Drugs in diabetes mellitus

Insulin

Occurrence

Insulin is a hormone secreted by the β-cells of the islets of Langerhans in the pancreas. Islet cells comprise about 1–3% of pancreatic cell mass and number 100 000–2 500 000. Islets also contain α-cells that secrete glucagon, delta-cells that secrete somatostatin and PP cells that secrete pancreatic polypeptide.

Biosynthesis

Insulin is synthesized in the rough endoplasmic reticulum as preproinsulin, a large precursor molecule. This is almost immediately split to form proinsulin, which is stored in the Golgi apparatus in small granules. The connecting or C peptide is also stored in these granules. The insulin molecule consists of two chains of amino acids: A with 21 amino acids and B with 30 amino acids (*Figure 4.7*). The insulins of different species are remarkably similar with human and porcine insulins differing only at the B30 position and human and beef insulins differing at the A8, A10 and B30 positions. The granules of insulin and C peptide are transported via the microtubular system to the cell surface where they are extruded by reverse pinocytosis.

Release

A number of different agents, including glucose, amino acids and gut hormones, act as insulin secretagogues. Neural regulation mechanisms also

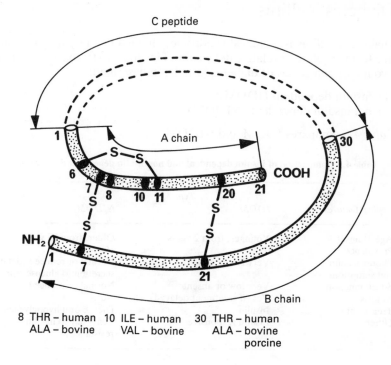

8 THR – human   10 ILE – human   30 THR – human
  ALA – bovine   VAL – bovine   ALA – bovine
                                         porcine

Figure 4.7 The structure of insulin

exist with sympathoadrenal activity inhibiting and parasympathetic activity stimulating insulin release. Insulin is secreted in anticipation of ingestion of food in the 'cephalic phase' of insulin secretion, which is thought to be mediated by the vagus nerve. After ingestion of food two further stages of release occur. The first is rapid and is due to release of preformed insulin from granules, the second involves the release of newly formed insulin. Insulin is secreted into the portal vein and is extensively metabolized in the liver and kidneys and has a short $t_{\frac{1}{2}}$ (4–5 min). This may be prolonged in patients with renal insufficiency.

Mechanism of action

Insulin binds to a specific receptor situated in the membranes of fat, muscle, liver and brain cells. The receptor–insulin complex is then internalized and acts to modify cellular synthetic processes. Receptor numbers are regulated by insulin concentrations and can be reduced in hyperinsulinaemic states as in obesity. Insulin facilitates entry of glucose into muscle and adipose tissue while inhibiting hepatic glycogenolysis and gluconeogenesis. In general it promotes anabolic and inhibits catabolic processes.

Diabetes mellitus

Diabetes mellitus is a clinical syndrome, characterized by hyperglycaemia due to an absolute or relative deficiency of insulin. On the basis of aetiology, two major categories of diabetes have been described:

(1) insulin dependent (IDDM);
(2) noninsulin dependent (NIDDM).

Table 4.9 compares IDDM and NIDDM.

Table 4.9 Comparison of insulin dependent and noninsulin dependent diabetes mellitus

	Type	
Typical features	*IDDM*	*NIDDM*
Age at onset	Younger, from 2 years	Older, from 25 years
Prevalence	0.2%	1%
Plasma insulin concentrations	Very low or absent	Normal or reduced (delayed secretion to glucose stimulus)
β-Cell function	Very low or absent	Normal or reduced
Ketosis	Yes (if treatment delayed)	No
Treatment	Insulin	Diet ± oral hypoglycaemics
Others	Insulin responsive	Tendency to insulin resistance

Treatment

Insulin treatment has remained the mainstay of treatment of IDDM patients over the last 60 years while patients with NIDDM may be treated with dietary control alone or in combination with oral hypoglycaemic agents or insulin. The role of insulin therapy in NIDDM is not clear and studies are in progress to assess this.

Insulin formulations

Insulin formulations can be classified in terms of duration of action (*Table 4.10*), source or purity. For clinical use, insulin has been formulated for short, intermediate or long duration of action. *Soluble insulin* consists of insulin in simple solution that is rapidly absorbed when injected. Insulin zinc suspensions can be prepared as insulin is relatively insoluble in a zinc acetate buffer. *Amorphous insulin zinc suspension* (semilente) has small particles and is absorbed more slowly than *soluble insulin*. *Crystalline insulin zinc suspension*, with larger particle size, is absorbed more slowly still and has a prolonged duration of action lasting up to 24 h. *Insulin zinc suspension* (lente) is a mixture of 30% amorphous and 70% crystalline insulin zinc suspensions.

Isophane insulin is another formulation from which insulin is released slowly. *Biphasic isophane insulin* is available containing both soluble and isophane insulins.

Table 4.10 Formulation and duration of action of insulins

Insulin	Other names	Time of onset (h)	Duration of effect
Soluble insulin	Soluble	$\frac{1}{2}$-1	Short
Isophane insulin		2	Intermediate
Insulin zinc suspension (amorphous)	Semilente	1–2	Intermediate
Insulin zinc suspension (mixed)	Lente	2–7	Intermediate
Insulin zinc suspension (crystalline)	Ultralente	4–7	Long

Purity and source of insulin

The duration of action of an insulin formulation can also vary with the purity and source of insulin. The highly purified insulins have a much shorter duration of action than the older insulins, which had a high content of antigenic 'contaminants' (proinsulin, pancreatic polypeptide, somatostatin). Similarly, the now popular human insulins have a more rapid onset and shorter duration of action than porcine or bovine insulins. These differences may be explained in part by the reduced formation of antibodies to the insulin.

Human insulin is produced by enzymatic modification of animal insulins or by using recombinant DNA techniques to induce *Escherichia coli* to synthesize human sequence insulin. Some patients have reported changes in the symptoms that warn of impending of hypoglycaemia after transfer to human insulin. This may be explained by the lower antibody binding to human insulin, which leads to rapid onset of action with rapid reduction in blood glucose concentration. In such instances, the release of the counter-regulatory hormones (for example, catecholamines) that produce the warning symptoms may not be sufficiently rapid. Controversy exists as to whether human insulins can cause sudden death by this mechanism. The vast majority of patients treated with human insulin experience no problems and those who do can be changed back to treatment with animal insulins.

Administration of insulin

Insulin is commonly administered as an sc injection using a disposable plastic syringe. However, increasing numbers of patients are now using pen devices instead of syringes. These devices resemble a fountain pen and contain cartridges of insulin. Visually handicapped patients may be helped by syringes that draw up a fixed dose or ones that give an audible click at each mark on the syringe, enabling them to do a 'click count' and vary the dose. Insulin may be delivered intraperitoneally in patients on continuous peritoneal dialysis. This method of insulin delivery is more physiological; insulin is absorbed into the portal circulation rather than the systemic circulation (as occurs with sc injection) and patients often find that control is easier. Continuous sc infusion of insulin by syringe pump is possible but a significant number of patients using such pumps develop ketoacidosis, electrolyte disturbances and infections.

Insulin regimens

In nondiabetic individuals, insulin is secreted at two rates, a basal rate in the fasting state and an accelerated rate in response to a meal. The aim of insulin replacement therapy is to mimic this as closely as possible. It is possible to achieve this using computerized glucose sensor/insulin delivery systems. However, these are used in research but are not yet suitable for routine use. A twice daily injection of a combination of short and intermediate acting insulins is commonly used. The intermediate acting component mimics the basal insulin secretion while the short acting component mimics the response to a meal. A near physiological pattern can also be achieved by using a single long acting injection with short acting insulin before each meal. The latter regimen is preferred by many younger patients as it permits a greater flexibility in life style.

In elderly patients and those whose compliance is suboptimal, a single daily injection of long acting insulin may be adequate to reduce or suppress symptoms.

Oral hypoglycaemic agents

The mainstay of treatment of NIDDM is weight reduction, diet and exercise. All NIDDM patients should have an adequate trial of these methods before drug treatment is considered. An appreciable proportion of NIDDM patients fail to achieve adequate control by these methods and oral hypoglycaemic agents are then indicated.

Sulphonylureas

These drugs require the presence of functioning β-cells in the pancreas for their action. They act in part by stimulating the release of insulin in response to a glucose load. This action on the β-cell may involve closure of membrane ATP-dependent K^+-channels, depolarization and consequential insulin release. They also enhance the effect of insulin on the liver and promote peripheral glucose utilization by increasing the number of insulin receptors. The net result is an improvement in glucose tolerance. Sulphonylurea drugs are indicated in patients at or near ideal body weight when diet and weight reduction alone are insufficient to produce satisfactory control of blood glucose. They are best avoided in overweight patients because sulphonylureas encourage weight gain. Data on the safety of sulphonylurea drugs in pregnancy are not sufficient and they are best avoided in females in the reproductive years.

The pharmacokinetic profiles of some sulphonylurea drugs are shown in *Table 4.11*.

These properties must be considered when selecting a drug for an individual patient. In the presence of impaired renal function, or if such impairment is likely as in the elderly, drugs with a long $t_{\frac{1}{2}}$ (*chlorpropramide*) and drugs excreted mainly by renal mechanisms (*glibenclamide*) are best avoided. Drugs excreted by hepatic pathways (**tolbutamide,** *gliclazide*) are less likely to cause dose related hypoglycaemia in these patients.

Table 4.11 Sulphonylurea oral hypoglycaemic agents

Drug	$t_{\frac{1}{2}}$ (h)	Dosage frequency per day	Effective dosage range (mg/day)
Tolbutamide	4	2	500–2000
Chlorpropamide	35–40	1	100–500
Glibenclamide	12	1–2	2.5–20

The principal adverse effect is hypoglycaemia. (Fatal hypoglycaemic episodes have occurred in elderly patients taking *chlorpropramide* or *glibenclamide*.) All patients must be advised about this danger and carry sugar or sweets to take when a warning is felt. Other adverse effects (gastrointestinal irritation, nausea, skin rashes, rarely blood dyscrasias and inappropriate diuretic hormone secretion) may occur. Some patients taking *chlorpropamide* may experience flushing with ingestion of alcohol due to a disulfiram-like interference with metabolism (page 249).

Biguanides

The action of the biguanide, *metformin*, requires the presence of functioning pancreatic tissue. It acts by increasing peripheral glucose utilization. As it does not stimulate endogenous insulin secretion it does not cause hypoglycaemia. *Metformin* is used mainly in the management of obese NIDDM patients. Lactic acidosis may occur in patients with impaired renal function and cardiac failure. *Metformin* is therefore best avoided in elderly patients in whom both renal impairment and cardiac failure are common.

Diabetogenic hormones and drugs

(1) Glucagon, a polypeptide secreted by the α-cells of the islets of Langerhans, is a very potent hormone that raises blood glucose concentration and increases free fatty acid release from adipocytes.
(2) GH promotes growth in the immature animal by laying down protein but in the adult is diabetogenic.
(3) Glucocorticoids have many actions that are opposite to those of insulin and when given at unphysiologically high doses are diabetogenic.
(4) Adrenaline inhibits insulin release (via α-adrenoceptors) and promotes glycogenolysis (via β-adrenoceptors).

Other diabetogenic agents are summarized in *Table 4.12.*

Table 4.12 Pharmacological agents that can produce or unmask diabetes

Agent	Mechanism of action
Antagonists at β-adrenoceptors	Inhibit insulin secretion
Thiazide diuretics, *diazoxide*, **phenytoin**	Inhibit insulin secretion
Combined oral contraceptive steroids	Gluconeogenesis, lipolysis (or tissue resistance to insulin)

Hypoglycaemia

Normal fasting blood glucose concentrations average 3.3–5.6 mmol/l; less than 2.6 mmol/l is termed hypoglycaemia. The signs and symptoms of hypoglycaemia fall into the following two groups:

(1) those due to adrenaline release. These include hunger, pallor, sweating, apprehension and tachycardia. The adrenaline response is sometimes sufficient to raise blood glucose concentration by mobilization of liver glycogen (mediated by β-adrenoceptors, *see above*).
(2) those due to neuroglycopenia. If the adrenaline response is insufficient then the signs and symptoms due to neuroglycopenia occur and include mental confusion, incoherent speech, retrograde amnesia and coma.

The main causes of hypoglycaemia are insulin administration and sulphonylurea drugs. Precipitating factors may be the omission of a meal or unaccustomed exercise.

Treatment

Glucose

When the patient recognizes the symptoms of hypoglycaemia he should swallow some sugar. If consciousness is lost glucose can be given iv.

Glucagon

Glucagon is given by injection and increases the output of glucose from the liver. The response is proportional to the glycogen reserve of the liver.

Diazoxide

Diazoxide is related to the thiazide diuretics (page 142). It is given orally and reserved for treating the chronic hypoglycaemia of excess insulin secretion (tumour – insulinoma). It may cause an increase in circulating catecholamine concentration, which indirectly alters glucose concentration or it may directly block insulin release from the β-cells.

Posterior pituitary hormones

Vasopressin

Synthesis, release and actions

Antidiuretic hormone (ADH, vasopressin) is a cyclic nonapeptide synthesized in the hypothalamus. Bound to neurophysin, it is transported to the posterior pituitary gland in the axons running between the two areas. The release of ADH into the circulation from the nerve terminals is Ca^{2+}-dependent and occurs in response to a rise in plasma osmotic pressure (including that due to diuretic agents) or haemorrhage. Release is also stimulated by nicotine and **morphine** and perhaps by *chlorpropamide* (alternatively this may sensitize the kidney to ADH) and is inhibited by ethanol.

The main physiological action of ADH is to increase the water permeability of the tubule membranes leading to reabsorption of water, unaccompanied by ions, in the collecting ducts of the kidney tubules to reduce the osmotic pressure of the plasma. In most circumstances this results in the production of a small volume of concentrated urine. The mechanism involves agonist action of ADH at a membrane V_2 vasopressin receptor, which produces activation of adenylate cyclase, generation of cAMP and an increase in the number of water channels.

Diabetes insipidus is characterized by the passage of large volumes of dilute urine (polyuria) with consequential thirst and water drinking (polydipsia). It results from either an absence of ADH release (pituitary diabetes insipidus) or a lack of responsiveness of the kidney tubule membranes to ADH (nephrogenic diabetes insipidus). Lithium salts may greatly reduce the sensitivity of the tubule to vasopressin leading to such adverse effects.

In much higher concentrations, vasopressin causes constriction of blood vessels, especially capillaries and venules, by agonist action at the V_1 vasopressin receptor, which promotes phosphatidylinositol breakdown and calcium mobilization.

Uses

As an antidiuretic agent

Diabetes insipidus of pituitary origin is treated with analogues of synthetic vasopressin (arginine vasopressin), *lypressin* (lysine vasopressin, lysine replacing arginine) or *desmopressin*. These latter two are longer acting than vasopressin, particularly *desmopressin*, which is also free of vasoconstrictor effects (it is a selective agonist at V_2 vasopressin receptors).

To prevent splitting of the peptide bonds in the stomach the compounds are administered by im, iv, sc or intranasal routes.

As a vasoconstrictor agent

Oesophagaeal varices. Vasopressin and terlipressin are given by iv infusion or injection in the control of the bleeding from oesophageal varicose veins that occurs in portal hypertension due to hepatic scarring, usually due to cirrhosis.

Local anaesthesia. Felypressin, an analogue that is a selective agonist at V_1 vasopressin receptors and has little or no antidiuretic action, is used to prolong the duration of local anaesthesia (page 121).

Oxytocin

Oxytocin, another hypothalamic nonapeptide, acts as an agonist at oxytocin (OT) receptors selectively to increase the frequency and duration of bursts of action potentials, leading to contraction of uterine smooth muscle and the myoepithelial cells of the mammary glands to produce milk ejection. High sensitivity of the two tissues to oxytocin is only seen in the appropriate hormonal environment, namely in late pregnancy (uterine action) or post partum (mammary action). This may reflect an increase in the numbers of myometrial OT receptors.

Uses

Beginning of labour

Oxytocin is used to augment labour or, along with rupture of the amniotic membranes, to induce labour at or near term by direct stimulation of phasic uterine contractions. Excessive response of the uterus to *oxytocin* consists of a maintained spasm which can result in fetal hypoxia, due to restriction of placental blood flow, or rupture of the uterus, particularly if the patient has had a previous Caesarean section. This narrow therapeutic range, as well as the short $t_{\frac{1}{2}}$ due to rapid metabolism, necessitates *oxytocin* administration by iv infusion (page 341) with dose rate titrated to uterine response. *Oxytocin* can interact with V_2 vasopressin receptors in the kidney (page 189) and so at high infusion dose rates *oxytocin* can produce water retention.

End of labour

The maintained spasm of the uterus produced by *oxytocin* is the basis of the use of the drug, by single bolus iv or im administration, after delivery for the prophylaxis of postpartum haemorrhage. More commonly *ergometrine* (with or without *oxytocin*) is used. This alkaloid selectively contracts uterine smooth muscle although some vasoconstriction and, therefore, rise in BP may be observed. *Ergometrine* has a longer duration of action than *oxytocin*.

Angiotensin

Occurrence, biosynthesis and metabolism

Angiotensin (angiotensin II) is an octapeptide formed by the action of the kidney enzyme, renin, on an inactive plasma α_2-globulin, angiotensinogen (*Figure 4.8*). A relatively inert intermediate, the decapeptide angiotensin I is formed initially. This is subsequently converted to angiotensin II by angiotensin converting enzyme (ACE). This enzyme, which is bound to endothelial cells and located mainly in the lungs, is identical to one of the two enzymes responsible for the breakdown of bradykinin.

Angiotensin II is rapidly destroyed (plasma $t_{\frac{1}{2}} = 1$–2 min) by angiotensinases (mainly aminopeptidases) to give angiotensin III and various inactive peptides.

Actions of angiotensin

Angiotensin II is the most potent pressor agent known (the equieffective molar dose ratio, angiotensin:NA is 1:40) causing arteriolar constriction and a rise in diastolic and systolic BP. This action is mainly exerted directly on the vessels via angiotensin receptors but facilitation of NA release from noradrenergic nerves may contribute.

Angiotensin also contracts the smooth muscle of the intestine, bronchioles and uterus and stimulates the adrenal medulla (to release catecholamines), parasympathetic and sympathetic ganglia.

Increased synthesis and release of aldosterone may be due to angiotensin III acting through specific receptors in the adrenal cortex.

Role in physiology and pathophysiology

The renin-angiotensin system is important in the maintenance of cardiovascular homeostasis and the control of electrolyte balance (page 178). It

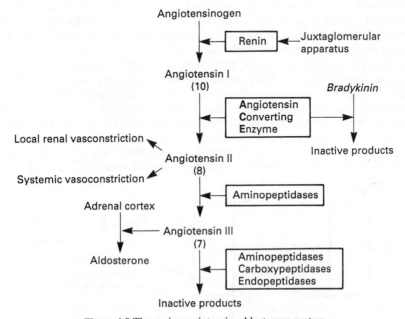

Figure 4.8 The renin–angiotensin–aldosterone system

may also play a modulatory role in the control of small blood vessel tone by virtue of its facilitatory effects on sympathetic nerve activity. A high renin concentration and hence high angiotensin concentration is a common finding in malignant (but not benign) hypertension (page 380).

Pharmacological and therapeutic exploitation

ACE inhibitors (**captopril** and *enalapril*) are useful in the treatment of hypertension (page 383) when antagonists at β-adrenoceptors and thiazide diuretics have failed or are contraindicated.

There are no antagonists at angiotensin receptors available for clinical use.

Local hormones

Histamine

Occurrence, biosynthesis and metabolism

Histamine, 2-(4-imidazolyl) ethylamine, is formed from the amino acid *l*-histidine by the action of histidine decarboxylase. It is present in many mammalian tissues with especially high concentrations in lung, skin and intestine. Most is stored in the granules of tissue mast cells (basophils in blood) bound electrostatically to the protein carboxyl groups of protein to form a heparin/protein complex (*Figure 4.9*).

The carboxyl groups binding the histamine are relatively weak. The much stronger acidic groups of the heparin molecule are fully neutralized by the basic groups of the protein. The bound form of histamine is inactive. This arrangement is significant for the mechanism of histamine release described below. Some histamine is located not in mast cells but in neurones in the CNS and in cells of the epidermis, gastric mucosa and growing or regenerating tissues where it turns over rapidly. More than 90% of an exogenous histamine load is metabolized either by deamination (enzyme: diamine

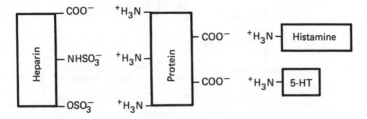

Figure 4.9 The granular storage of histamine in mast cells

oxidase, 'histaminase'; product: imidazolylacetic acid) or by a combination of N-methylation and deamination (enzymes: imidazole-N-methyltransferase and MAO; product: methylimidazolylacetic acid).

Release of histamine

The antigen/antibody reaction of anaphylaxis releases histamine from tissue stores (mast cells) as do trauma and certain compounds (*Table 4.13*).

Table 4.13 Agents that release histamine from mast cells

Type of activator	Examples
Tissue damage	Mechanical, chemical, heat
Complex macromolecules	Snake and wasp venoms Bacterial toxins
High MW polymers	*Dextran*
Detergents and surface active agents	Bile salts
Basic drugs	**Atropine** **Morphine** **Tubocurarine** Antagonists at H_1 receptors

The underlying principle of histamine release is that the heparin/protein complex acts as a weak cation exchange resin. Exposure of the granules to a cation containing medium results in an instantaneous exchange of histamine with the cation. Basic drugs and polypeptides with many basic groups displace the similarly basic histamine from its binding sites. Detergents, proteolytic enzymes and the antigen/antibody reaction of anaphylaxis cause cell disruption, with expulsion of granules into the extracellular cation-containing medium (degranulation), where instantaneous amine release by cation exchange occurs. Since the predominant extracellular cation is Na^+, the mechanism can be represented as in *Figure 4.10*.

Anaphylaxis develops by the following stages:

(1) exposure of animal or man to a foreign macromolecule (antigen) results in the formation of specific antibodies by B-lymphocytes;
(2) circulating antibodies are taken up and firmly bound on the surface of tissue cells;
(3) re-exposure to antigen results in combination with tissue-bound antibody and tissue damage;
(4) histamine (and other cell constituents) are released 'explosively': other mediators implicated in anaphylaxis include plasma kinins, 5-hydroxytryptamine (5-HT), prostaglandins (PGs) and leukotrienes (LTs).

Actions of histamine

In the cardiovascular system histamine dilates small arteries, capillaries and venules. Thus the BP falls but the heart rate increases due to reflex baroreceptor nerve stimulation (and a direct stimulant action of histamine on H_2

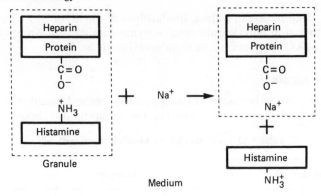

Figure 4.10 The cation exchange mechanism of mast cell degranulation

receptors in the heart, *Table 4.14*). Histamine increases the permeability of the endothelial lining of postcapillary venules to plasma protein. Cerebral vessels are especially sensitive to the dilator action of histamine. It also produces increased cerebrospinal fluid pressure and 'histamine headaches'.

Lewis's triple response consists of:

(1) a red mark due to capillary dilatation at injury site;
(2) a pink flare that is diffuse and surrounds the injury site due to arteriolar dilatation from an axon reflex triggered by sensory nerve stimulation;
(3) a wheal (a raised oedematous area close to the injury site), which is due to increased permeability of microcirculation to protein.

The response arises from injurious stimuli or from a small quantity of histamine injected intradermally.

Histamine stimulates the smooth muscle of intestine and bronchioles directly. It is a powerful stimulant of gastric secretion (mainly direct but also facilitates the secretogogue action of the vagus), both parietal and peptic gland cells are stimulated. In high doses, histamine stimulates the adrenal medulla and autonomic ganglia causing release of catecholamines. Histamine also stimulates sensory neurones to give itching and sometimes pain.

Role in physiology and pathophysiology

Histamine plays a role in the normal regulation of gastric secretion, in the body's protective mechanism at an injury site (triple response, acute inflammation) and as a mediator in allergic and anaphylactic conditions.

Pharmacological and therapeutic exploitation

Histamine itself has no therapeutic value. Compounds that are antagonists at histamine receptors or prevent the release of histamine are used therapeutically.

Histamine receptor antagonists

These selectively and competitively antagonize histamine whether it is injected or endogenously released. They can be divided into two groups as can histamine receptors (*Table 4.14*).

Table 4.14 Histamine receptors

H_1 receptors	H_2 receptors
Effects mediated	
Contraction of smooth muscle of:	Stimulation of gastric secretion
intestine	Stimulation of the heart
bronchioles	Inhibition of antigenic release of histamine from basophils
Most of depressor effects on BP	
Increased capillary permeability	
Stimulation of sensory neurones	
Selective competitive antagonist	
Chlorpheniramine	**Cimetidine**

Antagonists at H_1 receptors

Competitive antagonists at H_1 receptors are stable lipid soluble amines having in common the ethylamine chain of histamine. The group includes older (**chlorpheniramine,** *promethazine*) and newer drugs (*terfenadine*). Most drugs from both groups are absorbed rapidly after oral administration. All are metabolized by liver MFO enzymes and most have a duration of action of 4–6 h.

The antagonists at H_1 receptors block the action of histamine by reversible competitive antagonism at the H_1 receptor site (*Table 4.14*), however they also have actions that are not related to antagonism at H_1 receptors. Some of these other important actions are outlined in *Table 4.15*.

The main use of antagonists at H_1 receptors is the relief of histamine-mediated effects in allergic (seasonal rhinitis ['hayfever'], insect bites and stings) and anaphylactic reactions but they are largely ineffective in asthma, arthritic inflammation and systemic anaphylaxis where other local hormones are involved. Their other actions (*Table 4.15*) make them useful in motion sickness and as mild hypnotics (*promethazine*). Side-effects are frequent but tend to be mild. They include sedation, anorexia, nausea and vomiting, dizziness, blurred vision and dry mouth. Most of these effects are thought to be due to action in the CNS; some can be explained by antagonism at muscarinic cholinoceptors. The sedation may be such that the ability of users to drive or operate machinery is impaired. *Terfenadine* causes less sedation than the other antagonists at H_1 receptors and does not cause psychomotor disturbances because blood brain barrier penetration is slight.

Antagonists at H_2 histamine receptors

Competitive antagonists at H_2 receptors include **cimetidine** and *ranitidine*. Unlike the antagonists at H_1 receptors these are imidazole derivatives. They

Table 4.15 Other actions of some H_1 receptor antagonists

	Sedation	Antiemesis	Antagonism at muscarinic cholinoceptors
Promethazine	++++	+++	++
Chlorpheniramine	++	0	0
Terfenadine	0	0	0

++++ = strong; + = weak; 0 = no activity

inhibit cardiac stimulation evoked by histamine, and gastric acid secretion evoked by histamine, gastrin, physiological stimuli and agonists at muscarinic cholinoceptors. The latter three stimuli have histamine release as a final common pathway. **Cimetidine** and *ranitidine* are inhibitors of gastric secretion for use in the treatment of gastric and duodenal ulcer (page 371).

Cimetidine (but not *ranitidine*) binds to androgen receptors, occasionally causes gynaecomastia (page 161), and may potentiate such drugs as **phenytoin** and **warfarin** due to inhibition of cytochrome P_{450}.

Suppression of release

Sodium cromoglycate [cromolyn sodium] selectively suppresses the release of chemical mediators (histamine, LTs) arising from antigen/antibody reactions or degranulating agents. The precise mode of action is unknown but it may stabilize the mast cell membrane so that steps between antigen/antibody union and the release of chemical mediators are prevented. It does not affect the course of the response to mediator already released if given after the antigen/antibody interaction and has no direct anti-inflammatory activity.

Sodium cromoglycate is a very effective drug in allergic rhinitis and allergic conjunctivitis ('hay fever') and is moderately effective in food allergies in children and asthma. It is poorly absorbed from the gut and is administered by inhalation as an aerosol into the nose and respiratory tract or is applied topically, for example, to the conjunctiva in cases of allergic conjunctivitis.

5-Hydroxytryptamine

Occurrence, biosynthesis and metabolism

5-HT (serotonin) is present in many mammalian tissues with highest concentrations in the enterochromaffin cells of the gastrointestinal tract. 5-HT is complexed with heparin and protein in rodent mast cells. Elsewhere 5-HT is stored in association with ATP in intracellular storage particles within intestinal chromaffin cells, platelets and the specific 5-HT-containing (serotonergic) neurones of the brain (page 213).

The amino acid tryptophan is hydroxylated by tryptophan-5-hydroxylase to 5-hydroxytryptophan, which is then decarboxylated to 5-HT by aromatic amino acid decarboxylase.

The degradation of 5-HT occurs mainly in the liver where it is converted to 5-hydroxyindole acetaldehyde by MAO. This aldehyde is then rapidly converted to the excretory product 5-hydroxyindole acetic acid by aldehyde dehydrogenase.

Actions of 5-hydroxytryptamine

5-HT has complex cardiovascular actions. In general it acts directly to constrict arteries, which results in increased peripheral resistance.

5-HT stimulates intestinal and bronchial smooth muscle, the adrenal medulla and ganglia of the autonomic nervous system. It is a potent stimulant of sensory nerve endings and gives pain when applied to an exposed blister base. It is proaggregatory on platelets.

Recent nomenclature identifies at least three receptors for 5-HT and these have been designated 5-HT_1, 5-HT_2 and 5-HT_3. Most peripheral 5-HT receptors (in platelets and smooth muscle) appear to be of the 5-HT_2 type whereas 5-HT_1, 5-HT_2 and 5-HT_3 receptor types have been identified in the brain.

Role in physiology and pathophysiology

The selective localization of 5-HT in platelets and its vasoconstrictor properties suggest a role in blood clotting. 5-HT is a CNS neurotransmitter (page 213). A tumour of enterochromaffin or related cells (carcinoid) may develop in the gastrointestinal or respiratory tracts that secretes excessive quantities of 5-HT (in addition to polypeptides and PGs).

Pharmacological and therapeutic exploitation

There are no selective antagonists at 5-HT_1 or 5-HT_3 receptors available for clinical use.

Antagonists at 5-HT_2 receptors

Pizotifen is a potent antagonist at 5HT_2 receptors. It is an orally active, effective prophylactic in migraine (page 403). Its mechanism of action may involve inhibition of the local inflammatory response evoked by 5-HT.

Pizotifen also controls the increased intestinal motility but not the flushing (may be due to kinins or PGs) associated with carcinoid tumour. It also possesses antagonist activity at muscarinic cholinoceptors and is sedative. These adverse effects are frequent, as are increased appetite and weight gain.

Lysergic acid diethylamide (LSD) is an antagonist at 5-HT_2 and α-adrenoceptors but, like other ergot alkaloids, has partial agonist properties at central dopamine and 5-HT_1 receptors. These agonist actions may be relevant to its hallucinogenic properties (page 239).

Phenoxybenzamine and **phentolamine** are potent but not specific antagonists at 5-HT_2 receptors (page 111).

Eicosanoids

The term eicosanoid is used to describe a vast array of substances that includes the PGs (including prostacyclin), thromboxanes and the LTs since they are all derived from the same eicosanoic (eicosa = 20 carbon; enoic = containing double bonds) acid precursors.

Eicosanoid biosynthesis

The substrates for eicosanoid biosynthesis are generated mainly by the action of phospholipase A_2 on the phospholipid fraction of the cell (*Figure 4.11*). Some of the anti-inflammatory actions of glucocorticoids can be explained by their ability to induce the production of a group of proteins called lipocortins that are inhibitors of phospholipase A_2.

Released PG precursor (principally arachidonic acid) is acted upon by an enzyme (cyclo-oxygenase) resulting in the formation of the PG endoperoxides. Nonsteroidal anti-inflammatory drugs (**aspirin,** *indomethacin*) act by inhibiting cyclo-oxygenase (page 206).

The endoperoxides are then converted to one or other of the relatively stable PGs. A number of other derivatives is also formed from the endoperoxides, including prostacyclin and thromboxane A_2.

Arachidonic acid also acts as precursor for another group of biologically active substances, the LTs and certain hydroperoxide derivatives. The enzyme responsible for this conversion is 5-lipoxygenase (*Figure 4.11*).

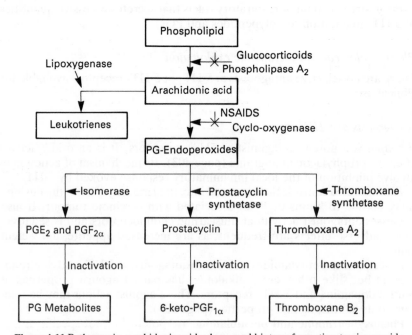

Figure 4.11 Pathways in arachidonic acid release and biotransformation to eicosanoids

The prostaglandins

The term PG is the generic name for a family of closely related cyclic, oxygenated, 20-carbon unsaturated fatty acids. The hypothetical basic 20-carbon skeleton of the PGs has been given the name 'prostanoic acid'. On the basis of their structures the PGs have been separated into nine groups, named A–I. All have in common a double bond at the 13,14 position and an OH— group at C_{15} (except PGG). In naming them the number of unsaturated carbon bonds is denoted by a subscript numeral and the subscript α or β denotes the orientation of an OH— group in position 9 below or above the molecular plane (*Figure 4.12*).

The PGs are synthesized and released by virtually every tissue in the body. Since there is no evidence for storage of PGs (except in the seminal fluid) the rate of release reflects that of biosynthesis. A wide variety of stimuli (trauma, allergies, inflammatory conditions) is capable of releasing PGs. Several of the PGs are very rapidly metabolized in the kidneys, lungs and liver.

Actions of prostaglandins

PGs have many and varied pharmacological actions that are mediated by several receptors. There are five receptors more or less selective for the natural prostanoids PGD_2, PGE_2, $PGF_{2\alpha}$, PGI_2 and TxA_2 named DP, EP, FP, IP and TP respectively. *Table 4.16* summarizes the effects of the E and F PGs and the receptors mediating these effects.

Table 4.16 Some effects of PGs typified by PGE_2 and $PGF_{2\alpha}$

	PGE_2 (receptor)	*$PGF_{2\alpha}$ (receptor)*
Blood vessels	Dilated (EP, DP)	Constricted (TP)
Capillary permeability	Increased (EP, DP)	Little effect
Gastric secretion	Decreased (EP)	Little effect
Bronchiolar smooth muscle	Relaxed (EP)	Contracted (FP, TP)
Uterine smooth muscle	Contracted* (FP)	Contracted (FP)
Sensory nerve fibres	Sensitized*	?

* Generalization – the responses produced are often complex.

The actions of PGs are usually exerted close to their site of release (local hormone action).

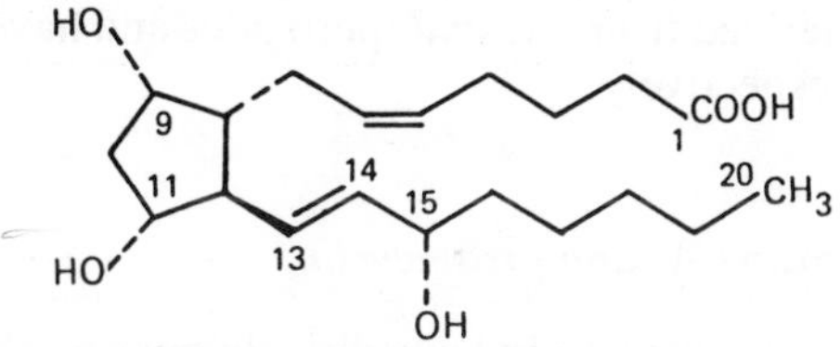

Figure 4.12 Prostaglandin $F_{2\alpha}$

Role in physiology and pathophysiology

The PGs are believed to be involved in many physiological processes. In female reproductive physiology they have been implicated in uterine and Fallopian tube contractility, labour (at term) and maintaining the patency of the fetal ductus arteriosus. There is good evidence that PGs play a role in gastric mucus secretion and modulation of renal blood flow.

Excessive production of PGs has been implicated in many pathological processes, in particular the acute inflammatory response (page 205), fever (page 241) and various female reproductive disorders (spasmodic dysmenorrhoea, habitual abortion and premature labour).

Pharmacological and therapeutic exploitation

Clinical application is based on either mimicking physiological effects by exogenous PGs or, in pathological situations, preventing their synthesis.

The uterine smooth muscle stimulating properties of PGE_2 and $PGF_{2\alpha}$ form the basis of their use clinically. Both PGE_2 (*dinoprostone*) and $PGF_{2\alpha}$ (*dinoprost*) are useful for induction of labour and second trimester pregnancy termination. Adverse effects are frequent but mild and include nausea, vomiting, diarrhoea, flushing, shivering, headache and dizziness and, when given iv, local tissue irritation and erythema, due to actions at other E-type and F-type receptors. Local application to the uterus helps to reduce these adverse effects. Another agent useful for the induction of labour (but not abortion) is *oxytocin*. Combinations of PGs and *oxytocin* have been used successfully for induction of labour and abortion with a reduction in the incidence of adverse effects due to the PG (a result of the lower dose now required).

PGE_1 (*alprostadil*) is used to maintain patency of the ductus arteriosus in neonates with congenital heart defects.

Misoprostol, a synthetic analogue of PGE_1, is relatively selective for the EP receptors that mediate decreased gastric secretion and is useful to promote healing of gastric and duodenal ulcers.

Thromboxane A_2 and prostacyclin

Occurrence, biosynthesis and metabolism

Thromboxane A_2 (TxA_2, synthesized predominantly by platelets) and prostacyclin (PGI_2, synthesized predominantly by heart, vascular endothelium and stomach) are derived from the endoperoxides and have short half-lives of 30 s and 2 min respectively.

Actions of thromboxane A_2 and prostacyclin

Thromboxane A_2 and prostacyclin have directly opposing pharmacological actions in many systems as shown in *Table 4.17*.

Table 4.17 Main actions of prostacyclin and thromboxane A_2

Prostacyclin (receptor)	Thromboxane A_2 (receptor)
Vasodilatation (IP)	Vasoconstriction (TP)
Inhibition of platelet aggregation (IP)	Platelet aggregation (TP)
Bronchodilatation (EP)	Bronchoconstriction (TP)
Cytoprotective (vascular endothelium)	Cytolysis

Role in physiology and pathophysiology

Generation of prostacyclin by vessel walls could be the biochemical mechanism underlying their unique ability to resist platelet adhesion. A balance between the formation of antiaggregatory vasodilator substances (prostacyclin) and proaggregatory vasoconstrictor substances (thromboxane A_2) could contribute to the maintenance of the integrity of vascular endothelium. An alteration of this balance may explain the mechanism of formation of intra-arterial thrombi in certain pathophysiological conditions.

Pharmacological and therapeutic exploitation

Synthetic prostacyclin (*epoprostenol*) is sometimes used during surgical procedures involving extracorporeal circulation of the blood to prevent platelet aggregation. There are no drugs available for clinical use that selectively modify the synthesis, actions or metabolism of prostacyclin or thromboxane A_2 (but *see* page 149).

Leukotrienes

Occurrence, biosynthesis and metabolism

Six groups of LTs have currently been identified and designated LTA–LTF. They can be synthesized from arachidonic acid by 5-lipoxygenase in a variety of tissues, in particular lung tissue and white blood cells.

Actions of leukotrienes

The LTs possess a wide variety of pharmacological actions but LTB_4 is a particularly potent chemotactic and chemokinetic agent on polymorphonuclear leucocytes. All LTs contract to varying degrees smooth muscle from the gut, bronchioles and various vascular beds, cause oedema formation and potentiate other inflammatory mediators.

Role in physiology and pathophysiology

The LTs are believed to be intimately involved in various inflammatory and allergic disorders, notably bronchial asthma, when LTC_4 and LTD_4 are the principal LTs generated during tissue anaphylaxis.

Exploitation

Compounds that selectively modify the synthesis, actions or metabolism of LTs are not clinically available.

The kinins

Occurrence, biosynthesis and metabolism

The kinins are bradykinin (a nonapeptide), kallidin (lysyl-bradykinin, a decapeptide) and related vasodilator peptides. Bradykinin and kallidin are formed from the same circulating α_2 globulins (kininogens/kallidinogens) by the action of specific proteolytic enzymes, kallidinogenases (kallikreins). Kallidinogenases are found in many organs and in urine, saliva, lymph, pancreatic secretions, blood, sweat and tears. Plasma kallidinogenase exists in the form of an inactive precursor (prekallidinogenase) but when plasma equilibrium is disturbed (change in pH, temperature or contact with water insoluble materials), various activators (including Factor XII, the Hageman factor of blood clotting) convert it to its active form, with subsequent formation of kinins. *Aprotinin* is an inhibitor of kallidinogenase, although not very specific. Its medical application rests on its ability also to inhibit plasmin.

Kinins are rapidly destroyed in blood ($t_\frac{1}{2}$ less than 1 min) by kininases, which remove one (carboxypeptidase-N) or two (kininase II or ACE, *see* page 191) amino acids from both bradykinin and kallidin.

Actions of kinins

The actions of bradykinin, which are mediated through interaction with at least two receptors, are typical of the vasodilator kinins.

On the cardiovascular system it is potent, both as a relaxant of vascular smooth muscle (causing a fall in systemic BP) and as a promoter of increased capillary permeability.

Bradykinin contracts the smooth muscle of the intestine and bronchioles, stimulates the release of transmitters via actions at the adrenal medulla and sympathetic ganglia and stimulates sensory nerve endings as demonstrated by the pain when applied to an exposed blister base.

Role in physiology and pathophysiology

Kinins have been implicated in many physiological functions including functional and reactive hyperaemia, regulation of tissue blood flow, BP control and neonatal circulatory changes.

They may be involved in various pathological states (shock, allergy, inflammation, pancreatitis) and the *pizotifen*-resistant flushing and bronchoconstriction seen with carcinoid tumour.

Pharmacological and therapeutic exploitation

No selective antagonist of bradykinin is available for clinical use.

Cytokines

Occurrence, biosynthesis and metabolism

Cytokines are a heterogeneous group of proteins, distinct from immunoglobulins, released by cells of the immune system and elsewhere (for example, endothelium). Alternative terms reflect the cell source (lymphokines from lymphocytes, monokines from monocytes). Individual cytokines have, or used to have, a descriptive name, sometimes several, based on the biological activity of interest (for example, tumour necrosis factor, TNF). The large number of descriptive names and related acronyms is now being reduced by the systematic allocation of interleukin (IL) numbers as the nature of each cytokine is established by its physicochemical, rather than its biological, properties.

Cytokines contain between 100 and 200 amino acids. They can be variably glycosylated and can form oligomers, hence conflicting reports on their molecular size. Production, controlled primarily at the level of transcription, is increased, usually in response to signals from the cell surface.

Internalization of cytokine/receptor complexes, enzymatic degradation, endogenous inhibitors, dilution in body fluids and excretion (for example, urine) contribute to a short $t_\frac{1}{2}$ for most cytokines.

Actions of cytokines

Cytokines bind to specific surface receptors. Most of their biological effects are localized near their site of release and confined to cells of the immune system. In general terms, these actions are concerned with;

(1) modulation of leucocyte margination and emigration (page 204);
(2) coordination of responses (including antibody formation and phagocytosis) from different kinds of leucocytes to infection and inflammatory stimuli;
(3) production and maturation of blood cells (haematopoiesis).

A few cytokines also appear to act as hormones affecting cells outside the immune system. For example, the monokine, interleukin-1 (IL-1), produces effects on the brain (fever), liver (synthesis of acute phase proteins) and skeletal muscle (proteolysis).

Role in physiology and pathophysiology

The immunomodulatory, cytotoxic, haematopoietic and other effects of cytokines are important in the maintenance of health, the defence against infection and the development of inflammation.

Pharmacological and therapeutic exploitation

Interferon-α (IFN-α), produced by recombinant DNA technology, has some antitumour effect in certain lymphomas and solid tumours. IFN-α has numerous biological effects. Adverse reactions include influenza-like symptoms, depression and lethargy.

There are no drugs available for clinical use that selectively antagonize cytokines. Some cytokine effects (for example, fever) are mediated indirectly by PGs and are blocked by NSAIDs (page 241).

Inflammation

Inflammation is an active defensive response from the body to injury of any kind. The inflammatory stimuli include chemical or physical trauma, infestation with helminths, infection with protozoa, fungi, bacteria, rickettsia or viruses and antigen/antibody interaction. In acute inflammation, a succession of changes takes place over a short period (minutes to days) which ends either by return of tissue to normal or by conversion to chronic inflammation. Chronic inflammation may last months or years and is characterized by periods of regression and repair, which may be punctuated by further acute inflammatory changes.

The inflammatory response

General characteristics

In the skin an inflammatory stimulus results in the area becoming warm and red due to increased blood flow, swollen due to leakage of plasma protein followed by salt and water into the interstitial space as a result of increased protein permeability of microcirculatory vessel walls and painful due to stimulation of sensory pain fibres. This is similar to Lewis's triple response (page 194). Loss of function may consequently occur. Similar inflammatory processes occur at all other sites.

Emigration of leucocytes and phagocytosis

In the early stages of inflammation, polymorphonuclear leucocytes (polymorphs) aggregate along the inner margins of vessel (mainly venule) walls (margination), then pass through into the interstitial space (emigration). At an inflamed site, polymorphs come within the chemotactic (chemical attractive) orbit of living or dead bacteria, or tissue or plasma factors (kinins, eicosanoids). Polymorphs move up the concentration gradient of the chemotactic stimulus and if not killed in the process ingest the invading organisms or tissue debris (phagocytosis).

Repair and regeneration

When an inflammatory lesion subsides, vasodilatation diminishes and oedema disappears due to exuded fluid being drained into lymphatics. Macrophages (monocytes and histiocytes) ingest dead polymorphs, bacteria and tissue debris. When loss or destruction of tissues has occurred, new capillaries and fibroblasts grow into previously inflamed tissues. Collagen is laid down (fibrosis) and the tissue becomes less vascular (granulation). Epithelium gradually extends over this granulation tissue. Blood vessels, nerves and lymphatics grow into the repair tissue, more collagen is formed and fibres already laid down by fibroblasts shorten, drawing the edges of the wound together and forming a scar (cicatrix).

Chemical mediators

The pattern of the response to various inflammatory stimuli is similar. This similarity indicates that certain chemicals commonly mediate the response. The following criteria should be satisfied by a putative endogenous chemical mediator of inflammation.

(1) It should be demonstrably present during the inflammatory reaction. The following have been demonstrated:
    (a) release of histamine from mast cells and 5-HT from platelets;
    (b) release of K^+ from all damaged cells and H^+ from hypoxic cells;
    (c) formation of bradykinin and kallidin from kallidinogen;
    (d) formation of eicosanoids from fatty acids (arachidonic acid);
    (e) activation of numerous enzymes including fibrinolysin, hyaluronidase and collagenase due to breakdown of lysosomes;
    (f) release of cytokines.
(2) It should produce effects that mimic one or more features of inflammation. The relevant effects of some putative chemical mediators are given in *Table 4.18*.

Table 4.18 Effects of putative mediators of acute inflammation

Putative mediator	Oedema	Increased blood flow	Pain	Cell damage
Histamine	+	+	+	
5-HT	+	+	+	
Kinins	+	+	+	
Eicosanoids*	+	+	+	
K^+			+	+
$H+$			+	+

* Effects vary depending on the individual eicosanoid involved. PGs enhance the effect of other painful stimuli rather than initiating pain themselves.

(3) Selective antagonists, that inhibit one or more of the effects of the postulated mediator, should inhibit similar components of the inflammatory reaction. Of the putative mediators, only specific antagonists for histamine are clinically available. Antagonists at H_1

histamine receptors inhibit the acute inflammatory response but only during the first 30–60 min, when histamine is detectable in the exudate.

(4) Depletion of tissues of the postulated mediator, or inhibition of its means of production and release, should suppress appropriate components of the inflammatory reaction. **Aspirin**-like drugs inhibit cyclo-oxygenase *in vitro* and suppress the secondary phase of inflammation associated with the presence of PGs in the exudate.

Thus many of the features of inflammation can be explained by a combination of histamine with one or more of the other compounds observed to be present. Histamine is thought to be significant only during the first 30–60 min of the response. Eicosanoids, kinins and cytokines are strong candidates for mediating the inflammatory response beyond this time.

Anti-inflammatory drugs

Defence reactions to trauma and infection are initially desirable but may become unacceptable or unhelpful to the patient. Inflammatory reactions to extrinsic (pollen – 'hay fever') or intrinsic (host tissue – rheumatoid arthritis) allergens may always be inappropriate. In both of these situations, the symptoms associated with acute inflammation can be suppressed by anti-inflammatory drugs.

The nonsteroidal anti-inflammatory drugs (NSAIDs)

This group includes **aspirin**, *ibuprofen*, *indomethacin*, *mefenamic acid* and *naproxen*. All relieve pain, reduce swelling and increase mobility in inflammatory diseases (acute rheumatic fever, osteoarthritis, rheumatoid arthritis). They do not alter the course of the underlying disease (chronic inflammation, fibrosis).

Anti-inflammatory effects

Their anti-inflammatory action is due to suppression of PG formation by inhibiting cyclo-oxygenase. Inhibition of cyclo-oxygenase may also explain the analgesic and antipyretic activity of the anti-inflammatory drugs (page 241). Although there appears to be a central component (page 241), the analgesic action of **aspirin** is a substantially peripheral effect. By preventing PG release in inflammation **aspirin** prevents the sensitization of the pain receptors to mechanical stimulation or to chemical mediators. This would also explain why **aspirin** is less effective as an analgesic in uninflamed tissues.

The relative activities of NSAIDs as anti-inflammatory, analgesic or antipyretic agents may depend on the susceptibility of different tissue cyclo-oxygenases to inhibition by these drugs. Thus in clinical concentrations **aspirin** and *indomethacin* inhibit cyclo-oxygenase in peripheral tissues and brain and each displays anti-inflammatory activity (a peripheral action) and antipyretic activity (a central action).

Uricosuric effect

The excretion of uric acid is increased by inhibition of renal tubular re-absorption.

Adverse effects

Major toxic effects of NSAIDs are uncommon but minor toxic effects are very common and shared by all the group.

Mucosal irritation due to the acidic nature of most NSAIDs and inhibition of production of a mucosal protective PGE lead to gastric erosion, epigastric discomfort and minor bleeding. With large doses major gastric bleeding or insidious chronic blood loss leading to iron-deficiency anaemia (page 426) is sometimes seen.

NSAIDs also produce allergic disorders or may precipitate asthma in susceptible individuals by inhibition of production of a bronchodilatory PG or diversion of free fatty acid precursors (arachidonic acid) towards LT production.

NSAIDs promote salt and water retention by the kidney by inhibiting the production of a PG regulating blood flow in the renal vasculature. They may also produce renal damage manifest as increased urinary excretion of epithelial cells and leucocytes.

Most NSAIDs are organic acids with affinity for plasma albumin binding sites. This may result in the diplacement of other drugs from plasma albumin with a consequent undesired increase in the free plasma concentration, leading to increased effect (page 41).

Adverse effects expressed primarily in the CNS are important features (*see* page 241).

Aspirin inhibits the formation of prothrombin, an effect which may result in haemorrhage and is reversible by injection of vitamin K.

Indomethacin is much more effective in rheumatoid arthritis and gout than salicylates but is a poorly tolerated drug. It is usually reserved for cases that are unresponsive to other drugs and then used only in short courses to reduce the risks.

Glucocorticoids

This group includes **prednisolone,** *beclomethasone, betamethasone, dexamethasone* and *hydrocortisone.* All suppress initial and secondary characteristics of the inflammatory response including emigration of polymorphs, phagocytosis and the process of repair and regeneration. They are used to suppress inflammation in a wide variety of disease processes including systemic lupus erythematosus, asthma (page 393), cranial arteritis, polyarteritis nodosa and some cases of rheumatoid arthritis (though chronic use is to be avoided, page 432). Their actions are palliative and the underlying cause of the lesion remains. Long-term therapy holds many hazards (page 180).

They stimulate the production of lipocortin which inhibits phospholipase A_2 thus decreasing the availability of substrate for eicosanoid synthesis. They also stabilize lysosomal membranes, thus preventing the liberation of enzymes, one of which is phospholipase A_2.

Antirheumatic drugs

These drugs, unlike NSAIDs and glucocorticoids, do influence the underlying disease process but are drugs of relatively low therapeutic index.

Chloroquine

Chloroquine may be indicated in those patients whose rheumatoid arthritis does not respond to the NSAIDs. The anti-inflammatory effect of *chloroquine* is brought about in part by inhibition of phospholipase A_2. Prolonged use of a dose larger than that effective in malaria is necessary (page 264), hence the risk of retinopathy is greater.

Penicillamine

Penicillamine is a reserve drug for severe rheumatoid arthritis that has not responded to other treatments. The mechanism may involve reduction of IgM concentration. Toxic effects are common and may be serious (page 431).

Organic gold compounds

Sodium aurothiomalate [gold sodium thiomalate] has long-lasting anti-inflammatory effects. This compound is chiefly employed against the early stages of rheumatoid arthritis. Its mode of action is unknown; current hypotheses attribute it to inhibition of mononuclear cell phagocytosis and suppressed immune responsiveness.

Despite this wide range of drugs the ideal anti-inflammatory and anti-rheumatic agent has yet to be discovered. The toxicity of these compounds (page 431) in effective doses often leaves NSAIDs as the mainstay of patient management.

5

Drug action on the central nervous system

Aims

- To describe those chemicals that have a neurotransmitter role in the CNS.
- To describe how imbalances in neurotransmitters can explain CNS disorders.
- To describe the range of mechanisms by which drugs can interfere with neurotransmission.
- To describe how transmitter imbalances can be restored by drugs leading to a rational treatment of CNS disorders.
- To anticipate how an understanding of neurotransmitter substances and of mechanisms of drug action can further lead to more selective treatment of brain disorders.

Introduction

The CNS has many functions and each involves an altered brain chemistry. Every thought, decision, perception and mood change is chemically mediated. In their simplest form the principles of drug action on the CNS are the same as those described for the peripheral nervous system. Drugs affect both peripheral and central neuronal functions by interfering with neurochemical transmission. Remember:

(1) neurotransmitters can be excitatory or inhibitory;
(2) drugs act by mimicking or antagonizing neurotransmitters;
(3) mimics may act directly (agonists at receptors) or indirectly (releasing agents, uptake inhibitors, enzyme inhibitors);
(4) antagonists may act directly (competitive and noncompetitive antagonists at receptors) or indirectly (preventing release, depleting transmitter stores).

However in the CNS the situation is infinitely more complex for several reasons including the following:

(1) the very large number of neurones in the brain;

(2) each neurone is in synaptic contact with thousands of other neurones;
(3) in addition to the two major transmitters of the periphery there are at least 50 other transmitters in the CNS and, as in the periphery, most may be excitatory or inhibitory depending on location;
(4) it is certain that some transmitters can interact with several different receptors (as in the periphery) and it is likely that receptors exist in the brain that have no peripheral equivalent;
(5) drug interaction with presynaptic receptors that then modulate the release of transmitters, is a more frequent explanation of drug action in the brain than in the periphery;
(6) there is growing evidence that at some synapses transmission is effected by the release of more than one transmitter from the same neurone ('cotransmission') but the relative inaccessibility of some brain areas hampers investigations.

To illustrate this complexity, consider the neurotransmission that governs the functioning of a particular brain area. The system is analogous to that in the autonomic nervous system where function is the result of a balance between inhibitory and excitatory inputs (*Figure 5.1*).

Presynaptic inhibitory neurones are shown. Four sites at which chemical transmission occurs are shown involving four different transmitters (A, B, C and D).

Assuming absolute selectivity of drug action, the overall phenomenon of excitation can be caused by mimics of transmitters A or D, or antagonists of B or C. Conversely, the phenomenon of inhibition will be caused by mimics of B or C, or by antagonists of A or D.

Accepting that this example is a massive oversimplification, and that most drugs interfere with more than one transmitter (for example, **chlorpromazine**, page 227), some idea of the complexity emerges. Nevertheless, because there is a range of chemical transmitters in the brain, which may be associated with certain brain areas (and therefore brain functions) and because some drugs have some selectivity of action, some degree of selective alteration of brain activity is possible. Good examples are found in the pharmacology of strychnine (page 215), **levodopa** (page 219) and **morphine** (page 231).

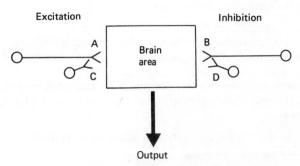

Excitation   Inhibition

Figure 5.1 Model of possible neuronal interconnections and sites of drug action

Chemical transmission in the CNS

Criteria for identification of a transmitter

(1) It must be present at the synapse.
(2) It should be stored in the presynaptic terminal.
(3) Processes for its synthesis should be present in the presynaptic neurone.
(4) It should be released on nerve stimulation.
(5) Postsynaptic application of the putative transmitter should mimic stimulation.
(6) Processes for its inactivation should be present at the synapse.

Many techniques are required to determine whether these criteria are satisfied, including:

(1) microelectrodes for recording from, or applying electrical stimuli to, neurones;
(2) micropipettes either for application of putative transmitters or for removal of ECF for analysis;
(3) biochemical and isotopic techniques for detection of transmitters or their precursors and metabolites;
(4) receptor binding techniques to map the distribution of a particular receptor in the CNS;
(5) histochemical fluorescence techniques for localization of putative amine transmitters;
(6) immunological techniques for the localization of enzymes involved in transmitter synthesis and breakdown, or for identification of putative peptide transmitters;
(7) lesion-making and neuroanatomy.

Substances acting as neurotransmitters

Many substances have been suggested to be chemical transmitters in the CNS, even though in many cases only a few of the above criteria have been satisfied and in some cases the only evidence available is that the substance appears to be present.

Our understanding of putative transmitters has generally depended on the availability of drugs that interfere with them.

The substances most commonly quoted as having a neurotransmitter role are those known to have transmitter function in the periphery, or those related to such compounds.

Monoamines

Dopamine, NA and 5-HT all have important neurotransmitter functions in the CNS. Three ascending monoamine tracts have been identified in

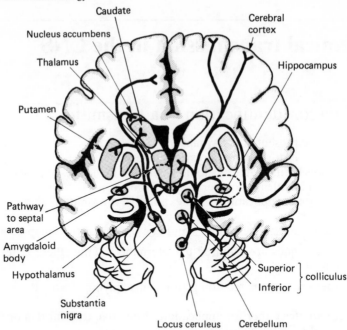

Caudate
Nucleus accumbens
Thalamus
Putamen
Cerebral cortex
Hippocampus
Pathway to septal area
Amygdaloid body
Hypothalamus
Substantia nigra
Superior ⎤
Inferior ⎦ colliculus
Locus ceruleus   Cerebellum

Figure 5.2 Ascending dopaminergic and noradrenergic tracts; dopaminergic tracts only shown on left half of diagram, noradrenergic on right

mammalian brain. Their cell bodies are located in specific areas of the midbrain and their axons transmit impulses to many brain areas (*Figures 5.2 and 5.3*).

The ascending nigrostriatal dopaminergic tract (*Figure 5.2*) plays an important role in the maintenance of gait and posture. Underactivity of this tract leads to a condition known as Parkinson's disease after the physician James Parkinson who first described it in 1817 (page 219).

The ascending NA and dopamine tracts to the limbic system are shown in *Figure 5.2*. The limbic system is a complex neuronal loop that connects the hippocampus, fornix bundle, mammillary body, thalamus, cingulate gyrus and amygdala. The limbic system plays an important role in the regulation of mood. Disorders of mood and behaviour are likely to have as their basis altered function of neurotransmitters in the limbic system. Many drugs that affect mood and behaviour can be shown to interact with either NA or dopamine.

Empirically this has led to the monoamine theory of nervous and mental disease, which suggests that clinical depression is related to a functional monoamine deficiency, whilst mania and other behavioural excitations are related to a functional monoamine excess. At present it is not possible to define a separate role for any one of the monoamines in any one mental disorder. However, the theory receives support when the effects of drugs on the CNS are compared with their known mechanism of action. Drugs that cause excitement are known to increase functional monoamine activity (*cocaine* inhibits uptake of monoamines into nerve terminals, page 104, and therefore delays inactivation; amphetamine releases stored monoamines

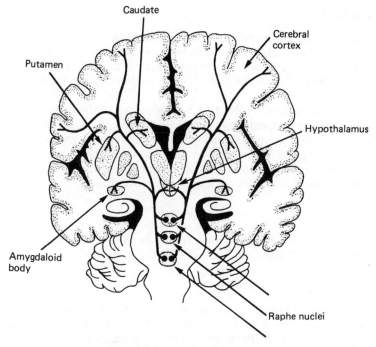

Figure 5.3 Ascending 5-HT tracts

from nerve terminals, page 99). Antidepressive drugs like **imipramine** are inhibitors of monoamine uptake. On the other hand, some drugs that cause sedation are known to decrease functional monoamine activity. Reserpine depletes neuronal stores (page 95) and **chlorpromazine** is an antagonist at monoamine receptors (page 227). Many drugs useful in treating disorders of mood are only effective on chronic treatment and acute pharmacological effects may not be relevant.

In the CNS α-adrenoceptors (α_2- and α_1-subtypes) and β-adrenoceptors are present. Chronic treatment with tricyclic antidepressive drugs causes β-adrenoceptors to become less responsive and α_1-adrenoceptors to become more responsive. Since antidepressive activity is slow to develop these changes may be more relevant to the therapeutic activity than inhibition of amine uptake.

Dopamine receptors have been subdivided depending on whether they are linked with adenylate cyclase (D_1) or not (D_2).

The ascending 5-HT tracts, which also innervate the limbic areas, are shown in *Figure 5.3*. It seems very likely that the monoamine theory of nervous and mental disease should be extended to include this amine, which has receptors situated both pre- and postsynaptically. There is some evidence to suggest that changes in 5-HT systems are linked to changes in sensitivity to painful stimuli, altered sexual behaviour, sleep patterns, anxiety and disorders of appetite.

Adrenaline and histamine may also have limited roles as neurotransmitters in the CNS.

Acetylcholine

ACh, its binding sites and the enzymes necessary for its synthesis and metabolism are distributed widely in most areas of the CNS. Notable concentrations of ACh are found in the thalamus, basal ganglia, brain stem and spinal cord. Both muscarinic and nicotinic cholinoceptors are found in the CNS.

The neurophysiological role of ACh in movement is the best documented. It is an excitatory transmitter in the basal ganglia. Agonists at muscarinic cholinoceptors are tremorogenic, whereas antagonists are useful in the management of pathological (Parkinson's disease) or drug-induced tremor.

There is a clear involvement of ACh in pain perception. Current research links cholinergic dysfunction with presenile dementia.

Amino acids

Several amino acids have been suggested to have neurotransmitter function but gamma-aminobutyric acid (GABA) is the most studied.

GABA

Concentrations of GABA in the brain are greater than those of any other neurotransmitter (by a factor of about 1000) though its presence as a metabolite linked with the Krebs cycle complicates interpretation of its distribution.

GABA is synthesized from glutamic acid by a decarboxylase. There is both an uptake system into neurones and glia and a metabolizing enzyme (GABA transaminase) producing succinic semialdehyde.

GABA is invariably inhibitory on neuronal activity.

GABA is involved in the control of movement and directly or indirectly acting GABAmimetics are effective in the treatment of epilepsy. **Phenytoin** and *phenobarbitone* enhance GABA transmission by a mechanism that is unclear. *Vigabatrin* is an inhibitor of GABA transaminase and **sodium valproate** inhibits this too, but succinic semialdehyde dehydrogenase more so (*Figure 5.4*). These inhibitions of its breakdown produce an accumulation of GABA and the motor inhibition that is associated with raised concentrations of GABA is utilized in the treatment of epilepsy. The benzodiazepines interact with a receptor that is linked with the GABA receptor, enhancing GABA transmission. Whilst this is likely to be the mechanism of their anticonvulsant activity, the specific role of GABA in mood and consciousness is unclear.

No direct agonist at GABA receptors has clinical use. Antagonists (bicuculline, picrotoxin) are convulsant poisons.

Glycine

Glycine is an inhibitory transmitter primarily in the spinal cord.

A collateral of the α-motoneurone synapses with the Renshaw cell within the ventral horn of the spinal cord as shown in *Figure 5.5*.

This collateral releases ACh, which depolarizes the Renshaw cell (via nicotinic cholinoceptors). The induced Renshaw cell activity liberates gly-

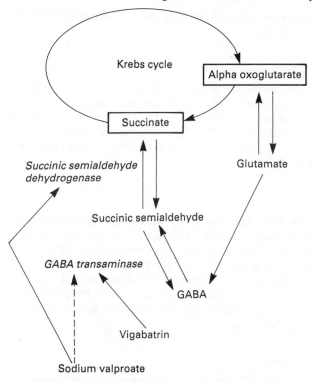

Figure 5.4 Sites of drug action on GABA metabolism

cine, which causes hyperpolarization of the α-motoneurone cell body. Thus, this forms a negative feedback loop, limiting activity in the α-motoneurone. Tetanus toxin prevents the release of glycine from the Renshaw cell, which explains the uncontrolled spasm of skeletal muscle seen after tetanus infection. Strychnine is an antagonist of glycine at its receptors on the

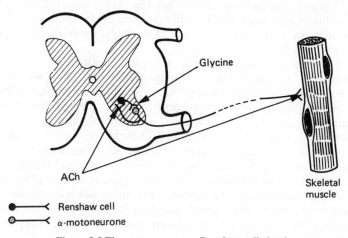

Figure 5.5 The α-motoneurone-Renshaw cell circuit

α-motoneurone, which explains why spasm of skeletal muscle is a feature of strychnine poisoning.

Excitatory amino acids

Glutamate and aspartate occur in high concentrations in the CNS but, as with GABA, their involvement in neuronal metabolism complicates the identification of neuronal tracts. The greatest evidence for a neurotransmitter role exists in the cortex. They are neurotoxins and excessive activation of their receptors has been suggested as a cause of the degenerative disease Huntington's chorea.

Peptides

Dozens of peptides have been implied to have neurotransmitter function. Peptide transmission seems to differ from that of other transmitters in that peptides are released from precursors at the nerve ending (*cf*. axonal transport of other transmitters to the nerve ending). Many coexist with other transmitters and may participate in cotransmission. Their action is terminated by metabolism. Many of them also exist in the periphery in neurones or elsewhere. Some related peptides have hormonal, in addition to neurotransmitter, function.

The opioid peptides

There are three families of opioid peptides – the enkephalins, endorphins and dynorphins.

The enkephalins are derived from a single precursor. They have the amino acid sequences of:

Tyr.Gly.Gly.Phe.Met – 'met-enkephalin'
Tyr.Gly.Gly.Phe.Leu – 'leu-enkephalin'

They are widely distributed throughout the CNS including those regions involved in pain perception – the substantia gelatinosa of the spinal cord, periaqueductal grey matter of the mid brain and the limbic system. They are also found in the periphery – neurones of the intestinal tract, in sympathetic ganglia and adrenals.

There are also several endorphins though it is not clear which are neurotransmitters or hormones and which are metabolites. Most widely studied is β-endorphin. β-Endorphin is a peptide of 31 amino acids, being a fragment of the arterior pituitary hormone β-lipotropin. The terminal five amino acids of β-endorphin are the same as those of met-enkephalin.

β-Endorphin is essentially a pituitary hormone and is released along with ACTH in stress (they share a common precursor). It is also present in a very limited number of CNS nuclei (hypothalamus and solitary tract).

The dynorphins are of intermediate size – typical is dynorphin-A, which has 17 amino acid residues. The terminal five amino acids are the same as the sequence of leu-enkephalin. The dynorphins are as widely distributed as the enkephalins but their concentrations are lower. However, they are more potent than the enkephalins.

Structural correlations

Figure 5.6 compares the structures of **morphine** and the enkephalins. The terminal tyrosine of enkephalin corresponds to the phenol group of **morphine** and the amino groups are held in the same spatial plane. The NH_2-terminal end of all endogenous opioid peptides commence: Tyr.Gly.Gly.Phe.

Opioid receptors

It is clear that there are different kinds of opioid receptor; the situation becomes progressively more complicated with more than 10 receptor types currently mooted.

The enkephalins are thought to interact preferentially with δ-receptors, the dynorphins with κ-receptors. The receptors for the endorphins may differ.

There is considerable overlap between these receptors and every opioid peptide or drug has at least some affinity for each receptor type. Similarly **naloxone** is active at each, though it is most effective at the μ-receptor. More selective antagonists are available.

Physiological role

Peripheral models. Instrumental in the discovery of these peptide transmitters and the research into their physiological role has been the existence of at least two peripheral neuroeffector junctions at which opioids and endorphins inhibit transmitter release. These are the guinea-pig ileum and mouse vas deferens (transmitters being ACh and NA respectively). These two sites have been extensively used as models of the central mechanism of action of opioids since:

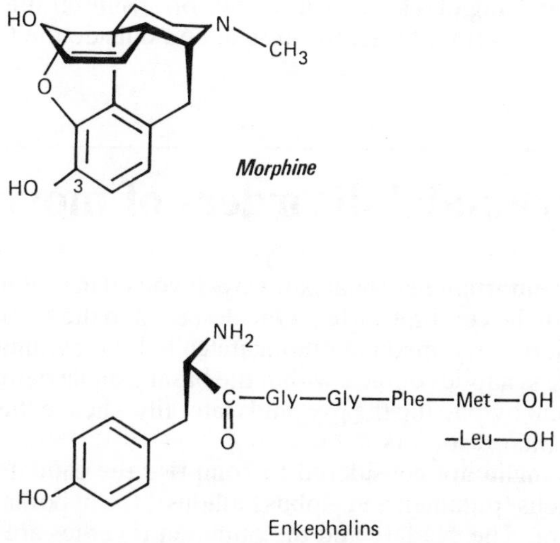

Morphine

Enkephalins

Figure 5.6 Structural analogy between morphine and the enkephalins

(1) potency ratios between agonists are the same as those for analgesic activity in man;
(2) antagonist as well as agonist activity can be demonstrated for some compounds at both sites as in the CNS.

It is known that in the CNS the opioids/transmitters can act presynaptically by inhibition of transmitter release (though not necessarily of ACh or NA).

Evidence for the physiological role of these peptides comes from our knowledge of the pharmacology of **morphine** and more importantly **naloxone,** the distribution of the peptides in the brain and the consequences of their local application.

In addition to pain perception, the peptides apparently have a role in modulation of hormone release, mood, consciousness and brain stem function – respiration, cough and vomiting. Coexistence with several other neurotransmitters has been reported in various brain regions. In the future opioid derivatives with actions not obviously related to those of **morphine** may have clinical use in the control of appetite, hypertension and psychotic disease.

Other peptides

Substance P is quite widely distributed, with high concentrations in the dorsal horn where it is been suggested to be involved in sensory perception. It coexists with 5-HT in the medullary raphe and with ACh in the pontine neurones.

A number of other peptides, many of which are well known for their hormonal activity, have been localized in CNS neurones. Neurotensin and neuropeptide Y commonly coexist with monoamines and thus their pharmacology may be associated with overall control of central monoamine transmission. Similar neuromodulator roles have been suggested for cholecystokinin, somatostatin, vasoactive intestinal peptide (VIP) and thyroid releasing hormone (TRH).

Bradykinin and angiotensin may have neurotransmitter function but they remain a more important target for drug action outside the CNS.

Extrapyramidal disorders of movement

There are two important neuronal pathways involved in motor coordination that originate in the cerebral cortex. One descends to the brain stem passing through a region of the medulla oblongata called the pyramids. The other makes multiple synaptic contacts within the basal ganglia before descending to the brain stem by-passing the pyramids laterally – hence the extrapyramidal tracts and their disorders.

The basal ganglia are considered to comprise the caudate nucleus, the lentiform nucleus (putamen and globus pallidus), the hypothalamus and the substantia nigra. The caudate and the putamen together are known as the striatum.

Important neurotransmitters in the basal ganglia are dopamine and GABA (which are inhibitory) and ACh (which is excitatory).

Because of clearly defined motor disorders that have been shown to be related to changes in neurotransmitter concentrations and an understanding of the drugs effective in the treatment of such disorders, we know more about this aspect of brain function than any other.

Parkinson's disease

This disease provides a good example of a nervous disease that can be attributed to a defect in a central neurotransmitter system. It is also of interest because it demonstrates how investigations of chemical transmission processes in the CNS ultimately led to the development of a rational therapy for the disease.

Parkinson's disease is characterized by tremor and rigidity in skeletal muscle and akinesia (lit. lack of movement – hypokinesia would be a more accurate description). There is a characteristic posture and gait. Severe depression commonly accompanies these motor change. When the disease is first recognized the signs and symptoms may be mild but the disease progresses and may ultimately lead to total incapacitation.

Treatment

Before 1960 empirical medical treatment involved the use of antagonists at muscarinic cholinoceptors. These drugs were more effective against tremor than against rigidity and a high proportion of cases showed little or no improvement. Originally belladonna (containing atropine) was used but this was superseded by synthetic atropine derivatives (*orphenadrine, benzhexol*).

In 1960 therapy was introduced based on the dopaminergic nature of the nigrostriatal tracts in animals and the lack of dopamine in the striatum of brains taken from Parkinsonian patients post mortem. It was postulated that in Parkinson's disease there was a functional deficiency in neurotransmitter dopamine and that correction of that deficiency should lead to an improvement in the condition. Dopamine administration was of no use because it does not pass the blood brain barrier and has a very short $t_{\frac{1}{2}}$. Therefore the precursor amino acid **levodopa** (*l*-DOPA) was used. This crosses the blood brain barrier and can be converted to dopamine within the brain by the enzyme *l*-aromatic amino acid decarboxylase. **Levodopa** is now the drug of choice in the medical treatment of Parkinson's disease.

This has led to the postulate that in the striatum there is a functional balance between ACh and dopamine and that any change causing a decrease in the activity of dopamine relative to ACh (*Figure 5.7*) will produce the Parkinsonian condition. The balance may be restored either by reducing the influence of ACh (by **atropine**-like drugs) or by increasing that of dopamine (**levodopa**).

Three of the undesirable actions of **levodopa** may also be explained in terms of overactivity in dopaminergic systems:

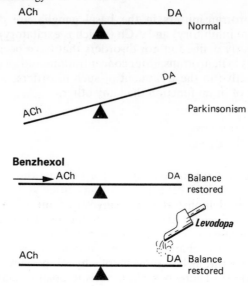

Figure 5.7 The functional balance between ACh and dopamine in the striatum, the imbalance in parkinsonism and its restoration by either antagonists at cholinoceptors or agonists at dopamine receptors

(1) vomiting – the chemosensitive trigger zone (CTZ) of the medullary vomiting centre (situated in the area postrema on the floor of the fourth cerebral ventricle close to the CO_2 sensing elements);
(2) involuntary muscle movements;
(3) some of the gastrointestinal and cardiovascular disturbances that occur during **levodopa** therapy may be peripheral in origin and related to the high doses required.

Since **levodopa** has a low therapeutic index partly because relatively little dopamine is rendered available to the striatum, two drug combinations are currently used to enhance drug availability where it is needed.

In combination with a decarboxylase inhibitor

Significant reduction in dosage may be obtained by combining **levodopa** with an inhibitor of aromatic *l*-amino acid decarboxylase that does not pass the blood brain barrier (*carbidopa, benserazide*). In this case little of the **levodopa** is metabolized in the periphery so that more is available for conversion to dopamine after penetrating the brain. Consequently lower oral doses are required.

In combination with a MAO-B inhibitor

Monoamine oxidases have been divided into two groups dependent on substrate and inhibitor specificities. That which exists in the striatum and oxidizes dopamine is termed MAO-B.

Selegiline (previously deprenyl) is a selective inhibitor of MAO-B and enhances striatal dopamine availability. There are no interactions with drugs or tyramine-containing foodstuffs.

Other agonists at dopamine receptors

Amantadine and *bromocriptine* are agonists at dopamine receptors. Neither appears to be as effective as **levodopa.** In most cases of Parkinson's disease selected for medical treatment **levodopa** and an antimuscarinic agent used together produce better results than either alone.

Parkinson's disease, along with the other extrapyramidal disorders, is an unpleasant and debilitating disease. The patient benefits from only a small improvement in condition.

Huntington's chorea

In this hereditary disease there is a progressive impairment of motor coordination with grimacing, distorted speech and bizarre movements of the limbs conveying a dance-like gait (hence chorea). There is accompanying dementia.

On examination post mortem, there is atrophy of components of the basal ganglia and a deficiency in GABA and the enzyme responsible for its synthesis, glutamic acid decarboxylase. There is also a deficiency of choline acetyltransferase and a functional excess of dopamine.

Treatment

Whilst the symptoms can be treated with antipsychotic drugs (*haloperidol*), the drug of choice is *tetrabenazine*.

Tetrabenazine causes a reserpine-like depletion of dopamine. Reserpine itself depletes catecholamines in the central and peripheral nervous systems and also drastically depletes brain 5-HT. Because of this nonspecificity it is a toxic drug that has no clinical use. In contrast, *tetrabenazine* causes more selective depletion of dopamine in the CNS without interfering with peripheral catecholamines or central 5-HT.

It does not cause the hypotension, depression and suicidal tendencies characteristic of reserpine.

Drug-induced extrapyramidal disorders

Iatrogenic motor disorders are common.

Drug-induced Parkinsonism

From consideration of *Figure 5.7* it is clear that drugs that either enhance central cholinergic activity or reduce dopamine activity will cause a parkinsonian state.

No centrally acting mimic of ACh has any long-term clinical use, which would otherwise result in drug-induced parkinsonism as a side-effect. However, physostigmine is known to cause tremor.

In contrast there is widespread use of antagonists at dopamine receptors, mainly in psychiatry.

The antipsychotic drugs are all capable of inducing such extrapyramidal disorders, though the incidence and severity differ within the group. Greatest incidence is with *fluphenazine* and *haloperidol*, moderate with **chlorpromazine** and least with *thioridazine*.

Treatment of this disorder is by reduction of dose and addition of antimuscarinic drugs.

Drug-induced tardive dyskinesia

This is also a characteristic side-effect of the antipsychotic drugs. The characteristics of tardive dyskinesia are a delayed impairment of motor coordination with typical movements notably of the face, tongue and neck. Paradoxically this is due to excess dopaminergic activity. During prolonged antagonism at dopamine receptors, there is compensatory supersensitivity to dopamine perhaps mediated by proliferation of dopamine receptors (cf. denervation supersensitivity).

Whilst it is clear that this extrapyramidal disorder could theoretically be treated by increasing the dose of the antipsychotic drug, in the long term this only aggravates the problem since it precipitates further supersensitivity.

Extrapyramidal disorders caused by drugs other than the antipsychotics

Antagonism at dopamine receptors is also the mechanism of action of many antiemetic drugs and these are also capable of causing extrapyramidal disorders. Some of these are prescribed either as antiemetics or antipsychotics (*perphenazine*), others are used solely as antiemetics (*metoclopramide*).

Antidepressive drugs

Depressive illness falls broadly into two kinds:

(1) neurotic (reactive) depression. Depression as a response to stress or problems particularly those involving loss of an 'emotional' attachment (for example, bereavement).
(2) psychotic (endogenous) depression. Manic-depressive psychosis is characterized by sustained phases of either excitement (hypomania, mania) or, more commonly, severe depression.

In contrast with psychotic depression, neurotic depression rarely requires drug therapy but between these extremes there may be a continuous spectrum of depressive illness. The use of drugs alone to treat depression is rarely sufficient; psychotherapy, electroconvulsive therapy and counselling may be required.

It is now clear that most cases of depression arise from a functional lack of NA and/or 5-HT within the limbic system.

The aim of chemotherapy in depressive illness is restoration of normal function by facilitating or stimulating transmission at central monoaminergic synapses.

Drugs that prevent enzymatic destruction of neurotransmitters

MAO enzymes can currently be classified into two kinds – MAO-A and MAO-B. NA and 5-HT are preferential substrates for MAO-A, dopamine for MAO-B.

MAO inhibitors are structurally related to amphetamine and may be reversible (*tranylcypromine*) or irreversible (**phenelzine**); both inhibit MAO-A and MAO-B. These drugs affect both NA and 5-HT. *Selegiline* selectively inhibits MAO-B but is ineffective in depression.

The ability of MAO inhibitors to attenuate the sedation and hypothermia induced in animals by reserpine can be used as an indication of the therapeutic potential of antidepressive drugs.

MAO inhibitors elevate the mood of depressed patients and this forms their primary use but there is about a 7–10 day delay before their clinical effect is seen, although inhibition of the enzyme is apparent within a few hours of administration. These drugs suppress REM sleep but alleviate sleep problems associated with depression.

It is still not certain that the antidepressive actions of these compounds rely solely on their ability to inhibit MAO.

Adverse effects

Acute overdosage may cause excitement, insomnia, pyrexia and convulsions. Chronic toxicity includes hepatotoxicity, orthostatic hypotension and excessive CNS stimulation that manifests itself as hypomania, tremor, insomnia and, in some instances, convulsions.

An important problem is the change produced in the response to exogenous substances present in food or administered as drugs (pages 42 and 102). The potentiation of tyramine in foodstuffs is the best publicized effect where, because of the inhibition of gut and liver MAO, dietary tyramine is not inactivated and achieves a high concentration in plasma. Tyramine is an indirectly acting sympathomimetic. **Phentolamine** is an effective antidote but patients receiving MAO inhibitors must be told which foodstuffs and drugs to avoid to obviate such a crisis. It is largely this problem that has led to the virtual disuse of these drugs in depressive illness. However, the recent development of reversible and selective MAO-A inhibitors that do not appear to exhibit a toxic interaction with tyramine has reawakened interest in MAO inhibitors.

Drugs that prevent amine reuptake into the nerve terminal

Drugs that preferentially inhibit the reuptake of NA and 5-HT, offer the possibility of selective action in the treatment of depressive illness.

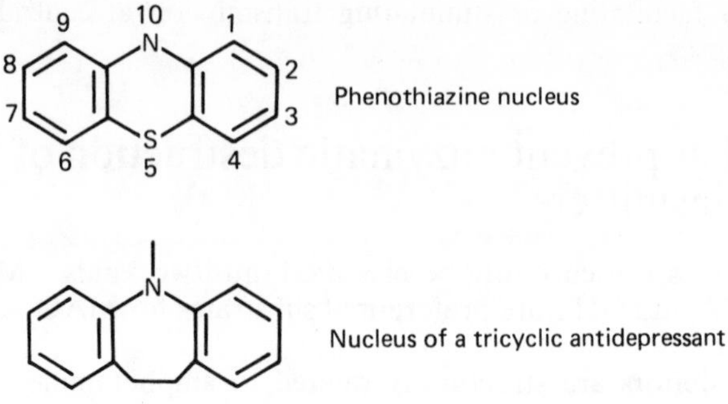

Figure 5.8 The phenothiazine antipsychotic and tricyclic antidepressive drug nuclei

Depression associated with violent and suicidal behaviour tends to respond better to drugs that preferentially inhibit 5-HT uptake.

Drugs that prevent NA reuptake

These compounds are structurally derived from the phenothiazine antipsychotic drugs (*Figure 5.8*). They are often referred to as 'tricyclic' antidepressive drugs. More recently 'quadricyclic' compounds have been introduced with similar pharmacology.

Tricyclic compounds include **imipramine** and **amitriptyline** while quadricyclic compounds are *mianserin* and maprotiline. All compounds in this category prevent the reuptake of NA by inhibition of the active uptake process that is in part responsible for the inactivation of neuronally released NA (page 103). These compounds also produce a competitive antagonism at central muscarinic cholinoceptors. Such antagonism may contribute to the elevation of mood and awareness.

Tricyclic compounds are broken down quickly in the body by demethylation. These metabolites also have antidepressive properties (desmethylimipramine, nortriptyline) and have approximately twice the potency of the parent compound. Although the action of these drugs within the synapse may be observed within 30 min of administration, the clinical effects, as with the inhibitors of MAO, develop only slowly over 2–3 weeks. The explanation for this is not known but may involve autoregulatory feedback mechanisms acting via presynaptic receptors.

Imipramine and **amitriptyline** are antagonists at muscarinic cholinoceptors and frequently give rise to serious cardiovascular problems. Other effects due to this property (dry mouth, urinary retention, blurred vision) are troublesome but may be minimized by giving a large single daily dose of the drug at night without loss of antidepressive effect. The antimuscarinic effect of **amitriptyline** in particular has been exploited to treat nocturnal enuresis in children.

Amitriptyline and *nortriptyline* are sedative and are used in psychotic depression accompanied by severe anxiety and agitation. **Imipramine** and compounds related to it are less sedative. Protriptyline, on the contrary, has stimulant properties and is used to treat 'somnolent' psychotic depression where motor retardation and inertia form part of the illness.

Quadricyclic antidepressive drugs also block NA reuptake but they have less antimuscarinic activity and may be more safely given to patients with cardiac problems. They have no active metabolites and are generally weaker antidepressive drugs.

Drugs that prevent 5-HT reuptake

These compounds show no basic similarities in chemical structure, other than the possession of one or more two-ring systems. However, such bicyclic compounds all share the property of primarily inhibiting reuptake of 5-HT into the nerve ending, in an analogous manner to the inhibition of NA reuptake by tricyclic compounds. Their effects on NA uptake are minimal.

Since their prime action is on 5-HT, bicyclic compounds are of benefit in depressive illness in which this transmitter plays a considerable part. Lack of antimuscarinic adverse effects and little effect on NA mean that they may be more safely prescribed in patients taking antihypertensive agents and in those with cardiac disease. *Trazodone* is currently used to treat mild neurotic depression.

Central agonists at 5-HT receptors

Iprindole has a chemical structure bearing slight similarities to 5-HT and it is believed to act as an antidepressive by an agonist action at central 5-HT receptors. Its efficacy in both mild neurotic depression and less severe psychotic depression suggests that it may have an action at central adrenoceptors. It is less sedative than the tricyclic antidepressive drugs and has weak antimuscarinic activity but it is hepatotoxic and is contraindicated in liver disease.

Drugs acting on electrolytes

Many patients suffering from affective illness show a grossly elevated concentration of intracellular Na^+. In depression this is typically doubled; in mania Na^+ retention is even higher. **Lithium carbonate** given as a slow release preparation is able to displace the Na^+ and allows intracellular Na^+ to return to normal. This is an effective way of treating mania but, in depression, the illness must first be eliminated using a tricyclic or other compound, following which **lithium carbonate** may be given prophylactically. By this means, recurring bouts of depressive illness, which often become part of a patient's lifestyle, can be entirely eliminated. The use of this compound is limited by its acute nephrotoxicity; dosage must be determined for each patient and regular checks on Li^+ clearance should be maintained.

Future developments

It has been suggested that the failure of noradrenergic transmission that is believed to underlie psychotic depression may be due to overactivity or oversensitivity of presysnaptic α-adrenoceptors. Similar mechanisms may operate to cause lowered 5-HT transmission. Presynaptic receptors may offer novel targets for drug treatment.

Antipsychotic drugs

Psychosis

Psychosis is a major mental disorder characterized by derangement, loss of contact with reality and often delusions, illusions and hallucinations.

In functional psychosis the brain appears macroscopically normal at post-mortem examination.

Schizophrenia embodies a group of functional psychotic disorders characterized by retreat from reality, bizarre or regressive behaviour, auditory hallucinations and, commonly, delusions of grandeur or persecution (paranoia).

Antipsychotic drugs are useful in the treatment of psychoses and in preanaesthetic medication. In the past they have misleadingly been termed neuroleptics ('mood regulating') or 'major tranquillizers'.

Current antipsychotic drugs originate from different chemical classes.

Phenothiazines

Phenothiazine has a tricyclic structure (*Figure 5.8*) and is the nucleus of numerous derivatives with antipsychotic activity (**chlorpromazine**).

Thioxanthines

Substitution of the N in position 10 of phenothiazine (*Figure 5.8*) by C produces thioxanthene. Some derivatives of thioxanthene have antipsychotic activity similar to that of **chlorpromazine** – *flupenthixol*.

Butyrophenones

Butyrophenones are tricyclic compounds but are unrelated chemically to either the phenothiazines or thioxanthenes. Some butyrophenones have antipsychotic activity similar to that of **chlorpromazine** – *haloperidol*.

Diphenylbutylpiperidines

Pimozide causes less sedation than **chlorpromazine** and may be the antipsychotic of choice in schizophrenia in apathetic withdrawn patients.

Antipsychotic drugs of different chemical classes produce qualitatively similar effects on mood and behaviour, differing only in potency. Butyrophenones are generally the most potent.

These drugs exert a relatively selective depressant effect on conditioned responses. In man, they reduce defensive hostility, attention and emotional responses. Intellectual activities are not altered appreciably. The most obvious effect of **chlorpromazine** is a dose related depression of behaviour. With low doses there is a taming effect in aggressive animals. As the dose is increased there is reduced locomotor activity and at higher doses the animals become immobile and catatonic. In the catatonic state the animal has increased muscle tone and will for a time maintain an abnormal posture imposed on it. Induction of catatonia distinguishes **chlorpromazine** from the barbiturates (page 250) and the anxiolytics (page 247). It is also possible to demonstrate inhibition of conditioned behaviour (for example, escape behaviour in response to a bell) with doses too low to modify an unconditioned response (for example, escape behaviour in response to a mild noxious stimulus). This again is in contrast to the effects of nonspecific depressants with which both conditioned and unconditioned responses are similarly affected.

These antipsychotics are the drugs of choice in the treatment of both functional psychoses (notably schizophrenia) and organic psychoses. Antipsychotics are also effective antagonists of the centrally acting sympathomimetics and hallucinogens and are the drugs of choice in poisoning from these drugs.

Mechanism of antipsychotic action

The similar effects of chemically different antipsychotics on behaviour and mood is ascribed to their common ability to block dopamine receptors in the mesolimbic system, a part of the brain controlling emotion, behaviour and mood. The antipsychotic action correlates better with antagonism at D_2 than D_1 dopamine receptors (page 213). This antipsychotic property suggests that psychoses are manifestations of excess dopaminergic activity in the mesolimbic system but such an abnormality has not been substantiated by nonpharmacological means.

Other effects due to dopamine antagonism

Blockade of D_1 and D_2 dopamine receptors in the brain by antipsychotics is not restricted to the mesolimbic system.

Antagonism of dopamine in the caudate and putamen causes rigidity and tremor of skeletal muscle (page 221, *Figure 5.9*). These extrapyramidal motor effects are most prominent with butyrophenones (*haloperidol*) and phenothiazines with a piperazine group at position 10 in the phenothiazine nucleus (*Figure 5.8, fluphenazine, prochlorperazine, trifluoperazine*).

Centrally acting antimuscarinic agents (*benzhexol*) that relieve Parkinson's disease (page 219) reduce antipsychotic drug-induced motor effects. Tranquillization with a piperidine-substituted phenothiazine (*thioridazine*) may be preferable therapy because this kind has a lower incidence of extrapyramidal motor disturbances. This is attributable to the ratio of antimuscarinic:antidopaminergic activity being greater in piperidine phenothiazines than in other antipsychotics.

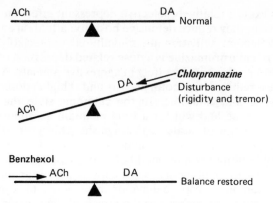

Figure 5.9 Functional balance between ACh and dopamine in the striatum, its disturbance by antipsychotics and its correction by antagonists at muscarinic cholinoceptors
(*cf. Figure 5.6*)

Since dopamine is an important neurotransmitter within the vomiting reflex, antagonists at dopamine receptors are important antiemetic drugs (page 230).

Antipsychotics antagonize dopamine-mediated inhibition of prolactin release from the anterior pituitary gland and may cause an excess flow of milk (galactorrhoea, page 157). Elevated dopamine content may cause increased libido in women and decreased libido and depression in men. Appetite can be stimulated with resultant obesity.

Effects not due to dopamine antagonism

Antipsychotic drugs can block central and peripheral receptors other than those for dopamine. Receptors that may be affected include muscarinic cholinoceptors, α-adrenoceptors and H_1 histamine receptors. Blockade of nondopamine receptors is most marked with phenothiazines and least with butyrophenones.

Clinically useful effects

Numerous effects can result from blockade of nondopamine receptors by antipsychotics, some of these are clinically useful, including:

(1) the antimuscarinic activity in alleviating motion sickness (*promethazine*);
(2) the antihistamine activity in alleviating allergic reactions (*promethazine*);
(3) the sedative activity in suppressing restlessness caused by mental disturbances or alleviating itching (pruritus) associated with jaundice (*promethazine*);
(4) the potentiating effect on the action of other central depressants particularly opioid analgesics (**chlorpromazine**).

Unwanted effects

Some effects resulting from blockade of nondopamine receptors are unwanted – on the cardiovascular system (orthostatic hypotension), the gastrointestinal tract (constipation) and the eye (blurring of vision).

Sensitization reactions to phenothiazines occur as blood dyscrasias, cholestatic jaundice and skin rashes.

Choice of antipsychotic drug

There is no convincing evidence that combinations of antipsychotic drugs are more beneficial than one drug alone. The choice of drug depends on the acceptability of a particular unwanted effect in individual patients. The differing abilities of antipsychotic drugs to induce extrapyramidal motor effects (page 222) and autonomic disturbances (*see above*) have been noted. Outpatient treatment of psychotic or agitated patients who may not take their tablets regularly is facilitated by the use of long-acting preparations (*fluphenazine decanoate* injection deep im) despite the common occurrence of extrapyramidal motor effects with piperazine substituted phenothiazine.

Vomiting, emetics and antiemetics

The output of the medullary vomiting centre, which lies laterally in the reticular formation, near the solitary tract, passes:

(1) to high centres to be perceived as the sensation of nausea;
(2) by parasympathetic outflows to the gut (relaxation of the cardiac or oesophagogastric sphincter) and the exocrine glands (sweating and salivation);
(3) by somatic efferent pathways to the expiratory (retching) and inspiratory (expulsion) muscles of respiration and postural muscles.

Linked with the vomiting centre is the CTZ. This area is sited on the floor of the fourth ventricle in the area postrema. It lies outside the blood brain barrier so can detect toxic substances in the blood.

Important neurotransmitters associated with the vomiting reflex are 5-HT (particularly mediated by 5-HT_3 receptors), dopamine (agonists at dopamine receptors are emetic) and ACh (note the increased parasympathetic activity that precedes and continues during vomiting).

Vomiting is usually preceded by parasympathetic activation and is effected by respiratory muscles.

There are parallel mechanisms for the initiation of the vomiting response to any stimulus. All therapeutically useful antiemetic drugs seem to act on the input circuitry of the emetic centre. The neural and humoral inputs are of four origins (at least) as follows:

(1) psychic – bombardment from higher centres generated by, for example, the sight, sound and smell of someone else vomiting or conditioned anticipation of a noxious stimulus, for example, cancer chemotherapy;
(2) gastrointestinal afferents – excited by, for instance, pharyngeal mechanical stimulation, chemical damage, irritation or disease in the gut;
(3) motion – which is only partly of vestibular (labyrinthine) origin, a significant part is visual and disagreement between the visual and proprioceptive versions of the position of the body in space is a particularly potent cause;
(4) chemical – many drugs can directly (CTZ) or indirectly (from gut) cause nausea and vomiting as a part of their acute toxicity: agonists at dopamine receptors (apomorphine, **levodopa**), agonists at opioid receptors (which may be related to dopaminergic activity), oestrogens, **digoxin,** *cisplatin* and the other alkylating agents used in cancer chemotherapy.

Antiemetics

Antiemetics are generally antagonists of 5-HT, dopamine, ACh, or all of these.

As with coughing, clinical situations in which vomiting serves a protective function should not be suppressed by drugs. In most clinical situations, however, emesis serves no useful purpose and may exacerbate the condition of the patient – early pregnancy, travel sickness, postoperative period, migraine, radiotherapy, cancer chemotherapy and drug therapy (for example, **morphine**).

Motion sickness

Hyoscine (page 88) is most effective, though sedative and producing all the expected **atropine**-like peripheral side-effects. Better tolerated (though still sedative) but less effective are some antihistamines (*cyclizine, promethazine*). The neural pathway carrying vestibular impulses to the emetic centre actually passes through the CTZ, though its neurones are not those excited by apomorphine and other chemical triggers. These two pathways converge on the emetic centre later. Not surprisingly, the drugs effective in motion sickness are effective in middle ear disease and to a lesser extent in Ménière's disease. They have some effect in postoperative (or postanaesthetic) vomiting and in the vomiting of early pregnancy. The opioids are much more emetic in ambulant than bedridden patients and this (vestibular) component is countered by the drugs for motion sickness.

Other conditions

In most other situations the phenothiazines (**chlorpromazine,** *trifluoperazine*) are effective, notably postoperatively, in radiotherapy, uraemia, carcinomatosis and pregnancy. In pregnancy drugs should be avoided if at all possible (page 33). They are also very effective against vomiting induced by ergot alkaloids, sympathomimetics and **levodopa** and at high doses against **digoxin** and opioid analgesics.

Metoclopramide, an antagonist at dopamine receptors and weak antagonist at $5\text{-}HT_3$ receptors, is an antiemetic relative of *procainamide* with peripheral (increased gastric emptying, reduced reflux) and central antiemetic actions. It has been found effective in the vomiting associated with migraine, pregnancy, Menière's disease, motion sickness, opioid analgesics, radiotherapy and postoperatively but it is not potent against cytotoxic chemotherapy. It shows extrapyramidal adverse effects, worse in children, that summate with those of phenothiazines. It causes prolactin release (galactorrhoea).

Anticipatory nausea and vomiting, for instance before cancer chemotherapy, may be alleviated by the benzodiazepines. Nausea and vomiting during chemotherapy may be partially relieved by high dose *metoclopramide* in combination with *dexamethasone*. The recently discovered selective antagonists at $5\text{-}HT_3$ receptors (ondansetron) show great promise in this area.

Opioid analgesics and their antagonists

All are structurally related to **morphine,** the most important of the alkaloids extracted from the latex of the opium poppy (*Papaver somniferum*). The term 'opioid' means acting like opium but they are also called opiates (derived from opium) or narcotic analgesics, because high doses can cause narcosis – a state of stupor and insensibility. They produce their effects by interacting with receptors for the peptide neurotransmitters, enkephalins, endorphins and dynorphins (*see* page 217).

Opioid analgesics

Derivatives of **morphine** possess two kinds of activity:

(1) they can act as agonists causing the well known effects of analgesia, respiratory depression, cough suppression, vomiting and constipation;
(2) they can act as antagonists of these agonists.

Some derivatives (**morphine**) are termed 'pure' agonists, whilst others are pure antagonists (**naloxone**). Yet further derivatives have both agonistic and antagonistic actions. The spectrum of agonist/antagonist activity at three of the opioid receptor types is summarized in *Table 5.1.*

Opioid actions are both central and peripheral.

Central agonist actions

The narcotic analgesics have very selective actions upon centres throughout the CNS. The receptors responsible for these different actions are currently being elucidated. Actions include analgesia, sedation, anaesthesia, respiratory

Table 5.1 Three kinds of opioid receptor

	mu (μ)	kappa (κ)	delta (δ)
Agonist	**Morphine**	**Pentazocine** (ketocyclazocine)	Some peptides
Antagonist	**Pentazocine** **Naloxone**	Norbinaltorphimine **Naloxone**	Naltrindole **Naloxone**

Note: **pentazocine** possesses both agonist and antagonist activities but at different receptors.

depression and cough suppression, hallucinations, convulsions, miosis and vomiting. The opioid analgesics also cause euphoria.

Which of these factors predominates depends on the drug and the animal species. *Pethidine* is more likely to cause convulsions than is **morphine** whilst *methadone* causes less sedation than **morphine** in man. **Morphine** is sedative in man but convulsant in cats.

Analgesia

Analgesia is produced both by an effect on the pain pathways, possibly at the spinal level (pain threshold), and on the reaction to the stimulus within the limbic system (pain tolerance). The latter is associated with the drug's euphoriant action. Patients state that the pain is still perceived but that it does not matter so much.

The opioids are more effective against dull constant pain though sharp stinging pain can be reduced. This suggests some selectivity of action on one of the two major pain pathways. Their analgesic action is enhanced by salicylates (summation) and antipsychotic drugs (unknown mechanism) but reduced by barbiturates, which lower pain threshold when given alone.

The individual drugs differ in the following ways.

Maximum analgesic efficacy. *Diamorphine* (heroin) has the greatest analgesic efficacy, then in descending order **morphine** (and *methadone* and *dextromoramide*), *pethidine*, *dihydrocodeine*, **codeine** and *dextropropoxyphene*.

Systemic bioavailability after oral administration. This is a function of lipid solubility. Note that **morphine** (*Figure 5.6*, page 217) has two hydroxyl groups and is relatively insoluble in lipid and therefore shows moderate oral efficacy, whilst *pethidine* is less polar and is more effective orally.

Duration of action. *Diamorphine* and *fentanyl* are short acting, most others act for longer.

Incidence of undesirable side-effects at satisfactory analgesic doses. Sedation may or may not be clinically undesirable. Vomiting is always undesirable in an analgesic. **Codeine** is capable of causing the same degree of analgesia as 10 mg **morphine** (im) but this would be accompanied by excessive vomiting.

Respiratory depression

Analgesia caused by any opioid is accompanied by depression of respiratory rate (changes in tidal volume may be variable). There is an elevation in the threshold of the medullary centres to the excitatory effects of CO_2: $PaCO_2$ rises. The resultant periodic breathing (*Figure 5.10*) is characteristic of narcotic poisoning.

Although respiratory depression is the cause of death in **morphine** poisoning, people can tolerate the consequences of severe respiratory depression caused by an opioid because it can occur without significant cardiovascular depression. This contrasts with that caused by most general anaesthetic agents when vasomotor depression and hypotension accompany hypoventilation.

Cough suppression

The derivatives of **morphine** are the only clinically useful drugs that depress the cough centre (situated in the medulla near the respiratory centres). Some derivatives of **morphine** possess similar antitussive activity relative to analgesic activity. Quantitative separation is seen in derivatives with bulky substituents at position 3 (*Figure 5.6*, page 217), hence **codeine** and pholcodine, which are effective antitussives at subanalgesic doses. Qualitative separation has also been achieved. Only those stereoisomers equivalent to *l*-morphine possess opioid-like activity (generally these are also *l*-rotatory but there are some exceptions). **Dextromethorphan** possesses no analgesic or respiratory depressant activity yet retains antitussive activity. It is equipotent with **codeine**.

Emetic action

All the derivatives of **morphine** can cause vomiting. The mechanism is by stimulation of the CTZ. Vomiting can be especially troublesome if the patient is ambulatory. Subsequently opiates can depress the vomiting centre. Thus, if vomiting is going to occur it will happen soon after injection. Vomiting can be controlled by antagonists at dopamine receptors (phenothiazines, *metoclopramide*).

Selectivity of emetic action is seen with **apomorphine,** which has few other **morphine**-like actions. **Apomorphine** is known to be a mimic of the neurotransmitter dopamine (page 230).

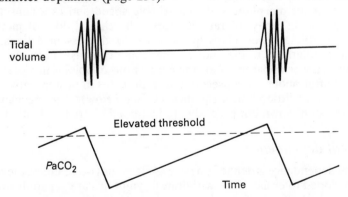

Figure 5.10 Periodic breathing induced by large doses of opioid drugs (due to an elevated threshold for the respiratory stimulant action of CO_2)

Miotic action

Most derivatives stimulate the oculomotor centre and cause pupillary constriction (parasympathetic innervation). This may complicate the use of pupil size as an index of depth of anaesthesia (page 245), though it is a useful symptom of opiate poisoning. Tolerance to this excitatory action occurs slowly; thus miosis is still present in addicts.

Peripheral agonist actions

Gastrointestinal effects

Morphine causes an increase in tone of the stomach, duodenum, small intestine and colon leading to decreased intestinal propulsion. Sphincters throughout the tract are particularly sensitive. Opiates also have a direct effect on mucosal ion transport reducing fluid accumulation in intestinal contents. Both these mechanisms contribute to the constipative action of opiates. Hence the use of kaolin and morphine for diarrhoea of assorted causes. A selective opioid constipative agent is **loperamide.** This drug is poorly absorbed and acts locally in the intestine so it lacks analgesic and respiratory depressant actions at constipative doses. It is available as an over-the-counter preparation.

Histamine release

Morphine, in common with other basic drugs (**tubocurarine, atropine**), can displace endogenous histamine from its binding site. This is of clinical importance if the patient has a history of allergic conditions. The consequences are irritation at the site of injection, bronchospasm (which may be fatal in an asthmatic patient) and peripheral vasodilatation leading to postural hypotension.

Tolerance

Tolerance is a decreased response to continued drug use, which is generally surmountable by increasing the dose of the drug. Tolerance develops to some actions of **morphine** with remarkable speed and to a considerable extent. An addict may tolerate 500 times the clinical dose of **morphine.** Generally, tolerance develops quickest to the depressant actions, there being little tolerance to the miotic, emetic and convulsant actions. Whilst tolerance may be apparent after single injections of opioids in a person and certainly after about six consecutive injections (as in postoperative pain), this may be of little clinical significance (*see below*). The mechanism of tolerance is unknown but is not due to increased biotransformation.

Physical dependence

Physical dependence is defined on page 44. It cannot occur unless the subject has developed tolerance. The withdrawal symptoms are generally opposite to the original effects of agonists (diarrhoea, hyperventilation, mydriasis) though vomiting occurs.

The symptoms develop at the time the next regular dose is due, reach peak severity in 36–72 h and last for about 1 week.

If opioids are used to relieve acute pain (for example, six injections), withdrawal symptoms, though detectable, may pass unnoticed if the patient is not anticipating any reaction.

The treatment of dependence is theoretically simple and effective. Hospitalization is essential. The injected addictive drug (commonly *diamorphine*) is withdrawn and a derivative that has a longer duration of action, that causes less euphoria and has adequate oral bioavailability is substituted (commonly *methadone*). The dose given is just sufficient to prevent withdrawal symptoms. Over a period of weeks (governed by the severity) the dose of the substitute is reduced gradually, during which time whatever biochemical imbalance was responsible for the syndrome returns to normal (page 45). Intense psychiatric supervision is necessary. Following this the patient is clinically cured. The difficult part is the rehabilitation that must follow.

It should be stressed that the risk of inducing severe dependence in a patient during treatment for acute pain (the 'therapeutic addict') is remote. Treatment of dependence is more relevant to illicitly obtained drugs and in these instances there are complicating factors – pathological, psychological and sociological.

The opioid antagonists

The narcotic antagonists should be considered from two view points:

(1) their use in the treatment of agonist overdose;
(2) the use of mixed agonist antagonist drugs as analgesics in their own right.

Use as antagonists (naloxone)

Naloxone is a more effective antagonist at μ-receptors than at κ- or δ-receptors. Thus 10 times less **naloxone** is needed to antagonize **morphine** than to antagonize **pentazocine.** The characteristics of the antagonism in all cases are competitive. The major use of **naloxone** is in reversal of postoperative respiratory depression, notably in the neonate. **Naloxone** has a short duration of action (30 min).

All derivatives possessing antagonist activity will precipitate the withdrawal syndrome in narcotic addicts. The symptoms thus precipitated will appear within seconds and last for 24 h (*cf.* the withdrawal syndrome precipitated by abstinence).

Use of mixed agonist antagonists as analgesics (pentazocine)

The antagonist analgesics share with the pure agonists analgesic, respiratory depressant, cough suppressant, constipative and emetic activities. They differ in that they normally cause dysphoria, they can cause hallucinations (which are normally of a persecutory nature) and they do not cause dependence of the pure μ-receptor agonist type.

Several derivatives are currently available. The two most commonly used are **pentazocine** and **buprenorphine**.

Pentazocine

Pentazocine, an agonist at κ-opioid receptors and antagonist at μ-receptors, has analgesic efficacy similar to *pethidine* and causes dysphoria though hallucinations are uncommon. A very rare form of dependence has been described – it is different from dependence on pure agonists at μ-receptors (even weak agonists like **codeine**). Withdrawal symptoms are abdominal pain, sweating, lacrimation and rhinorrhoea and can be tolerated without medication.

Buprenorphine

Buprenorphine differs from **pentazocine** in that it has a greater efficacy and a much longer duration of action. In addition, both the agonist and antagonist actions of *buprenorphine* appear to be mediated at one opioid receptor type, the μ-receptor. It is therefore a partial agonist. It is strongly sedative and causes neither euphoria nor dysphoria. Psychotic effects have not been reported. Vomiting (especially in the ambulatory patient) may be more frequent than that characteristic of the group. The drug may be administered parenterally, sublingually and orally. **Naloxone** is not an effective antagonist when injected after *buprenorphine*, though it can prevent its action when given before. *Doxapram* (page 238) is an effective antidote to *buprenorphine* overdosage.

Stimulants and hallucinogens

Though one transmitter may be excitatory at one site and inhibitory at another, it is possible to generalize that some transmitters are more likely to be excitatory and others inhibitory – glycine and GABA generally inhibit neuronal activity in the CNS.

Stimulants either enhance excitation or antagonize inhibition. Following drug-induced excitation there is commonly a phase of depression.

Stimulants

Centrally acting sympathomimetics

Amphetamine causes stimulation throughout the CNS, particularly of the reticular formation. This, in combination with other actions (*see below*) results in prolonged alertness, postponement of fatigue, motor stimulation, suppression of appetite (anorexia), confusion and anxiety. Hallucinations are rare. It is a potent peripheral sympathomimetic amine (page 99).

Its central mechanisms of action include release of NA and dopamine (it causes a behaviour pattern characteristic of other agonists at dopamine receptors), release of 5-HT, inhibition of monoamine uptake and inhibition of MAO.

Whilst the *d*- and *l*-isomers have equal potency in the periphery, dexamphetamine [dextroamphetamine] is twice as potent as a central stimulant.

Acute poisoning is characterized by delirium and autonomic symptoms. Treatment involves acidification of urine to promote excretion (page 364) and **chlorpromazine** (its antipsychotic and α-adrenoceptor blocking actions are of benefit). Death is due to cardiovascular collapse.

Chronic toxicity poses problems of tolerance, severe psychic dependence and a psychosis almost identical to paranoid schizophrenia.

Common clinical use was as an appetite suppressant, though it is no longer used because newer derivatives cause less central and cardiovascular stimulation and have a low dependence liability. Current use is restricted to the rare condition of narcolepsy.

Structural manipulation of the amphetamine molecule affords more selective derivatives. *Tranylcypromine* has MAO inhibitory activity but causes less stimulation of the autonomic and central nervous systems than amphetamine.

Fenfluramine has anorectic activity but causes no central or autonomic stimulant action. Its mechanism of anorectic action involves 5-HT rather than catecholamines.

Convulsants

Drugs can cause convulsions by many different mechanisms at sites between the spinal cord and cerebral cortex.

Strychnine

Strychnine poisoning is treated with short-acting neuromuscular blocking agents and sedatives (the mechanism of action of strychnine is described on page 215).

Bicuculline and picrotoxin

Bicuculline is a competitive and picrotoxin a functional antagonist of the inhibitory transmitter GABA.

Nikethamide

The mechanism of action of nikethamide is not known. Since the respiratory stimulant dose is lower than the convulsant dose in conscious subjects, it was once used in the treatment of barbiturate poisoning. However, the dose necessary to stimulate respiration in a comatose subject is a convulsant dose and this has led to the abandonment of such drugs. Since then the prognosis for barbiturate poisoning has significantly improved and its incidence decreased.

Doxapram

Unlike nikethamide, the ratio between respiratory stimulant and convulsant doses is acceptable and *doxapram* is used as a respiratory stimulant when no more specific method is available. Its relative selectivity of action may be related to peripheral stimulation of chemoceptors.

Whilst some of the above drugs have negligible clinical use, several are valuable in neurophysiological and pharmacological research.

Methylxanthines

The related alkaloids *caffeine* and *theophylline* have useful central and peripheral actions. They stimulate the CNS, skeletal and cardiac muscle, relax smooth muscle and cause diuresis.

For central stimulation *caffeine* is much more potent than *theophylline*. At oral doses of 200 mg, *caffeine* postpones fatigue, with no adverse effects. A cup of strong tea or coffee contains about 150 mg *caffeine*. The lethal dose in man is so high as to be unknown.

For cardiac stimulation, smooth muscle relaxation and diuresis *theophylline* is more potent than *caffeine*. *See* page 136 for a further description of their peripheral actions and mechanisms of action.

Appetite and centrally acting anorectic drugs

The complex control of appetite involves many regions of the brain but is integrated from the hypothalamus. Of the neurotransmitters that have direct or indirect involvement in feeding behaviour, the most studied are the catecholamines and 5-HT but more recently attention has been focused on some peptides, notably the opioid peptides.

In the past amphetamine was widely used to suppress appetite. It is a potent and effective drug. Now its use is not recommended because it causes pronounced peripheral sympathetic stimulation, often unsurmountable difficulties in sleep and chronic CNS toxicity, notably dependence and psychosis. Several derivatives of amphetamine are available that are less effective though are proportionately safer. Their mechanism of anorectic action is mediated by catecholamines.

The anorectic action of **fenfluramine,** though it is chemically related to amphetamine, is mediated by the release of 5-HT. **Fenfluramine** is almost as effective as amphetamine but causes negligible sympathetic change (acute poisoning is unaccompanied by significant cardiovascular change) and the drug has a generally sedative profile.

If a drug is deemed necessary to assist a patient to follow a reducing diet, **fenfluramine** remains the only recommended drug.

Appetite stimulation is produced as an adverse effect by the antipsychotic drugs (antagonism of catecholamines and 5-HT) and by the anxiolytics (which may imply a role for GABA in the feeding centres).

Hallucinogens

A hallucination is a sense perception not based on objective reality. Though normally thought of as visual, drugs can alter all the senses (tactile, auditory, taste, pain).

Many drugs cause hallucinations by affecting various neurotransmitters. In few cases is the mechanism of action fully understood. In effect, however, hallucinogens cause a failure of sensory input control resulting in a flooding of the perception and stimulation, via collaterals, of the reticular formation but note that not all hallucinogens in the following list can be classified as 'stimulants'. Hallucinogens also enhance attentional processes (*Figure 5.11*).

Centrally acting sympathomimetics

Whilst amphetamine (page 236) can occasionally cause hallucinations following parenteral administration, its methoxylated derivatives (mescaline, dimethoxymethylamphetamine) are potent hallucinogens. They cause vivid visual hallucinations, though the mechanism is unknown.

Lysergic acid diethylamide

LSD causes vivid visual hallucinations. The mechanism is presumed to stem from its ability to interact with the central neurotransmitter 5-HT.

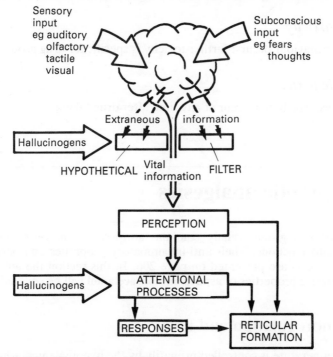

Figure 5.11 Possible aetiology of hallucinations: in this model for the processing of information in the brain, hallucinogens cause both a breakdown of the input filter and heightened attentional process

Cocaine

Cocaine causes euphoria, indifference to pain and tactile hallucinations. The mechanism is presumed to be related to inhibition of central neurotransmitter uptake (page 104).

Narcotic antagonist analgesics

Pentazocine causes dysphoria and visual hallucinations that are commonly persecutory. The mechanism is presumed to be interference with endorphins and enkephalins.

Nitrous oxide

Nitrous oxide lowers the sensory threshold causing notably auditory distortion. The mechanism is unknown: it may involve interaction with endorphins and enkephalins.

Cannabis

The main active constituent of cannabis is δ^9-tetrahydrocannabinol. It lowers the sensory threshold and causes euphoria and time distortion.

Hallucinogens have no therapeutic use as such.

Acute toxicity

Bizarre behaviour occurs; further toxicity is specific for drug group.

Chronic toxicity

Psychoses, which may occur at any time after drug taking.

Antipyretic analgesics

Drugs of this group usually combine antipyretic, analgesic and anti-inflammatory actions. Their anti-inflammatory properties and peripheral adverse effects are presented on page 206. In this section the antipyretic and analgesic properties of **aspirin** and **paracetamol** will be covered.

Thermoregulation and fever

Body temperature is controlled primarily by the hypothalamus, which acts like a thermostat and also as an integration centre for sensory information from deep body (core) and environmental (cutaneous) thermoceptors.

Hypothalamic outflow to peripheral effector systems controls body temperature. Thermoregulation is initially by either heat conservation (cutaneous vasoconstriction, piloerection) or a reduction in thermogenesis (rest). If further adjustment is necessary to maintain body temperature, increased thermogenesis (voluntary exercise, shivering) or active heat loss (cutaneous vasodilatation, sweating, panting in animals) is initiated.

In fever (for example, as a result of infection or after injection of pyrogenic substances) the hypothalamic thermostat behaves as if it had been reset at a higher temperature. Thus effectors raise the core temperature so that it is higher than normal (febrile state). Peptides (for example, interleukin-1 and tumour necrosis factor), released from macrophages involved in the immune response to infection, mediate fever. These endogenous pyrogens increase synthesis of PGs of the E series, which appear to be the final chemical mediators of fever. PGs have been detected in the cerebrospinal fluid (CSF) of febrile animals and hypothalamic injection of PGEs causes fever.

Pain

The role of the various central neurotransmitters in the response to pain is as yet poorly understood. Enkephalins (page 216) may be involved but other substances including substance P and the PGs, particularly when the pain involves a peripheral inflammatory response, have been implicated.

Aspirin

Antipyretic action

Aspirin acts as though to reset the central thermostat to its prefebrile level so that the abnormally high core temperature is detected and heat loss effectors (for example, sweating) are brought into play. **Aspirin** does not reduce core temperature when the thermostat is operating normally or when the body temperature is otherwise elevated (for example, during excessive physical exercise).

Aspirin inhibits a febrile response and at the same time prevents the appearance of PGs in the CSF. Thus it has been argued that by inhibiting cyclo-oxygenase aspirin prevents the production of the eicosanoid mediators of fever.

Analgesic action

Aspirin analgesia has a peripheral component particularly when inflammation is the origin of pain. In addition, a central component seems likely (*see* **paracetamol**) and **aspirin** is useful for the relief of many kinds of mild pain.

Other CNS actions

In high doses **aspirin** first causes stimulation and then depression of the CNS. Stimulation of respiration leads to a fall in $PaCO_2$ (respiratory alkalosis). Compensation occurs by bicarbonate loss in the urine so that the plasma bicarbonate concentration falls. Later, in more severe poisoning, lactic and ketoacids accumulate in the blood due to interference with normal carbohydrate and fat metabolism (metabolic acidosis). Confusion, dizziness, tinnitus (ringing in the ears) and high-tone deafness can occur and as the dose is increased delirium, psychosis, stupor and coma may ensue. Nausea and vomiting may occur, and though there is a peripheral component (gastric irritation), a central effect is also involved since iv **aspirin** can cause vomiting that is abolished by ablation of the medullary CTZ. Dehydration from vomiting, sweating and overbreathing is severe.

Aspirin is thought to cause a rare, but often fatal, syndrome (Reye's) of liver and brain damage in children with chicken pox or influenza. Consequently **paracetamol,** not **aspirin,** is the antipyretic analgesic drug of choice in children aged under 12 years, unless **aspirin** is specifically indicated (for example, juvenile rheumatoid arthritis).

Paracetamol

Antipyretic and analgesic actions

Paracetamol is approximately equipotent with **aspirin** as an antipyretic and analgesic but differs from **aspirin** in that it lacks anti-inflammatory action. This is because **paracetamol** inhibits peripheral cyclo-oxygenase less than it does the central enzyme. This indicates that **paracetamol** has a central component to its analgesic action. The mechanism of the central action is not known but differs from that of opioid analgesics.

Other CNS actions

In some individuals relaxation, drowsiness and euphoria have been reported following ingestion of **paracetamol** but this may be related to relief from pain rather than a direct action on the CNS. After very high doses CNS stimulation, excitement and delirium may occur followed by sedation and stupor.

Other toxic effects are mainly peripheral in origin with delayed liver damage being the most serious consequence of acute overdosage and renal damage being possible after chronic abuse. Liver damage may be less with *benorylate* (aspirin-paracetamol ester) or concurrent administration of *acetylcysteine* (alternative source of —SH groups for toxic metabolite of **paracetamol** – page 327).

Many proprietary mixtures that include **aspirin** or **paracetamol** are available as are preparations in which **aspirin** is presented in a soluble form. The application of such preparations is discussed on pages 402 and 431.

The state of consciousness and the general anaesthetic agents

When given in large enough doses the structurally nonspecific drugs are capable of depressing the activity of all excitable cells. Some general observations concerning the activity of structurally nonspecific drugs are outlined elsewhere (page 4). The state of anaesthesia, which occurs with lower doses of these agents, involves a loss of consciousness with minimal depression of other brain functions. A simplistic approach is to say that anaesthesia is a depression of neuronal functions, those responsible for consciousness being the most vulnerable. However, there is a lack of understanding of the basic mechanisms of consciousness and thus of its modification by drugs. It may be that recent developments identifying enhanced neurotransmission by the inhibitory transmitter GABA or antagonism of excitatory transmission as selective actions of some agents in this group are relevant to the mechanism of anaesthetic action.

Table 5.2 Structurally nonspecific drugs

Organic solvents		
Clinically useful	General anaesthetic agents:	diethyl ether, *isoflurane*, **halothane**
Socially used	Ethanol	
Clinically useless	Acetone, petrol	
Iv anaesthetic agents	**Thiopentone**	
Sedatives and hypnotics	*Chloral hydrate*, **diazepam**, some barbiturates	

The physiological basis of sleep and consciousness

The reticular formation contains areas responsible for the sleep/wake cycle (reticular activating system). The sleep and wake centres have inherent rhythmicity and are mutually inhibitory. The wake centre is dominant. Their regular control of the cycle is influenced by many factors which can:

(1) maintain wakefulness – unusual sensory stimuli (noise, light, pain), excessive limbic activity (anxiousness), mental disorders (anxiety, depression), a will to stay awake and various unsatisfied urges;
(2) encourage sleep – absence of the above.

Consciousness, on the other hand, is believed to be the responsibility of the cortex. Sleep/wake cycles are still observed in animals or children in whom the cortex is absent or virtually destroyed. Automatic responses occur but no signs are shown of awareness of self and environment. It is likely, but impossible to prove, that such animals or humans lack consciousness.

Sleep and insomnia

The depth of sleep can be measured by electroencephalogram recordings (*Figure 5.12* illustrates typical records) although behavioural changes do not always correlate with the EEG record.

Note the fast electrical activity of 'alertness'; α-rhythm (typical of drowsiness, eyes closed); the bursts of activity during sleep (spindling) and the δ-waves (high voltage, low frequency) of deep sleep.

There is an additional stage of sleep called paradoxical sleep. This is

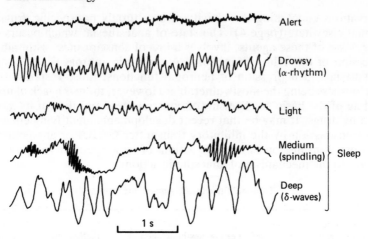

Figure 5.12 Electroencephalogram patterns

characterized by rapid eye movements (REM sleep), an increase in electrical activity, difficulty in arousing the subject and dreaming.

The course of a night's sleep is usually constant with deep sleep occurring early and the incidence and duration of paradoxical sleep increasing as the course of sleep progresses. Paradoxical sleep is thought to be a psychological necessity and its reduction (by drugs) undesirable.

Anxiety is the most common cause of insomnia characterized by difficulty in getting to sleep, followed by ingestion of caffeine-containing drinks and then pain. The pattern of insomnia in patients suffering from depression is, instead, early awakening.

There is no drug that causes natural sleep. The drugs usually used to treat insomnia are the relatively selective anxiolytics (**temazepam**), which reduce the cause of insomnia and encourage more natural sleep. Insomnia due to pain can rationally be treated with analgesics and that due to depression responds to antidepressive drugs.

Anaesthesia

Anaesthesia refers to a reversible drug-induced absence of all awareness and sensation.

Anaesthetic agents reduce the overall activity of all parts of the brain in a predictable order. A progressive depression descends through the CNS, the cortex (loss of inhibition leading to excitation), the mid brain (sedation leading to anaesthesia), the spinal cord (loss of reflexes) and finally medulla (respiratory and vasomotor depression leading to death).

Stages and planes of anaesthesia

These were defined many years ago for diethyl ether without premedication and were based on observations of peripheral manifestations of the progressive depression of the CNS, notably change in pupil size, skeletal muscle tone, respiratory pattern, eye movements and the presence or absence of various reflexes (corneal, laryngeal, pharyngeal). With the replacement of diethyl ether by other anaesthetic agents and the use of preanaesthetic medication the historic stages and planes are less relevant to modern anaesthesia.

The most useful index of the stage of surgical anaesthesia is the absence (or near absence) of sympathetic responses to pain (BP, heart rate, pupil size). Pupil size (constricted) and respiratory pattern (diaphragmatic assuming the patient is breathing spontaneously) are also confirmatory indices.

Each anaesthetic agent produces a different pattern of EEG changes, although, in general, there is an increase in electrical activity equivalent to the stage of excitation, a distortion of rhythm equivalent to surgical anaesthesia and electrical silence indicating brain death. The distortion of rhythm during anaesthesia may range from cortical depression to something resembling seizure activity. It has been suggested that there may be a number of different nonconscious CNS states.

The general anaesthetic agents

Since the site of action of these agents is within a lipid phase in the brain, a most important consideration is their ability to reach that phase. This governs the speed of induction of and the recovery from anaesthesia (page 356). Since most lipid soluble compounds (organic solvents) are potentially anaesthetic agents, the only difference between clinically useful and useless agents is whether anaesthesia is or is not accompanied by undesirable effects – petrol is a general anaesthetic agent but causes bronchial irritation, liver and kidney damage.

Inhalational anaesthetic agents

Though a homogeneous group the clinically useful anaesthetic agents differ in the following properties.

Physical properties

Nitrous oxide is a gas at normal temperature and pressure. Some agents are highly inflammable (diethyl ether). **Halothane,** *enflurane* and *isoflurane* have ideal physical properties (they are inert).

Speed of induction

Nitrous oxide is the fastest (the least soluble in blood, page 358), diethyl ether the slowest. **Halothane** is intermediate.

Potency

The volatile anaesthetic agents are more potent than the gases. For example, anaesthetic concentrations are: **nitrous oxide,** > 100%; **halothane,** 2%.

Analgesic activity

It is not an inevitable property of an anaesthetic agent that it is also an analgesic at subanaesthetic concentrations. **Nitrous oxide** is a potent analgesic while **halothane** has no selective analgesic properties. Alone among anaesthetic agents **nitrous oxide** is used as an analgesic (for example, in labour and in emergency pain relief before hospital admission) at concentrations of about 50%. The mechanism of its analgesic action is release of opioid peptides.

Muscle relaxation

Major surgery requires neuromuscular blocking agents, though diethyl ether causes some peripheral neuromuscular blockade (*Table 2.3*, page 77).

Production of cardiac dysrhythmias

Most anaesthetic agents containing a halogen can sensitize the myocardium to the actions of catecholamines causing dysrhythmias. *Enflurane* and *isoflurane* are less likely to cause dysrhythmias than **halothane.**

Hypotension and respiratory depression

Medullary depression occurs with high doses of all anaesthetic agents, though if respiration is maintained artificially medullary depression is usually unimportant.

Liver damage

Liver damage is a common toxic action of organic solvents. Modern anaesthetic agents are relatively free from this toxicity but those that are extensively biotransformed (**halothane**) may be hepatotoxic particularly following repeated administrations. *Isoflurane* is not extensively biotransformed.

Summary

The most commonly used inhalational anaesthetic is a mixture of **nitrous oxide** (50–70%) and **halothane** (1%) although the use of alternatives to **halothane** is increasing.

Intravenous anaesthetic agents

The advantages of iv anaesthesia are: rapid (a few seconds) and pleasant induction, simple equipment, little postoperative vomiting, short duration, no respiratory irritation.

The disadvantages are: inability to control depth of anaesthesia easily, severe respiratory and vasomotor depression (especially in the shocked patient) and local irritation at the injection site.

Note that the anaesthetic agents are at the limits of solubility since they must be both lipid in nature (to act) and miscible with blood. Some unusual solvents are necessary to effect solution and these may contribute to local inflammation or more general toxicity (anaphylaxis).

Thiopentone sodium and *methohexitone sodium* are barbiturate derivatives whilst *propofol* is a hindered phenol. They are widely used. Specific disadvantages of barbiturates are necrosis on extravascular injection and fatal exacerbation of acute intermittent porphyria (page 31). This disease is an absolute contraindication to administration of any barbiturate. *Propofol* may cause pain on injection. Recovery from the iv anaesthetic agents currently available is due to drug redistribution (page 313). The speed of subsequent metabolism is *propofol* > *methohexitone sodium* > **thiopentone sodium.**

Diazepam (*see below*) and *midazolam* are not really classified as anaesthetic agents but are used extensively by the iv route to cause deep sedation. *Midazolam*, unlike **diazepam,** is water soluble and causes less irritation at the injection site.

Preanaesthetic and postanaesthetic medication

Drugs commonly used before, during and after anaesthesia include: antagonists at muscarinic cholinoceptors (**atropine**) to reduce secretions and stop excess bradycardia; anxiolytics (**temazepam**) to allay anxiety and cause amnesia; antipsychotic drugs (droperidol) to sedate and minimize the risk of vomiting; neuromuscular blocking agents (**suxamethonium, pancuronium**) to cause skeletal muscle relaxation; opioid analgesics (**morphine, pentazocine**) and antagonists of some of the above (**neostigmine, naloxone**).

Neuroleptanalgesia

A technique of preparing a patient for major surgery using a combination of a potent short-acting narcotic analgesic (*fentanyl*) with an antipsychotic (neuroleptic) agent (droperidol). Whilst the patient remains conscious and can (up to a point) follow instructions, such is his 'indifference' to his circumstances that surgery can be performed.

Anxiolytic, sedative and hypnotic agents

Derivatives of the benzodiazepines constitute the vast majority of anxiolytic agents that are, in increasing dose, clinically useful as sedative and hypnotic agents.

Benzodiazepines

These drugs enhance the activity of the inhibitory transmitter GABA by interacting with a receptor associated with, though distinct from, the GABA receptor (page 214). Several endogenous ligands for this receptor have been proposed. Endogenous benzodiazepines have been detected in several animal species and it is clear that plants, if not the animals themselves, can synthesize the structure. Some proposed ligands (those related to β-carbo-line and a large protein known as diazepam binding inhibitor) bind to benzodiazepine receptors but exert pharmacological actions generally op-posite to those of the benzodiazepines (inverse agonists).

Diazepam has a relatively selective action on components of the limbic system (septum, amygdala and hippocampus) thereby reducing anxiety at doses that have little effect on the reticular activating system (that is, little sedative effect). It also has a relaxant effect on skeletal muscle (mediated centrally) of value in the treatment of anxiety in which skeletal muscle tone is increased.

It causes amnesia and whilst this is undesirable in patients taking the drug long term, it can be valuable in preanaesthetic medication (for example, in dentistry).

It possesses anticonvulsant activity (page 417), has a long $t_\frac{1}{2}$ and the drug can accumulate.

As is characteristic of the drug group **diazepam** has neither antidepressive nor antipsychotic properties.

Unwanted effects are common to similar drugs: lapses in attention, drowsiness and sedation (caution – performance at use of machinery or driving may be adversely affected). Its actions summate with similar drugs (*Table 5.2*). Psychic and physical dependence can develop (page 44).

More than a dozen benzodiazepine depressants are currently available. The clinical differences between these are negligible. The custom of using some (chlordiazepoxide) for day time alleviation of anxiety and others (*nitrazepam*) for night time sedation probably reflects either marketing policy or the relative doses in available preparations (page 406).

Actual differences are as follows.

Duration of action

For anxiolytic use long durations of action are generally preferred (**diazepam,** chlordiazepoxide). For insomnia drugs with shorter durations are generally preferred causing less hangover effect and less motor impairment the following morning (**temazepam**). This distinction is important in the elderly with impaired liver function.

Cost

The longer established derivatives (**diazepam**) are about 10 times less expen-sive than the newer drugs. This difference is important in view of the 20 million or so prescriptions for the drugs dispensed each year.

Benzodiazepine antagonists

Antagonists at the benzodiazepine receptor antagonize both the benzodia-zepine agonists and the inverse agonists. The most widely studied is **flumaze-nil.** It antagonizes **diazepam** in volunteers and has been used clinically in the management of benzodiazepine poisoning. It also finds a use in reversing the deep sedation of iv benzodiazepines used in anaesthesia. **Flumazenil** vir-tually lacks pharmacological activity when given alone.

The alcohols

The alcohols are nonspecific depressants – ethanol being the derivative with fewest adverse effects. It is widely used in self medication, for social purposes and as an anxiolytic.

The sequence of events is illustrated by ethanol (a weak general anaesthetic agent):

 (1) tranquillization (removal of anxiety);
 (2) excitation (loquaciousness, recklessness);
 (3) dysarthria (slurring of speech);
 (4) ataxia (staggering);
 (5) sedation;
 (6) hypnosis (loss of consciousness);
 (7) anaesthesia;
 (8) coma;
 (9) medullary depression (respiratory and vasomotor centres);
(10) death.

This sequence of events applies to all nonspecific depressants (anxiolytic, sedative, hypnotic and inhalational and iv anaesthetic agents). The only differences are speed of induction and margin of safety. The terms 'anxiolytic', 'sedative', 'hypnotic' and 'anaesthetic' drugs have been used but it is more accurate to think in terms of anxiolytic, sedative, hypnotic or anaesthetic doses of drugs.

Excessive consumption of ethanol leads to dependence (page 44), psychosis and liver damage.

Dose of ethanol in available beverages

Approximately the same amount of ethanol (7 g) is contained in a half pint of bitter beer, a single measure of spirits, a glass of sherry or of wine. The apparent volume of distribution, V, is about 0.7 l/kg, that in males being greater than that in females. Elimination is normally by zero order kinetics at a rate of 15 (mg/dl)/h.

The drug is oxidized in the liver by the route shown in *Figure 7.9* (page 315). Note the toxic acetaldehyde in the pathway but as the aldehyde dehydrogenase step is normally rapid it does not accumulate.

Some drugs (**metronidazole,** page 263 and *chlorpropamide*, page 187) are inhibitors of aldehyde dehydrogenase and ethanol consumption is contraindicated during therapy with them. Disulfiram is an inhibitor of aldehyde dehydrogenase and is useful in the aversion treatment of ethanol addiction. During disulfiram treatment, if the patient takes ethanol, acetaldehyde accumulates and causes unpleasant effects including nausea and vomiting.

The central pharmacology of methanol is identical to that of ethanol. It is also biotransformed via the same pathway (*see Figure 7.9*) but the enzymes are less capable of handling formaldehyde and formic acid. These accumulate and cause blindness (chronic toxicity) or severe acidosis (acute toxicity).

Poisoning by a third commercially available alcohol, ethylene glycol (antifreeze), is characterized by CNS depression (coma, respiratory depression) and severe nephrotoxicity.

Chloral and its derivatives

The pharmacological properties of chloral and its derivatives are due to their biotransformation to trichloroethanol.

They are used at sedative and hypnotic doses, are relatively safe and are useful as sedatives in children.

Chloral hydrate is potentially an anaesthetic agent but its safety margin is too low for this usage. Gastric irritation often occurs and the drug should always be taken in dilute form and never on an empty stomach. Allergic reactions (urticaria, erythema) sometimes occur.

Triclofos sodium is a more palatable complex of *chloral hydrate* and gastric irritation rarely occurs.

Patterns of dependence on chloral derivatives are similar to ethanol dependence. Poisoning is treated in the same way as barbiturate poisoning.

The barbiturates

Structural modification of barbituric acid (itself without CNS activity) leads to hypnotic, sedative and anaesthetic agents that differ only in their time to onset and duration of activity.

The only justifiable clinical uses of barbiturates are:

(1) the specific use of *phenobarbitone* as an antiepileptic drug (page 416);
(2) the use of **thiopentone sodium** and *methohexitone sodium* as iv anaesthetic agents (page 246).

Although many barbiturate derivatives of intermediate duration of action have been used as sedatives and hypnotics in the past and are still commercially available (amylobarbitone, butobarbitone) they are no longer recommended. Since 1985 these barbiturates have been included in the Misuse of Drugs Act.

Barbiturate poisoning and its treatment

The characteristics of barbiturate poisoning are: coma; hypothermia; shallow, regular and infrequent breathing; hypotension, imperceptible pulse. Death is usually due to inhalation of vomit.

The treatment of poisoning is artificial ventilation, forced diuresis and intensive care. The practice of using nonspecific CNS stimulants (*nikethamide*, amphetamine) has been virtually abandoned.

Antagonists at β-adrenoceptors

In patients in whom acute anxiety might impair performance drastically and crucially, the reduction in sympathetic symptoms can cause welcome relief. This particularly applies in 'one off' occasions (interviews, examinations, auditions). In these instances antagonists at β-adrenoceptors are preferable to benzodiazepines if medication is deemed necessary.

Antagonists at H₁ histamine receptors

Phenothiazine antihistamines with sedative action are used as sedatives. *Promethazine* is available without prescription.

Tolerance and dependence

The definitions of tolerance and dependence are given elsewhere (pages 234 and 44).

Tolerance is due to two components:

(1) induction of liver MFO enzymes that accelerate drug biotransformation – most of the depressants are biotransformed to an appreciable extent even if this is not the mechanism of recovery (**thiopentone sodium, halothane**);

(2) an unknown mechanism other than the above, which is presumably at the level of the biophase in the CNS. Note that this tolerance is apparent during the time course of action of a single dose. For instance, the blood ethanol concentration at recovery of normal gait is significantly higher than that at the onset of observable intoxication (for example, ataxia). On full recovery from massive **diazepam** overdose, very high plasma concentrations of drug may persist.

Cross tolerance exists between all members of the group though cross tolerance is most marked between members of the same chemical group (for example, barbiturates).

All of the members of this group are drugs of psychic and physical dependence and are the most common cause of addiction in the UK (there are about 500 000 ethanol addicts). The severity of dependence is a function of the potency of the drugs (barbiturates the greatest, benzodiazepines the least); the incidence is a function of availability (ethanol the greatest). More than a million people in the UK have been taking benzodiazepines for over a year.

Symptoms of dependence are tolerance, adjustment of life style around periods of drug taking, anxiety, amnesia, sluggishness, nutritional deficiencies and ataxia.

Symptoms of withdrawal are craving, tremor, anxiety, hallucinations and, if severe, grand mal convulsions. Deaths have occurred during withdrawal.

Assuming regular drug taking, the time for development of dependence is a function of potency (barbiturates a few months, ethanol and benzodiazepines longer).

Treatment involves hospitalization, gradual reduction in drug intake (and where applicable switching to a less potent drug) and intensive psychiatric supervision.

Anticonvulsant drugs

Epileptic seizures are due to the presence in a part of the brain of unstable neuronal membranes (an ectopic focus) that can fire off spontaneously at high frequency (100 Hz). The attack is self potentiating by positive feedback (post-tetanic potentiation). The result depends on the location of the lesion – momentary loss of consciousness, restricted movement of a limb, pain (trigeminal neuralgia) or generalized motor and autonomic changes.

Anticonvulsant drugs act by reducing the post-tetanic potentiation, rather than by stabilizing the membranes of the ectopic focus.

Since antagonists of GABA cause convulsions and mimics are anticonvulsant, recent attention has concentrated on this neurotransmitter but this should not be to the exclusion of other neurotransmitter involvement.

Anticonvulsant drugs range from *phenobarbitone* (a fairly nonspecific depressant of brain function), the benzodiazepines (which enhance GABA systems by a receptor mediated mechanism) to **sodium valproate**, which is an inhibitor of GABA aminotransferase (page 214). In the grey area between is **phenytoin**. The fact that **phenytoin** additionally has antidysrhythmic activity may suggest a membrane stabilizing action.

The kinds of epilepsy and methods of treatment are described in detail on page 414.

6

Antiparasitic chemotherapy

Aims

After studying this section you should be able to:

- name each of the principal current agents useful in antiparasitic chemotherapy and chemoprophylaxis;
- describe the mechanism of its cytotoxic action;
- describe the basis of its selectivity (a) towards parasite rather than host cells, and (b) towards some parasites rather than others;
- indicate something of its useful place in therapeutics;
- indicate something of its adverse effects and disadvantages.

Introduction

The first part of this section deals with how the selectivity of action of agents useful in antiparasitic chemotherapy has been achieved. On pages 254–264 those antiparasitic chemotherapeutic agents exhibiting biochemically based selectivity are classified according to their mechanisms of primary cytotoxic action with cross-reference to their therapeutic use. On pages 264–268 those antiparasitic chemotherapeutic agents exhibiting distributionally based selectivity are classified according to their mechanisms of differential disposition with cross-reference both to their mechanism of primary cytotoxic action and to their therapeutic use. The remainder of the section places these same drugs, and others found empirically to be selective but by as yet unknown mechanisms, in a therapeutic context by classifying the parasitisms with back reference to the mechanisms of toxicity and selectivity of the useful antiparasitic drugs.

Definitions

Antiparasitic chemotherapy is the treatment of symptomatic parasitism with chemicals of known constitution. Human parasitisms fall into three groups:

(1) infestation of organs with metazoa (insects, arachnids, worms);
(2) infection of tissues or cells with unicellular organisms (protozoa, fungi, bacteria, Rickettsiae, Chlamydiae, viruses);

(3) invasion of organs or tissues by aberrant human cells (malignant neoplasms).

Cytotoxicity means direct injury to, or disturbance of function of, cells. The injury may be reversible or irreversible, structural or functional. The cytotoxic action may result in the death of cells (cytocidal effect) or prevention of their multiplication (cytostatic effect) without cell death. In the latter case the body's chemical (antibody) and cellular (phagocytic) defence mechanisms can usually clear the residual static infecting population. Most antiparasitic drugs can be cytocidal in high concentration and cytostatic in lower concentration: which is seen in practice depends on the body concentration attained with normal therapeutic doses.

The scale of measurement of cytotoxic action is really a continuous quantitative one (median cytotoxic concentration) but is often expressed less numerately as sensitivity or resistance of a parasite to clinically attainable concentrations of a chemotherapeutic agent. If a parasite population acquires increased resistance (reduced sensitivity) to a chemotherapeutic agent it also shows cross-resistance to other agents sharing the same mechanism of cytotoxic action.

When we say that the cytotoxic action of a drug exhibits selectivity we mean that the drug affects one kind of cell more than another. The cytotoxic action of a drug is said to be qualitatively selective when that drug affects one kind of cell but does not affect a second kind of cell. The cytotoxic action of a drug is said to be quantitatively selective when the drug at a given dose injures one kind of cell more that a second kind of cell or the drug injures one kind of cell at a dose lower than that required to injure a second kind of cell.

The scale of measurement of selective toxicity is the chemotherapeutic index, which in animal models of parasitism =

$$\frac{\text{the median toxic dose to the host}}{\text{the median curative dose}}$$

More conservatively expressed in patient terms,
the chemotherapeutic index =

$$\frac{\text{the threshold dose toxic to some patients}}{\text{the minimum dose curative for most patients}}$$

The basic assumption of human antiparasitic chemotherapy is that parasite cells differ from human cells. By chemical exploitation of these differences, toxicity to the parasite can be achieved without harm to the host. There are many ways of classifying these differences (and hence the origin of selectivity). We shall adopt a two-way classification into biochemical and distributional bases of selectivity.

Biochemical selectivity

The action of a chemotherapeutic agent exhibits biochemical selectivity when that agent is more toxic to parasite than to host cells, even when the sites of toxic action in both are exposed to the same drug concentration. This may be a qualitative difference (cell wall synthesis, page 255; dihydropteroate synthetase, page 256; anaerobic energy metabolism, page 263) or only a quantitative one (dihydrofolate reductase, page 257; thymidine kinase, page 258; DNA polymerase, page 260; RNA polymerase, page 260; cytoplasmic membrane, page 262).

Mechanism of toxic action

This may be one that makes the chemotherapeutic agent cytotoxic to all phases of the parasite's life cycle, including the adult resting phase (cytoplasmic membrane, page 262; energy-yielding metabolism, page 263; muscle, page 263).

Alternatively, it may be one that makes the chemotherapeutic agent cytotoxic only to parasites in the rapid growth and multiplication phase of their life cycle (cell wall synthesis, page 255; nucleic acid synthesis and replication, page 259; protein synthesis, page 260).

Mechanisms of cytotoxicity in cells undergoing rapid growth and multiplication

Inhibition of cell wall synthesis

Bacterial and fungal, unlike mammalian, cells provide themselves with an exoskeletal cell wall. The cell wall performs the important function of protecting the cell from osmotic damage. When cell wall synthesis is prevented, dividing bacterial and fungal cells swell and lyse if growing in a hypotonic medium. Drugs that interfere with the synthesis of cell wall material therefore show a qualitative, biochemically selective action.

Penicillins, cephalosporins and *vancomycin* inhibit the formation of the insoluble mucopeptide peptidoglycan (murein), which is a major constituent of the cell wall of Gram-positive bacteria and Gram-negative cocci (*Figure 6.1*). It is in part formed of *d*-alanine.

Penicillins, (**benzylpenicillin** [penicillin G], page 286) and the closely related cephalosporins (*cephradine*, page 289) are structural analogues of *d*-alanyl-*d*-alanine. These drugs act exterior to the cell membrane. They inhibit the process of transpeptidation, a cross-linking reaction in which soluble peptidoglycan precursors emerging from the cell membrane are linked to the insoluble, growing peptidoglycan chain. They have similar spectra of antibacterial activity, basically all Gram-positive bacteria and Gram-negative cocci are sensitive. They are the most biochemically selective antimicrobial agents available. Resistant bacteria secrete a β-lactamase enzyme (penicillinase or cephalosporase) that hydrolyses and inactivates the drug. Individual members of this group have significant differences in properties and use.

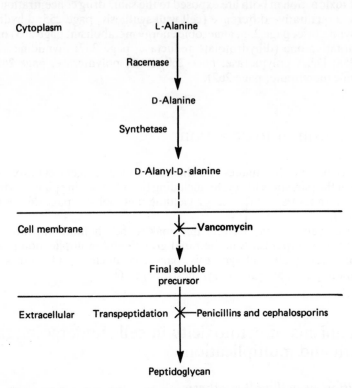

Figure 6.1 Overview of the synthetic pathway from alanine to peptidoglycan

Vancomycin binds to the *d*-alanyl-*d*-alanine portion of the final soluble precursor of peptidoglycan and inhibits its cleavage from a membrane phospholipid carrier. Exteriorization of the peptidoglycan precursor and its cross-linking to the growing peptidoglycan chain are therefore prevented. It is bactericidal to Gram-positive organisms.

Inhibition of nucleic acid synthesis

Interference with supply of precursors

Pteridine coenzyme precursors are essential for the synthesis of purine and pyrimidine bases. Because cells have stores of preformed intermediates there is a long lag time between an attack upon an early stage of this replicative metabolic pathway and the resulting inhibition of growth and multiplication.

Many bacteria, unlike mammalian cells, cannot absorb folate and so utilize aminobenzoate to synthesize dihydrofolate (DHF) (*Figure 6.2*).

Drugs that interfere with the synthesis of DHF from aminobenzoate

Since mammalian cells do not synthesize DHF from aminobenzoate,

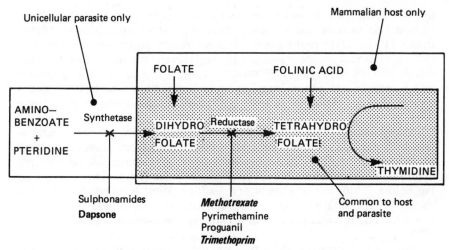

Figure 6.2 The folate pathway and its inhibitors

inhibitors of dihydropteroate synthetase necessarily show qualitative biochemical selectivity. Such inhibitors include sulphonamides and sulphones.

All are structural analogues of aminobenzoate (*Figure 6.3*) and compete with it for dihydropteroate synthetase; the enzymes make a functionless DHF analogue from sulphonamides.

Sulphonamides (sulphamethoxazole) have a patchy spectrum of bacteriostatic and antimalarial activity. They may cause renal toxicity unrelated to their effect on aminobenzoate metabolism (page 292). Sulphones (*dapsone*) are exploited in the treatment of the bacterial infection leprosy and of the protozoal infection malaria.

Drugs that interfere with the synthesis of tetrahydrofolate (THF) from DHF

Methotrexate, pyrimethamine, *proguanil* and **trimethoprim** can only show a quantitative biochemical selectivity. They are all structural analogues of DHF that inhibit DHF reductase (*Figure 6.2*).

Methotrexate is a large and complex analogue that cannot penetrate into bacteria and protozoa. However, it enters mammalian cells by the folate

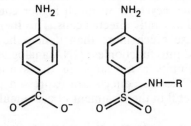

Para-aminobenzoate   A sulphonamide

Figure 6.3 Structural analogy of sulphonamides to para-aminobenzoate

uptake mechanism. It only shows quantitative selectivity for cells with the highest THF turnover (most rapid cell division). It has a much higher affinity than DHF for DHF hydrogenase so it is virtually an irreversible inhibitor (folic acid cannot compete successfully and thereby overcome its effects but folinic acid, by supplying THF directly, can). It can cure choriocarcinoma and is useful (with other drugs) in acute leukaemias. The host toxicity is typical of drugs acting on cell populations with rapid multiplication (page 299).

Pyrimethamine has a simpler structure that allows passive penetration into parasites. It inhibits DHF hydrogenase from malaria parasites much more than the homologous enzymes from mammalian or bacterial sources (it shows quantitative biochemical selectivity). There is a long lag before inhibition of growth and multiplication is effected. Thus it is useless in the treatment of clinical malaria but a valuable prophylactic agent for nonimmune persons in an area where malaria is endemic (page 277).

Proguanil is a prodrug; the active principle formed from it in the body has properties very like those of pyrimethamine.

Trimethoprim is another simple DHF analogue that is able to diffuse into parasite cells. It inhibits DHF hydrogenase from bacterial sources (and malaria parasites) much more than the homologous enzyme from mammalian sources (it shows quantitative biochemical selectivity). There is a long lag before inhibition of growth and multiplication is effected. It is combined with a sulphonamide (sulphamethoxazole) as *co-trimoxazole* to achieve very efficient synergism by sequential blockade of the THF synthetic pathway (*Figure 6.2*).

Drugs that interfere with the supply of nucleoside and nucleotide precursors of DNA

Some structural analogues of purines and pyrimidines are incorporated into the cell's metabolic pathways causing the synthesis of functionless intermediates that suppress nucleic acid synthesis.

Purine analogues

Acyclovir is a guanine analogue (acycloguanosine) that has much higher affinity for virally coded than mammalian thymidine kinase isoenzyme. This enzyme phosphorylates **acyclovir** so much higher concentrations of acycloGTP are produced in virally infected cells. This then selectively inhibits viral DNA polymerase much more than it does host polymerase, and becomes incorporated into functionless DNA analogues.

Mercaptopurine inhibits many steps in the synthesis and interconversion of purines. Cytotoxic effects are expressed in the most rapidly dividing cells. It is useful in the treatment of acute leukaemias (with other agents).

Azathioprine is a prodrug from which mercaptopurine is released in the body. It is particularly employed as an immunosuppressant in organ transplant recipients.

Pyrimidine analogues

Fluorouracil is incorporated into a false nucleotide that blocks deoxyribonu-cleotide (especially thymidylate) synthesis.

Flucytosine is a prodrug deaminated intracellularly to fluorouracil. It shows distributional selectivity (page 265) for fungi.

Cytarabine generates derivatives that compete with cytidine derivatives and cause profound inhibition of DNA synthesis. Like *fluorouracil*, it shows toxicity limited to rapidly multiplying cell populations and is useful in the palliative treatment of malignant neoplasms.

Drugs that directly interfere with nucleic acid synthesis

Alkylating agents

Nitrogen mustards (**cyclophosphamide,** *chlorambucil*). All effective anti-neoplastic drugs in this class possess two alkylating groups (*cf.* **phenoxyben-zamine** – page 111). The highly reactive cyclic cations formed spontaneously in watery solution (*Figure 6.4*) bind to side-chains of large molecules, especially the guanine codon of DNA. This causes functional damage to the DNA, perhaps by cross-linking it to other macromolecules. Any unbound cyclic cation is spontaneously hydrolysed to an inactive alcohol. The members of this group differ in the rate of the two reactions (production and inactivation of the cyclic cation). They show toxicity limited to rapidly multiplying cell populations and the expected problems for the host (page 299).

Cyclophosphamide is a prodrug metabolically activated by ring cleavage in the liver.

Cisplatin diffuses into cells. The molecule dissociates yielding Cl$^-$ ions

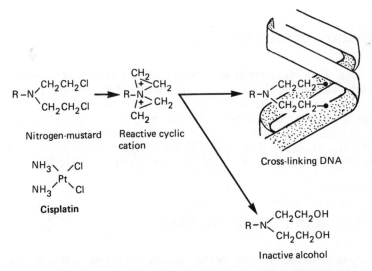

Figure 6.4 (a) The chemical changes in a nitrogen mustard which lead to alkylation and cross-linking of DNA; (b) *cisplatin* also can cross-link adjacent DNA strands

and revealing two reactive sites (*Figure 6.4b*), which bind particularly to the guanine base of DNA cross linking both within and between strands.

Busulphan does not ionize; it alkylates —SH in cysteine and is the treatment of choice in chronic myelogenous leukaemia.

Procarbazine is a hydrazine derivative that binds covalently to DNA.

Intercalating agents

Doxorubicin is a basic antibiotic with a flat ring system that intercalates into DNA between layers of base pairs of the double helix. This disturbs the structure and function of the starter DNA employed by DNA polymerase. It inhibits DNA synthesis at the same high concentration in isolated systems from all cells.

Inhibition of DNA-polymerase

Acyclovir can be regarded as a prodrug from which is generated the selective viral DNA-polymerase inhibitor acycloGTP (page 258).

Inhibition of RNA-polymerase

Rifampicin combines with and inhibits the RNA-polymerase in bacteria but not that in mammalian cells. It is bactericidal to Gram-positive bacteria and *M. tuberculosis* and *leprae* and has low host toxicity. Gram-negative bacteria have a low permeability to rifampicin. It is reserved for use in tuberculosis (page 292) and leprosy.

Inhibition of mitosis

The vinca alkaloids (**vincristine,** *vinblastine*) and *etoposide* (related to podophyllotoxin) bring about an arrest of mitosis in metaphase. In each case this is due to specific and reversible combination with the protein tubulin, though the binding sites differ. This prevents polymerization into microtubules and hence formation of a mitotic spindle. Abnormal nuclear structures result and cell function is so disturbed that cell death often ensues. Cells with the highest replication rate are the most and earliest affected.

Inhibition of protein synthesis

To help in the understanding of this section you should revise the stages of protein synthesis on ribosomes. Most mammalian protein turnover is slow (fibrinogen apart) compared with that associated with cellular multiplication. Quantitative biochemical selectivity, for bacterial rather than mammalian protein synthesis, is possible because bacteria contain only 70S (a measure of their density) ribosomes whereas most mammalian ribosomes are 80S.

Drugs that inhibit tRNA binding to ribosomes

Aminoglycoside antibiotics (**gentamicin**, *streptomycin*) bind irreversibly to the acceptor part of the 30S subunit (*Figure 6.5a*) and distort it so that aminoacyl-tRNA cannot bind to its acceptor site. Some bacteria resistant to these antibiotics have ribosomes that do not bind them. Aminoglycoside antibiotics are highly polar water soluble bases not absorbed from the gut. All show ototoxicity (damage to the hair cells of the inner ear) resulting in

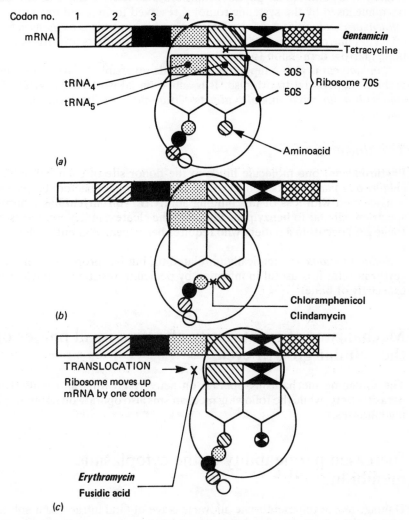

(a)

(b)

(c)

Figure 6.5 The three stages of elongation of the growing polypeptide chain in protein synthesis on the ribosome

impaired balance and hearing. They have a fairly broad spectrum that includes *M. tuberculosis*. Resistance develops readily so another drug should be given at the same time.

Gentamicin is useful in treating life-threatening infections by Gram-negative bacilli. Its spectrum includes *Pseudomonas (Ps.)*. It shows renal toxicity.

Streptomycin is mainly useful as a second line drug in tuberculosis (page 293).

Peptide bond formation

Chloramphenicol is a dipeptide. One molecule binds to each 50S subunit (*Figure 6.5b*) and blocks peptidyl transferase activity. It has a broad spectrum but, used by the systemic route, is reserved for typhoid fever and *H. influenzae* meningitis. A dose related reversible anaemia is a common toxic effect but one patient in 40 000 is hypersensitive and suffers total irreversible bone marrow depression (page 32).

Clindamycin is also a dipeptide that binds reversibly to the 50S subunit and blocks peptidyl transferase. It is active on all isolated bacterial ribosomes but *in vivo* mainly affects Gram-positive bacteria including *Bacteroides*.

Translocation

Erythromycin: one molecule binds to the donor site of each 50S subunit (*Figure 6.5c*) and blocks translocation. Development of bacterial resistance is associated with loss of this binding ability. **Erythromycin** has a narrow spectrum, similar to **benzylpenicillin,** and the clearest indication for its use (page 289) occurs in a patient who requires **benzylpenicillin** but is allergic to it.

Sodium fusidate is chemically unrelated to, but has properties very like, **erythromycin;** it is useful in infection by penicillin-resistant staphylococci, especially of bone.

Mechanisms of cytotoxicity effective in all phases of the cellular growth cycle

The foregoing mechanisms operate on actively growing and multiplying parasites only, while the following mechanisms also operate on nonmultiplying parasites.

Increased permeability of the cytoplasmic membrane

Damage to the cell membrane allows leakage of vital intracellular solutes. This mechanism makes a wide spectrum of parasites susceptible and exerts a cytocidal effect on nongrowing cells but limits selectivity.

Polyene antibiotics

Amphotericin binds to sterols in the cell membrane. These are abundant in fungal membranes and largely comprise ergosterol. Intermediate amounts of sterols are found in mammalian membranes and mainly comprise cholesterol. Sterols are absent from bacterial membranes. The drug molecule enters the membrane to form an artificial pore or ionophore, increasing the membrane's outward permeability to low MW intracellular solutes especially ions. The drugs show useful selectivity for certain fungi (not those of ringworm) but also substantial host toxicity (page 281).

Imidazoles

Imidazoles (**miconazole**) exhibit some biochemical selectivity. They show *in vitro* antifungal activity (fungicidal at high concentrations) but also attack certain bacteria and protozoa. They impair the synthesis of membrane ergosterols. The affected fungal cell membranes become disorganized and show secondary impairment of the uptake of nutrients.

Miscellaneous

Aminoglycosides (page 261) also damage cell membranes. This aspect of their action contributes to the bactericidal effect but also to the host toxicity.

Energy yielding metabolism

Most aerobic organisms derive their energy by similar mechanisms, so that interference with this process has not been a fruitful source of selectively toxic drugs. Anaerobes differ significantly from the human host so selective interference with their anaerobic pathways is possible.

Nitroimidazoles (**metronidazole**) interfere with the function of ferredoxin (a Fe-S-protein acting as an electron transfer agent in plants, anaerobic bacteria and protozoa) by acting as an electron acceptor. **Metronidazole** is a prodrug in that it is its reduced form that is lethal to anaerobic protozoa (*Trichomonas*, page 279; *Giardia*; *Entamoeba*, page 278) and bacteria (*Bacteroides, Cl. difficile* and *Borrelia vincenti*, page 291). The cell is also deprived of reducing power by this diversion of electrons from their normal recipient. The drug shows very little host toxicity.

Muscle

Roundworms (*Ascaris*) and threadworms (*Enterobius*) need their motility to stay in their intestinal environment; paralysis therefore leads to their expulsion (page 273). **Piperazine** is a functional antagonist of ACh at worm neuromuscular junctions with little effect at those of mammals. It is well absorbed from the gut and host toxicity is negligible.

Distributional selectivity

Even a drug that is equally toxic at its biochemical sites of action in host and parasite cells may nevertheless be useful as a chemotherapeutic agent if the sites of action in the parasitizing cells can be exposed to a higher concentration than those in the host cells. There are three ways in which this can come about.

Selective accumulation by the parasite

Tetracyclines

Tetracyclines (oxytetracycline) are cytotoxic to a wide range of parasites. Those affected include many bacteria (but not *Pseudomonas* or *Proteus*), *Rickettsia* and *Chlamydia* (large viruses). These organisms accumulate tetracyclines to a high intracellular concentration by a carrier-mediated transport process requiring ATP. Tetracycline-resistant cells (fungi, mammalian cells and resistant bacteria) do not do this.

After selective intracellular accumulation tetracyclines bind reversibly to the acceptor part of the smaller subunit of the ribosome and prevent the binding of aminoacyl-tRNA and therefore protein synthesis (*cf.* page 261). Unlike aminoglycoside antibiotics, tetracyclines do this in both 70S and 80S isolated ribosomes.

Tetracyclines are broad spectrum antibiotics with low host toxicity (page 290).

4-Aminoquinolines

Chloroquine and *quinine* are concentrated in all nucleated cells but more concentrated by malaria parasites. **Chloroquine** resistance in malaria is associated with a loss of this concentrating mechanism.

After selective intracellular concentration these basic drugs (their molecular structures incorporate flat ring systems) intercalate into DNA between layers of base pairs of the double helix. This disturbs the structure and function of the starter DNA employed by DNA polymerase. They inhibit DNA synthesis at the same high concentration in isolated systems from all cells.

These are the drugs of choice for patients clinically ill with malaria. They clear the blood though they do not clear the liver of malaria parasites (page

276). In amoebic liver abscess (page 278) the accumulation by liver cell nuclei can be regarded as a selective distribution into the parasites' environment (below). The amoebae selectively further accumulate the **chloroquine** by engulfing nuclear material. **Chloroquine** shows little toxicity in antiparasitic doses; large doses have an anti-inflammatory action utilized in rheumatoid arthritis (page 208) but such high doses can cause retinal toxicity.

Prodrugs

Acyclovir is a prodrug selectively activated (page 258) in cells infected with herpes virus. It is in this sense that the drug formed from it, acycloGTP, accumulates in the viral parasite and also within infected host cells – that is the parasites' environment.

Flucytosine is a prodrug that is accumulated by certain fungi. Once within the fungal cell it is selectively deaminated to the pyrimidine analogue, fluorouracil (page 259). It is a narrow spectrum antifungal drug.

Malathion is a prodrug activated to the organophosphorus anticholinesterase compound malaoxon selectively by insects, which also inactivate malaoxon more slowly than mammals. Thus, it is the malaoxon rather than the prodrug that is selectively 'accumulated' by the parasite. **Malathion** is useful in treating louse infestations (page 270).

Selective distribution into a limited compartment that forms the parasites' environment

Liver

The liver cells accumulate **chloroquine,** which intercalates into their nuclei (page 264). When *Entamoeba histolytica* infection becomes localized in the liver (page 277) opening up an abscess, the amoebae engulf liver cells and their nuclei and hence further accumulate **chloroquine.**

Skin

Griseofulvin is very poorly absorbed from the gut but that small proportion of the dose that is absorbed is selectively concentrated in the keratin precursor cells of skin. As these differentiate it is strongly bound to keratin. It is a mitotic inhibitor and it is fungistatic to ringworm fungi that parasitize keratin – skin, nails, hair. It is also accumulated by these fungi. The keratin formed during treatment resists invasion by fungal hyphae but treatment must be continued until static fungus and infected keratin have been shed. It is reserved for hair and nail infections with dermatophytes (page 280).

Urinary tract – urinary antiseptics

Nalidixic acid is rapidly and completely absorbed from the gut. Healthy kidneys clear the drug quickly by glomerular filtration. Normal therapeutic doses do not produce accumulation to an antibacterial blood concentration but renal tubular abstraction of water from the nascent urine results in a bactericidal concentration in the urine.

Nalidixic acid shows some biochemical selectivity (it inhibits DNA synthesis, by inhibition of DNA gyrase, which reverses the supercoiling of DNA strands, in Gram-negative bacilli), which is reinforced in use by distributional selectivity based on the concentrating activity of the kidney. Bacterial resistance develops readily.

Selective administration to a limited compartment that forms the parasites' environment

Lumen of gut

All of these drugs, when swallowed, are poorly absorbed from the gut either because they are water, but not lipid, soluble or because they are water insoluble. They therefore provide a high exposure to parasites within the gut lumen.

The aminoglycoside antibiotic *neomycin* is toxic to bacteria (page 261) but when given systemically is toxic to the host too. Gut absorption is negligible because it is highly polar (page 345). It is used in bowel preparation for intestinal surgery to reduce the bacterial content of any spills and of wall seams with the intention of reducing postoperative infective complications. Along with dietary protein restriction, it reduces the bacterial ammonia and amine production that is responsible for the encephalopathy (disturbance of consciousness, coma) of liver failure (*Figure 6.6*).

Nystatin is a polyene antibiotic (page 263) that is too toxic for systemic use. It is not absorbed because it is only slightly soluble in water. It is useful orally for candidiasis (page 281) of the gut.

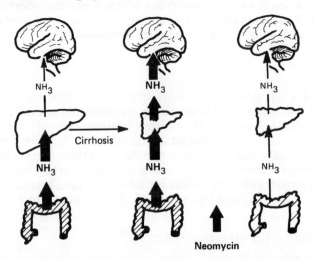

Figure 6.6 The liver normally clears the portal blood burden of ammoniacal compounds arising from gut commensal bacteria. In liver failure the brain is reached and affected; neomycin restricts the gastrointestinal production of ammoniacal compounds

Niclosamide is a water-insoluble drug that kills intestinal metazoa, probably by damaging their cell membranes. It is useful for tapeworm infestations (page 271).

Mebendazole is a water-soluble drug that kills intestinal metazoa, probably by interference with glucose uptake. It is useful for threadworm infestations (page 273).

Pyrantel is a water-insoluble agonist at nicotinic receptors of muscle, causing depolarizing neuromuscular blockade (like **suxamethonium,** page 74) and spastic paralysis of worms (page 273).

Skin

Antibacterial antibiotics

So little of a drug applied to the unbroken skin is absorbed into the systemic circulation that the more systemically toxic antibiotics can safely be used on the skin – *framycetin, neomycin, chlortetracycline*. The advantages of such a reliance on distributional selectivity are that pathogens are less likely to develop resistance to systemically valuable antibiotics and it avoids the need for penicillins, sulphonamides, *streptomycin* or *chloramphenicol* to be applied to the skin (all have a strong tendency to induce skin allergy, page 436).

Antiseptics

Chlorhexidine and *cetrimide* are cationic detergents that act at all cell membranes and rely for any selectivity they may have on poor penetration of the unbroken skin.

Hexachlorophane is a chlorinated phenol that is bactericidal to Gram-positive bacteria. Regularly applied to the skin it gradually accumulates; the number of organisms in the surface layers is gradually but substantially reduced. Misuse, by whole body immersion of babies in strong solutions, allows sufficient to be absorbed through the skin to give CNS toxicity, even death.

Antifungal drugs

Nystatin is useful for mucocutaneous candidiasis (page 281).
    Imidazoles can be applied locally in fungicidal doses.

Arachnicides and insecticides

These include *carbaryl* and *lindane*. Selectivity is great and while some show a biochemical component the dominant basis is distributional. Spread on the skin as powder or emulsion, the dose per unit of body mass received by the ectoparasite is much greater than that received by the host. This is due both to the differing body mass:surface area ratios of the host and parasite and also to the more ready penetration of the chitinous exoskeleton of the ectoparasite than of the intact human skin. In addition the parasite engulfs some of the material.

Eye

Similar considerations apply as to the choice of antibiotics for skin use (page 267). *Framycetin, neomycin, chlortetracycline* and *chloramphenicol* are examples.

Idoxuridine is a pyrimidine analogue that shows slight biochemical selectivity based on metabolic acceptance as a pyrimidine and incorporation into a functionless DNA. Its main selectivity is based on distributional considerations (site of administration – eye, skin). It inhibits the replication of certain DNA viruses (page 295).

Drug resistance in parasites

Origin

The development of drug resistance in microbial parasites usually has its origins in spontaneous mutation. This occurs at a frequency of 1 per 10^6–10^7 cell divisions.

Selection

Mutants have no advantage, and may be at a disadvantage compared with the wild type, in a drug-free environment. However, they are better able to survive and multiply in a drug-containing environment, having been naturally selected by the administration of a drug to which the wild type is sensitive but the mutant strain is resistant. A single mutation may confer a high degree of resistance (one step) or just a small increment of resistance to which others can be added (multistep) with selection to a high degree of resistance by prolonged or repeated inadequate drug dosage.

Spread

Spread of drug resistance is by cross-infection or by transfer of genetic material (usually extrachromosomal DNA – plasmids) by:

(1) transduction – by a bacteriophage (*Staph. aureus*): plasmids are carried from one (resistant) bacterium to another (which was sensitive but becomes resistant on receipt and expression of the plasmid);
(2) conjugation (*Shigella* and *E. coli*): plasmids are conveyed between bacteria along with the donated chromosomal DNA during sexual reproduction.

Mechanisms

(1) Inactivation of the drug:
    (a) β-lactamase inactivation of penicillins and cephalosporins. *Staph.*

aureus is most often discussed but this occurs in other species too, including Gram-negative bacteria, but not in *Streptococcus* (*Str*). The gene confers the ability to synthesize the β-lactamase enzyme, production of which is induced by contact with the antibiotic;
  (b) acetylation of *chloramphenicol*;
  (c) acylation of aminoglycoside antibiotics.
(2) Loss of permeability to, or uptake process for drug:
  (a) bacterial resistance to tetracyclines (page 264);
  (b) neoplastic cell resistance to antimetabolites;
  (c) plasmodial resistance to **chloroquine** (page 264).
(3) Increased production of a metabolite that competes with the drug: aminobenzoate production is increased in some sulphonamide-resistant cells; DHF in *Plasmodium* resistant to pyrimethamine (page 277).
(4) Enhanced activity of alternative metabolic route by-passing the inhibited pathway:
  neoplastic cell resistance to purine or pyrimidine analogues.
(5) Increased production of drug-sensitive enzyme:
  methotrexate resistance in neoplastic cells – increased production of DHF hydrogenase.
(6) Modification of drug sensitive site:
  (a) ribosome loses ability to bind **gentamicin**, **erythromycin**;
  (b) RNA polymerase loses ability to bind **rifampicin**;
  (c) DHF synthetase decreases affinity for sulphonamides.

Chemotherapy of metazoal infestations

Ectoparasites

Scabies

Scabies is a highly contagious infestation by the skin-dwelling mite (arachnid) *Sarcoptes scabiei* (*Figure 6.7*). The fertilized females burrow into the horny layer of the skin. This is symptomless at first but an allergic, itching rash develops later. Fortunately scabies infestation rarely involves the head.

Treatment involves completely covering the body surface (except the head) with a preparation containing *lindane* or **malathion**. The treatment should be repeated on several days and should be extended to all members of the patient's household. The mites are killed by this process but the rash takes several weeks to clear. Renewal of symptoms is due to reinfestation.

Lindane damages neuronal membranes inducing repetitive action potential discharge and hence the convulsive death of the scabies mite. The basis of the selectivity is entirely distributional.

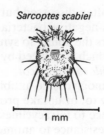

Sarcoptes scabiei

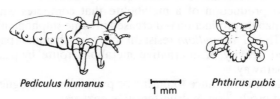

Pediculus humanus   1 mm   *Phthirus pubis*

Figure 6.7 Metazoal ectoparasites

Louse infestation

Pediculosis is infestation with the head or body louse (*Pediculus humanus*, races *capitis* and *humanus*; *Figure 6.7*) whilst phthiriasis is infestation with the crab louse (*Phthirus pubis*; *Figure 6.7*). Pediculosis is transmitted by bodily contact or by the sharing of combs, hairbrushes or clothing. The lice infest head or body hair in circumstances of poor personal hygiene and are the vector of typhus. Phthiriasis is transmitted during sexual intercourse and the lice generally infest the pubic hair.

Louse infestation can be eradicated using a lotion containing *carbaryl* or **malathion**. Ideally the treatment should be extended to all members of the patient's household. During treatment the infested hair should be assiduously combed to remove the dying lice and their eggs (nits).

Carbaryl and the prodrug **malathion** (page 265) act to inhibit cholinesterase enzymes. When used topically to eradicate lice, both drugs exhibit a high degree of distributional selectivity.

Endoparasites – worms

Classification of parasitic worms:

(1) Flatworms:
    (a) tapeworms;
    (b) flukes (includes schistosomes);
(2) Roundworms:
    (a) Ascaris (often called 'roundworm');
    (b) threadworms;
    (c) hookworms;
    (d) filariae.

Infestation with adult worms can occur in two basic sites:

(1) The worms live in the tissues of the host:

(a) lymphatics, skin, connective tissue – filariae;
(b) liver, bile ducts, lungs – flukes and some schistosomes;
(c) blood vessels – schistosomes.

(2) The worms live in the lumen of the alimentary canal (which has a low PO_2) and are therefore anaerobes:
(a) tapeworms;
(b) all roundworms except filarie.

Infestations with tissue-dwelling worms (*Table 6.1*) are not endemic in the UK and present great problems in the design of efficacious drugs or vaccines, the creation of a laboratory model of the infestation and field trials (including worm counts). Some effective, if rather toxic, drugs have been developed empirically but their mechanisms of toxicity have been little studied.

Table 6.1 Metazoal infestations not endemic in the UK

Worm	Vector	Drug
Tissue infestation		
Schistosoma (Bilharzia)	Fresh water snail	*Praziquantel*
Filariae	Biting flies	*Diethylcarbamazine*
Intestinal infestation		
Ancylostoma (hookworm)		*Pyrantel*
Strongyloides		*Thiabendazole*

Anaerobic worms inhabiting the gut lumen are more readily controlled by chemotherapy. Most worms in the infesting population are adult, so interference with nucleic acid or protein synthesis, which so successfully achieves selective toxicity in bacteria (because they are rapidly growing and multiplying) is an inappropriate mechanism of vermicidal action. Since intestinal worms depend on muscle activity to maintain their position in the gut, biochemically selective interference with the function of worm musculature (**piperazine**) is valuable. However, distributional selectivity underlies the action of most useful vermifugal drugs because:

(1) the worms are located in a limited compartment;
(2) the factors limiting absorption of chemicals from this compartment into the systemic circulation are known;
(3) unlike the intestinal mucosa, the worm's pellicle is highly permeable.

Infestation with beef tapeworm

In the UK beef tapeworm (*Taenia saginata*; *Figure 6.8*) infestation is of low incidence and in most cases is asymptomatic. The adult tapeworm clings to the intestinal mucosa (upper jejunum) by means of suckers found on its scolex (head). Successful treatment depends on the scolex being made to relinquish its hold on the mucosa.

Niclosamide kills the tapeworm, possibly by interfering with its anaerobic production of ATP. Since *niclosamide* is not absorbed from gut, this

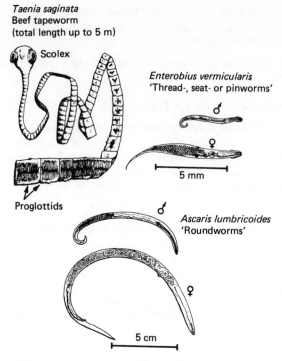

Figure 6.8 Metazoal endoparasites

biochemical selectivity receives great distributional reinforcement. Since the killed worm is not passed whole but partially digested, the scolex may be unrecognizable. The criterion of cure is 12 weeks without recurrence of segments in the stool.

Roundworm infestation

Threadworms (*Enterobius vermicularis*; *Figure 6.8*) inhabit the colon and rectum. Threadworm infestation is very common in the UK (particularly in children) causing perianal irritation and sleeplessness when the females emerge from the anus at night to lay eggs. Reinfestation is common so good hygiene practice (to break the ano-oral transmission process) and chemotherapy should be adopted by all members of the patient's household.

Roundworm (*Ascaris lumbricoides*; *Figure 6.8*) infestation is less common in the UK. Ingestion of contaminated food or water leads to egg hatching in the intestinal lumen. Microscopic larval worms burrow through the intestinal wall and are carried in the blood stream to the lungs. Worm larvae enter the alveoli, ascend to the glottis, are swallowed and develop as adults in the small intestine. The pathological consequences of Ascaris infestation are variable (very mild to fatal), may depend on the number of infesting worms and can include tissue damage caused by larval invasion.

Enterobius and Ascaris both hold their position in the intestinal lumen by swimming against intestinal peristalsis. Enterobius may also anchor to the intestinal mucosa using the fluke-like appendages located near its buccal orifice.

Mebendazole is effective against both Enterobius and Ascaris. It kills the worms by interfering with their uptake or utilization of glucose. Interference with blood glucose concentration is not seen in humans so *mebendazole* may exhibit some biochemical selectivity. However *mebendazole* is poorly absorbed from the gut so that its selectivity as a vermifuge undoubtedly has a large distributional component.

Piperazine, too, is effective against both Enterobius and Ascaris. It acts as an inhibitory agonist on the musculature of the worms, directly evoking relaxation. The living, flaccidly paralysed worms are then expelled from the host's intestine by peristalic activity. **Piperazine** is well absorbed from the gut. However, it has little or no relaxant activity in human muscle (page 264) and is relatively free from unwanted effects. The vermifugal action of **piperazine** thus exhibits good biochemical selectivity.

Pyrantel is effective against both Ascaris and Enterobius. *Pyrantel* acts as an excitatory agonist at the cholinoceptors of the muscle of Ascaris and Enterobius causing the spastic paralysis of the worms. Tested on isolated mammalian muscle *pyrantel* has significant **suxamethonium**-like activity. *Pyrantel* is water insoluble so little is absorbed by the host. Hence its vermifugal action exhibits distributional selectivity.

Chemotherapy of protozoal infections

Malaria

Tens of millions of people worldwide are infected by the malarial parasite. About 2250 cases of malaria are reported annually in the UK, with an increasing proportion being due to infection with *Plasmodium falciparum* (*see below*). Several of these patients die because of delayed or incorrect diagnosis or treatment.

Human malaria is caused by four species of the protozoon *Plasmodium* (*Table 6.2*) transmitted by the female anopheline mosquito. Approximately 50% of cases are due to *P. falciparum* and 40–45% to *P. vivax*.

The main clinical features of malaria are fever, anaemia, enlarged spleen and jaundice. In *P. falciparum* malaria the sequestration of parasitized red blood cells in the cerebral capillaries leads to cerebral malaria, which has a high mortality rate. The fever is due to the periodic rupture of red cells containing parasites. The older names for the various forms of malaria are derived in part from the periodicity of this rupture and fever, namely 'tertian' malaria, as for *P. vivax* and *P. ovale* when the fever occurs on every third day (counting the onset of fever as day 1) and 'quartan' as for *P. malariae* where the fever occurs on every fourth day. In *P. falciparum* infections the fever may be tertian but is often continuous or irregular.

The life cycle is depicted in *Figure 6.9*. When an infected female mosquito takes a blood meal, sporozoites are inoculated from the saliva. These are

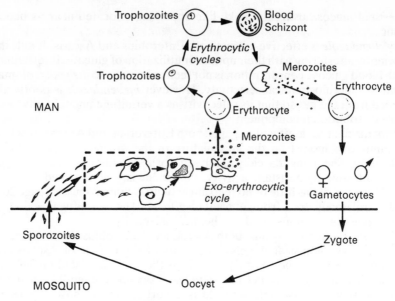

Figure 6.9 Malaria: life cycle

Table 6.2 The characteristics of human malaria infections

Infecting species	P. falciparum	P. vivax	P. ovale	P. malariae
Time to onset of symptoms	6 days	8 days	9 days	14 days
Fever cycle	2 days or irregular	2 days	2 days	3 days
Severity of attack	Severe	Mild/severe	Mild	Mild
Relapse (due to hypnozoites)	No	Yes	Yes	No
Recrudescence (due to persistent blood forms)	Yes	Yes	Yes	Yes
Older name	Malignant malaria	Benign tertian	Benign tertian	Benign quartan

rapidly transferred from the blood to the liver parenchymal cells (hepato-cytes) where they divide (tissue schizogony) to form tissue schizonts. On completion of this pre- or exo-erythrocytic cycle, several thousand mero-zoites are released to infect the blood. Some of these enter red blood cells and undergo a series of divisions and periods of growth to form trophozoites and subsequently schizonts. It is the rupture of these schizonts and the release of merozoites, malaria pigment and other cellular contents that induces the fever (*see above*). Each released merozoite is capable of in-fecting another erythrocyte to repeat the process of schizogony. Some of the trophozoites develop into male and female gametocytes. These are trans-ferred to the mosquito (primary host) during a blood meal and undergo a sexual phase of division (sporogony) yielding sporozoites.

In *P. vivax* and *P. ovale* but not *P. falciparum* and *P. malariae* malaria some parasites (hypnozoites) remain dormant in the liver cells (exoerythrocytic). Reactivation of these over varying periods is responsible for clinical relapses. In *falciparum* and *malariae* malaria the development of immunity or treatment with a drug that clears the blood (**chloroquine**) can genuinely rid the body of the parasites (radical cure). In *vivax* and *ovale* malaria, however, the symptoms are temporarily suppressed (clinical cure) but parasites can subsequently emerge from the liver causing relapse. Recrudescence, reappearance of the clinical disease due to the persistence of erythrocytic forms, can occur in all four forms of malaria.

Drugs providing radical cure: tissue schizontocides

Radical cure of malaria implies clearing the liver of exoerythrocytic parasites (hypnozoites) in *P. vivax* and *P. ovale*. Since the only drug available (**primaquine**) is potentially toxic (*see below*), radical cure should not be attempted until a clinical cure has been achieved (using a blood schizontocide) and the patient is fit enough to withstand the treatment.

Primaquine, an 8-aminoquinoline, is rapidly absorbed from the gut but neither the antimalarial activity nor the host toxicity is directly related to the blood concentration of **primaquine.** It is a prodrug transformed in the liver to oxidizing agents (quinoline-quinone derivatives). These oxidizing agents are cytotoxic and responsible for both the antimalarial effect and host toxicity. The malarial parasite and human erythrocytes depend on the activity of the pentose-phosphate biochemical pathway for the production of reduced glutathione, which protects cellular proteins from oxidation. If this pathway is compromised the cells become very vulnerable to oxidative damage. Gametocytes and the liver-dwelling (but not blood-dwelling) forms of the malarial parasites have a deficiency of an enzyme or cofactor in the pentose-phosphate pathway and are thus killed by the oxidizing action of **primaquine** metabolites.

In most patients the antimalarial action of **primaquine** exhibits moderate biochemical selectivity. However, in patients with a genetically determined deficiency of glucose-6-phosphate dehydrogenase (page 32), the pentose-phosphate pathway of erythrocytes is compromised and the cells become very susceptible to oxidative damage. **Primaquine** thus evokes intravascular haemolysis. Glucose-6-phosphate dehydrogenase deficiency has a high incidence in areas where malaria is endemic. This abnormality may have been naturally selected there because it is speculated to confer some natural immunity to malaria. Labile erythrocytes are severely damaged by parasite entry and are destroyed by the reticuloendothelial system before the parasite can grow to maturity. In all patients, **primaquine** can cause methaemoglobinaemia. Patients deficient in methaemoglobin reductase (page 30) are prone to this problem as they cannot rapidly reverse the reaction.

Drugs providing clinical cure: blood schizontocides

Clinical cure implies clearing the blood of parasites and thus suppressing symptoms. Since *P. falciparum* and *P. malariae* display no exoerythrocytic hypnozoites, clinical cure provides radical cure. For other Plasmodia it does not and relapse can occur.

4-Aminoquinoline and 4-quinolinemethanol derivatives

These include **chloroquine,** *quinine* and *mefloquine*, which can clear the blood of parasites within 24 h. The mechanism of this action is not clearly understood although a number of mechanisms have been suggested including intercalation into DNA, suppression of DNA replication (page 264), inhibition of polyamine synthesis and formation of haemolytic complexes with ferriprotoporphyrin IX derived from host cell haemoglobin. The mechanism of selectivity is distributional. These drugs are selectively concentrated by the erythrocytic parasites, therefore only in these is a concentration adequate to produce the toxic effect achieved.

Resistance to **chloroquine,** particularly in *P. falciparum*, due to failure of the parasite to concentrate the drug is now widespread, probably as a consequence of its prophylactic use. Resistance to *quinine* and *mefloquine* does occur but these drugs are still effective in many **chloroquine**-resistant strains and provide alternative (albeit more toxic in the case of *quinine*) treatments.

Antiparasitic doses of **chloroquine** do not usually produce serious unwanted effects (but *see* pages 208 and 431). *Quinine* exhibits unwanted effects collectively known as cinchonism. These include depression of muscular force (unwanted hypotension but relief of nocturnal leg cramps), tinnitus, visual disturbances, rashes, abdominal pain and nausea. *Mefloquine* causes a number of adverse effects including dizziness, loss of balance and more rarely neuropsychiatric disturbances. On prolonged treatment or frequent use there may be accumulation because of the long $t_{\frac{1}{2}}$.

Drug combinations providing sequential inhibition of DHF synthetase and DHF reductase

Combinations of pyrimethamine with either sulfadoxine or dapsone are slow-acting schizontocides. This action is too slow to be used alone in clinical cure (*see* prophylaxis *below*) but may be used as an adjunct to *quinine* in the treatment of **chloroquine** resistant *P. falciparum*. The antimalarial action represents sequential inhibition of nucleic acid synthesis with biochemical selectivity (page 258).

Resistance to pyrimethamine is widespread, including many **chloroquine**-resistant strains of *P. falciparum*.

High doses or long-term use of pyrimethamine may cause bone marrow depression, which can be offset by discontinuing the drug or administration of folinic acid. This by-passes inhibited enzyme in the host cells but does not impair the antiplasmodial action because folinic acid cannot be taken up by *Plasmodium*.

Prophylaxis of malaria

No drugs or vaccines provide true causal prophylaxis, that is prevention of pre-erythrocytic liver infection, against all four species of infecting sporozoites. **Primaquine** is too toxic for routine prophylactic use.

Drugs currently available provide imperfect suppressive treatment. They do not stop the contraction of malaria, or its establishment in the liver. Signs and symptoms of malaria may break through during the treatment course or may appear after termination of therapy.

Drugs for prophylaxis include **chloroquine,** *mefloquine*, pyrimethamine combined with dapsone, and *proguanil* (which has the same mechanism of action as pyrimethamine, page 258). Resistance to *proguanil* develops readily and there is cross-resistance to pyrimethamine. The mechanism of this resistance involves increased synthesis of DHF, so resistant parasites are more dependent on DHF synthetase and hence more susceptible to sulphonamides. In this situation the pyrimethamine and dapsone combination is valuable.

Prophylaxis should be commenced before visiting a malaria-endemic area and should be continued for at least 1 month after returning from it. *Mefloquine* should be used only for short stays (3 weeks) in endemic areas. The choice of an appropriate agent should take into account a number of factors including the risk of exposure to malaria, the extent of drug resistance, the efficacy and adverse effects of the drug and patient-related criteria such as age, pregnancy, hepatic and renal function. Specialist centres listed in the *BNF* can provide up-to-date advice.

Entamoeba histolytica amoebiasis

Entamoeba histolytica (*Figures 6.10b* and *6.11*) is one of several species of anaerobic amoebae that can colonize the lumen of the human intestine. Distribution of the infection is worldwide and about 10% of the world population harbour Entamoebae as harmless commensals. Symptoms of the infection are infrequent in the UK but occur when, for an unknown reason, the Entamoebae invade the wall of the large intestine, causing ulcers and phagocytosing red blood cells (amoebic dysentery). Amoebae may also be carried via the portal vein to the liver. Here they cause tissue necrosis (bacteriologically 'sterile' abscesses) and hepatitis.

When conditions in the intestine are unfavourable the amoebae form

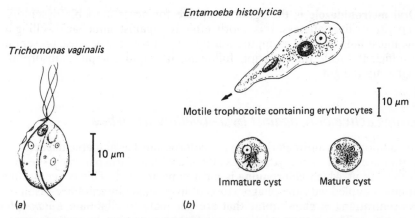

Entamoeba histolytica

Trichomonas vaginalis

Motile trophozoite containing erythrocytes   10 μm

10 μm

Immature cyst   Mature cyst

(a)   (b)

Figure 6.10 Protozoal parasites; (a) *Trichomonas vaginalis* (b) *Entamoeba histolytica*

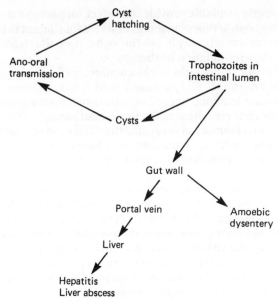

Figure 6.11 *Entamoeba histolytica:* life cycle

cysts, which are excreted in the faeces. Ingestion of food or water contaminated with cysts completes the ano-oral transmission process and cysts hatch in the small intestine.

Good sanitation and hygienic food preparation successfully prevents transmission of Entamoebae. Amoebicidal drugs can eradicate infection both in patients exhibiting symptoms and in asymptomatic cyst-passers. Amoebicides may be classified according to the body compartments from which the parasite is removed.

Drugs active against amoebae invading the gut wall and liver

Oral **metronidazole** is the agent of choice for acute amoebic dysentery, hepatitis or liver abscess. It is poorly effective against amoebae dwelling in the intestinal lumen of asymptomatic patients, probably because present in insufficient local concentration following its rapid complete absorption higher up the gut.

Drugs active only against liver-dwelling amoebae

In addition to its antimalarial activity, **chloroquine** has amoebicidal activity. With the exception of erythrocytes infected with malaria parasites, the liver is the site at which **chloroquine** is most concentrated. This concentrating ability, coupled with the phagocytosis of liver nuclei by amoebae results in concentrations of **chloroquine** that are adequate to eliminate *Entamoeba histolytica*. The amoebicidal action of **chloroquine** in liver abscess and hepatitis may involve interference with nucleic acid replication (page 264) but its selectivity has a distributional basis.

Drugs active only against amoebae dwelling in the intestinal lumen

Diloxanide furoate is used after all signs and symptoms of infection have subsided to prevent or terminate the carrier state. It is directly amoebicidal to the luminal trophozoites but the mechanism is unknown; it is presumed to be biochemically selective since most of the oral dose is absorbed and excreted in the urine but causes little host toxicity.

Antibiotic use

Incompletely absorbed antibiotics (tetracyclines), may be used as an adjunct to **metronidazole** in the treatment of intestinal amoebiasis. The antibacterial action leads to less favourable conditions for development of the amoebae and reduces secondary bacterial infections of lesions. Additionally tetracycline has some minor direct amoebicidal activity.

Trichomoniasis

Trichomonas vaginalis (*Figure 6.10a*) is an anaerobic flagellated protozoon that commonly inhabits the genitourinary tract. When conditions are favourable (for example, suppressed vaginal flora, more alkaline vaginal mucus) *Trichomonas* undergoes opportunist overgrowth causing vaginal inflammation. In men the infection is usually symptom-free though urethritis may occur. Transmission of infection results from sexual intercourse.

Nitroimidazole derivatives (**metronidazole**) orally are safe and effective trichomonacides. They are prodrugs selectively activated to short-lived cytotoxic intermediates (which possibly release superoxide anions) in anaerobic cells (page 263).

Recurrence of trichomonal vaginitis is usually the result of reinfection so that it is wise to treat the sexual partner even if symptom-free. **Metronidazole** shows an interaction, like *disulfiram*, with ethanol (page 249). Metabolites of **metronidazole** may cause dark coloration of the urine.

Chemotherapy of fungal infections

Compared with the development of antibacterial chemotherapy, the development of antifungal chemotherapy has been slow. There are two main reason for this:

(1) unlike bacteria, fungal cells are eukaryotic – biologically much more

akin to mammalian cells. This similarity militates against selective toxicity – and the currently available antifungal drugs are in general more
toxic than antibacterial agents;
(2) the stimulus for antifungal drug research has only become powerful
within the last few decades – since radiotherapy and the use of immunosuppressant drugs has created an immunocompromised population of
patients whose lives are threatened by systemic fungal infection.

Infections of keratin (dermatophytoses)

Various microscopic fungi utilize keratinized tissue (skin, hair, nail) as a
medium for growth. The initial skin infection tends to spread outwards as a
disc. The centre of the disc may heal so that the lesion takes on the
appearance of a ring – hence the name 'ringworm'. Ringworm is often
named according to the locus of the infection, for example, tinea pedis
(athlete's foot).

Localized ringworm infection of skin

Superficial infection is controlled by attention to personal hygiene reinforced by topical administration of antifungal agents.

Imidazole derivatives (**miconazole**) have a broad spectrum of fungicidal
activity being effective against both dermatophytes and yeast-like fungi. The
mechanism may involve an action on the fungal cell membrane whereby the
uptake of essential nutrients is inhibited. Applied topically in the treatment
of ringworm the modest biochemical selectivity is reinforced by selective
administration.

Compound benzoic acid ointment (Whitfield's Ointment) contains benzoic acid and salicylic acid. Salicylic acid is keratolytic and assists both the
shedding of fungus-laden tissue and the penetration of benzoic acid to
deeper-lying tissue. Benzoic acid has a fungistatic action whose mechanism
remains unclear. In topical treatment of ringworm *compound benzoic acid
ointment* has efficacy comparable to that of the preparations containing
imidazoles but is cosmetically less acceptable.

Tolnaftate is a narrow spectrum (dermatophytes only) fungicide.

Undecenoates, the acid and its esters or salts are used in the topical
treatment of ringworm but, like *tolnaftate*, are less effective than the
imidazoles.

Widespread or intractable ringworm

Widespread ringworm infection of the skin or infection of hair or nails is best
treated systemically.

Griseofulvin is the agent of choice when hair or nails are involved. It has a
narrow spectrum (dermatophytes only) of fungistatic activity. The mechanism is interference with the function of fungal tubilin. The selectivity of
the action has a distributional basis (page 265). The small fraction of each
oral dose that is absorbed is taken up selectively by cells synthesizing the
precursors of keratin. Growing dermatophytes concentrate the drug by

absorption of griseofulvin-containing keratin. Since treatment must be continued until all infected keratin has been shed (can be more than 1 year in the case of toe nails), unwanted effects (headache, skin rashes, nausea, impairment of memory, increased porphyrin excretion) assume greater significance.

Imidazoles

Oral *ketoconazole* is effective in widespread ringworm infection. However, *ketoconazole* has been associated with fatal hepatotoxicity and the potential benefits of oral *ketoconazole* should be carefully weighed against this risk.

Mucocutaneous infections by yeasts

The yeast *Candida albicans* is a normal inhabitant of the skin and mucous membranes of the gut and genitourinary tract. Opportunist overgrowth (candidiasis) occurs when competitive flora are suppressed (broad spectrum antibiotics), when normal defences are suppressed (glucocorticoids, cytotoxic drugs), and when biochemical changes occur in the fungal habitat (pregnancy, diabetes, debilitation). Candidiasis most frequently occurs in the mouth and throat (thrush) and in the vagina.

The polyene antibiotic *nystatin* (page 263) is fungicidal to many species of fungus by damaging their ergosterol-containing cell membranes. It is too toxic for systemic use so in practice its selectivity is distributional and it is only useful against mucocutaneous candidiasis. It is not absorbed from the gut so the oral route is useful for alimentary tract infection and local application (pessaries) for vaginitis.

Imidazole derivatives may be administered topically (**miconazole**) or orally (**miconazole**, *fluconazole*) in the treatment of superficial candidiasis.

Fungal infection of deep tissues

This tends to occur only in patients whose defences have been seriously impaired by glucocorticoids or cytotoxic drugs. The pathogens are a wide variety of fungi of low pathogenicity in immunocompetent patients.

The polyene antibiotic **amphotericin** is a close chemical relative of *nystatin* but sufficiently less toxic to allow its slow iv infusion. Adverse effects are common and include irritation at the injection site (pain and thrombophlebitis), nausea, vomiting, tinnitus and blurred vision. Renal toxicity is dose related, reversible at lower doses and seen in 80% of patients.

Flucytosine is a prodrug (page 265) with a narrow spectrum (yeasts) of antifungal activity. Following oral administration it is well absorbed from the gut and is selectively accumulated by susceptible fungi. Within the fungal cell *flucytosine* is deaminated to form fluorouracil, a pyrimidine analogue that interferes with DNA synthesis. The selectivity of action largely has a distributional basis and blood counts are necessary during prolonged administration.

Simultaneous administration of **amphotericin** and *flucytosine* can widen the antifungal spectrum of the chemotherapy and reduce the likelihood of fungal resistance.

Imidazole derivatives, too, are useful in the therapy of systemic fungal infections – *ketoconazole* can be given orally and **miconazole** by iv infusion but the injection vehicle (polyethoxylated castor oil) may cause hypersensitivity reactions.

Chemotherapy of bacterial infections

Principles of treatment

Before committing a patient to a course of antibiotic therapy ask – is it necessary?

The basis of rational treatment is the bacteriological diagnosis. The clinical diagnosis from the patient's history and physical signs often allows a provisional bacteriological diagnosis (exacerbation of chronic bronchitis – *Haemophilus (H.) influenzae*: lobar pneumonia – Pneumococcus: urinary tract infection – *Escherichia (E.) coli*) on which basis an antibiotic is chosen. A definitive bacteriological diagnosis requires isolation of the organism responsible. The time required depends on the test employed (Gram stain – 30 min; culture and identification of pathogens – 12–24 h; sensitivities to antibacterial drugs 24–48 h). When the bacteriological diagnosis and sensitivities are known, the initially chosen therapy may require modification but not if the patient is improving, for example, falling temperature and resolving of inflammation. *Table 6.3* lists some common infecting organisms and appropriate antibacterial agents.

Table 6.3 Common pathogenic bacteria, infections and drugs of choice

		Antibacterial agents	
Genus/species	*Infection*	*1st choice*	*2nd choice*
Gram-positive cocci			
Staph. aureus	Pneumonia	**Flucloxacillin**	**Erythromycin**
	Wound		**Gentamicin**
Str. pyogenes	Throat	*Phenoxymethyl-*	**Erythromycin**
	Middle ear	*penicillin*	
Str. pneumoniae	Pneumonia	**Benzylpenicillin**	**Erythromycin**
	Meningitis	**Benzylpenicillin**	*Chloramphenicol*
Gram-positive bacilli			
C. diphtheriae	Diphtheria	Antitoxin	**Benzylpenicillin**
Cl. perfringens	Gas gangrene	**Benzylpenicillin**	**Erythromycin**
Cl. difficile	Pseudomembranous colitis	*Vancomycin*	**Metronidazole**

Gram-negative cocci
  N. meningitidis   Meningitis   **Benzylpenicillin**
  N. gonorrhoeae   Gonorrhoea   **Amoxycillin**   *Ciprofloxacin*

Gram-negative bacilli
  H. influenzae   Bronchitis   **Ampi-/amoxycillin**   **Trimethoprim**
                Meningitis   *Chloramphenicol*   **Ampi-/amoxycillin**
  E. coli   Urinary tract   **Trimethoprim**   **Ampi-/amoxycillin**
                                              Cephradine
                                              Gentamicin
  Klebsiella   Urinary tract   *Cephradine*   **Gentamicin**
                Pneumonia   *Cefuroxime*
  Proteus   Urinary tract   **Ampi-/amoxycillin**   *Cephradine*
  Ps. aeruginosa   Urinary tract   **Gentamicin**   *Ciprofloxacin*
                Septicaemia   **Gentamicin**+*ceftazadime*
  S. typhi   Typhoid   *Chloramphenicol*   *Ciprofloxacin*

Others
  Tr. pallidum   Syphilis   **Benzylpenicillin**   **Erythromycin**
  Bacteroides   Various   **Metronidazole**   **Erythromycin**
  M. tuberculosis   Tuberculosis   **Rifampicin**
                                Isoniazid
                                Ethambutol   *Streptomycin*
                                Pyrazinamide
  Mycoplasma   Pneumonia   **Erythromycin**   Oxytetracycline
  Legionella   Pneumonia   **Erythromycin**   **Rifampicin**
  Pneumocystis   Pneumonia   *Co-trimoxazole*

Table 6.4 Sensitivity of important pathogenic bacteria to some of the principal antibiotics: usual minimum inhibitory concentration (mg/l) and average serum concentration

Bacterium	Antibiotic					
	BP	*A*	*FC*	*CE*	*E*	*G*
Staph. aureus[1]	0.03	0.06	0.12	0.12	0.12	0.06
Staph. aureus[2]	R	R	0.25	5	0.12	0.06
Str. pyogenes	0.01	0.03			0.03	
Str. pneumoniae	0.01	0.06				
Cl. perfringens	0.12	0.25				R
N. gonorrhoea	0.01	0.04				1
N. meningitidis	0.03	0.06	0.5			1
H. influenzae	0.5–2	0.25	16	8	1–8	1
E. coli[3]	R	8	R	3	R	0.5
Klebsiella	R	16–R	R	2–R	R	0.25
Proteus	R	R	R	R	R	0.5
Bacteroides	8–R	R	R		1–4	R
Serum concentration (mg/l)[4]	0.5	2.5	2.5	5	1.5	5

BP = **benzylpenicillin**   A = **ampicillin/amoxycillin**   FC = **flucloxacillin**
CE = *cephradine*   E = **erythromycin**   G = **gentamicin**
R = resistant

[1] = strains sensitive to **benzylpenicillin**; [2] = strains producing β-lactamase;
[3] = sensitivity varies considerably with species; [4] = approximate mean concentration achieved with recommended dose.

The object of chemotherapy is to attain an antibacterial concentration in the infected tissues to assist host defences in eradicating infection. In general the serum concentration should exceed the minimum inhibitory concentration *in vitro* (mic) by a factor of four. *Table 6.4* is a reference table. *Table 6.5* summarizes prescribing information on some commonly used antibiotics.

Routes of administration

Antibiotics are usually administered by mouth but inadequate doses and infrequent administration encourage the emergence of resistant organisms. In a severe infection the antibiotic should be given parenterally at a dose and dosage interval that provides subtoxic peak concentrations and antibacterial trough concentrations. Iv administration ensures that the necessary dose is received – to avoid chemical neutralization avoid mixing one antibiotic solution with another or with iv infusion fluid.

Duration of therapy

This should be decided at the outset but may be amended in response to objective clinical observations – temperature, pulse rate, resolution of signs. Five days is commonly sufficient. Chest infections may require 7 days' treatment. Prolonged therapy in the asymptomatic patient is occasionally necessary – relapsing urinary tract infections, pulmonary tuberculosis, infective endocarditis.

Table 6.5 Prescribing of some commonly used antibiotics

Drug	*Serum $t_{\frac{1}{2}}(h)$	Elimination	Usual dose (mg)	Route of admin.	Dosage interval (h)
Benzylpenicillin	0.5	ts	600	im iv	6
Phenoxymethyl-penicillin	0.5	ts	500	oral	6
Ampicillin	0.5	ts	250	oral im/iv	6
Amoxycillin	2	ts	250	oral	8
Flucloxacillin	0.5	ts	250	oral im/iv	6
Cephradine	1	ts	250	oral im/iv	8
Erythromycin	3	m	500	oral iv	8
Gentamicin	2.5	gf	80–160	im iv	8
Oxytetracycline	8.5	gf m	250	oral	8
Co-trimoxazole	8	ts	S 400 T 80	oral	12
Metronidazole	8	m gf	200–400	oral iv rectal	12
Ciprofloxacin	4	gf ts	250–750	oral iv	12

gf = glomerular filtration; m = metabolism; ts = tubular secretion; * = mean values for normal individuals; S = sulphamethoxazole; T = **trimethoprim.**

In severe infections the above doses may need to be increased.

Additional therapy

Chemotherapy may deal with the bacteria but other measures may be necessary to improve the patient's condition (respiratory infection – physiotherapy for improved drainage of the airways; abscess – drainage; osteomyelitis – removal of sequestrum; wounds – debridement).

Prophylactic use

This is permissible only in a restricted range of clearly defined circumstances. There must be a specific target infection to be prevented, due to a specific organism that is reliably sensitive to the proposed prophylactic antibacterial drug. Objective methods must have demonstrated effectiveness of the prophylaxis in reducing the incidence of the target infection. *See* pages 287–288, 289 and 291 for examples.

Failure to respond

If the patient does not improve consider the following factors.

Pharmacokinetic factors

(1) Inadequate dose – check mic (*Table 6.4*).
(2) Incorrect route – a pleural abscess may require intrapleural administration or a poorly absorbed drug has been given by the oral route.
(3) Inadequate duration of treatment may lead to early relapse.

Pharmacodynamic factors

(1) Failure of patient to take the drug (poor compliance); commonly occurs in patients on long-term therapy – tuberculosis.
(2) Additional measures required – drainage of pus.
(3) Response modified because of coexisting disease (anaemia, immune deficiency, malignancy) or other drug therapy (glucocorticoids, cytotoxic drugs).
(4) Development of antibiotic resistance (*see* page 268).

Laboratory factors

(1) Inadequate, inappropriate or delayed specimens may not allow the laboratory to identify the pathogen.
(2) Inadequate laboratory technique. Some organisms (*Cl. difficile*) are difficult to isolate and unless the laboratory is warned 'standard techniques' will fail to identify such organisms.

Factors modifying the response

(1) Age: newborn infants, especially those delivered preterm, have immature livers and cannot detoxify certain drugs (*chloramphenicol*, sulphonamides). Poor renal excretion may result in drug accumulation (**gentamicin**). Renal function declines in old age and dose adjustment may be necessary.

(2) Pregnancy: the possibility of harm to the fetus (for example, deposition of tetracyclines in developing bones and teeth).
(3) Renal impairment: causes accumulation (aminoglycoside antibiotics). Tetracyclines are contraindicated.

Antibacterial drug combinations

There are certain rules governing use of antibiotic combinations. Three are possible.

(1) Bacteriostatic with bactericidal – this combination should be avoided. Bactericidal drugs only kill growing bacteria. If growth is prevented by a bacteriostatic drug antagonism of the bactericidal drug may be important; for example, there is a higher mortality in pneumococcal meningitis when a tetracycline is given in addition to **benzylpenicillin.**
(2) Bacteriostatic with bacteriostatic – these are simply additive with the exception of **trimethoprim** and sulphamethoxazole (*co-trimoxazole*) in which synergism converts two bacteriostatic drugs into one bactericidal combination.
(3) Bactericidal with bactericidal – usually synergistic (**benzylpenicillin** plus **gentamicin** in patients with infective endocarditis). Synergistic combinations are useful in patients with severe neutropenia who readily develop a septicaemia.

The advantages of combination therapy are to:

(1) reduce the emergence of resistant strains during long-term therapy, as in tuberculosis;
(2) increase the antibacterial spectrum (severely ill patients, patients with impaired host defences, multiple infecting organisms);
(3) increase bactericidal activity (**benzylpenicillin** plus **gentamicin** in *Str. faecalis* endocarditis).

Penicillins

All penicillins have in common fused lactam and thiazolidine rings (*Figure 6.12*). Alteration of the side-chain improves the performance of the drug in different situations but results in a reduction of potency against organisms normally sensitive to **benzylpenicillin** (*Table 6.4*). The basic structure can be altered so that it:

(1) becomes resistant to hydrolysis by gastric acid but absorption from the gut remains incomplete although adequate for most clinical purposes;
(2) is made resistant to β-lactamase;
(3) has a broader spectrum of antibacterial activity.

For mechanisms of toxicity and selectivity *see* page 255. **Benzylpenicillin** [penicillin G] is very potent (*Table 6.4*) and is the drug of choice in certain infections. It is inactivated (hydrolysed) by gastric acid so it must be administered parenterally. After im injection absorption is rapid and the drug is widely distributed throughout the body but does not readily pass the blood brain barrier (unless very high doses are used and the meninges are in-

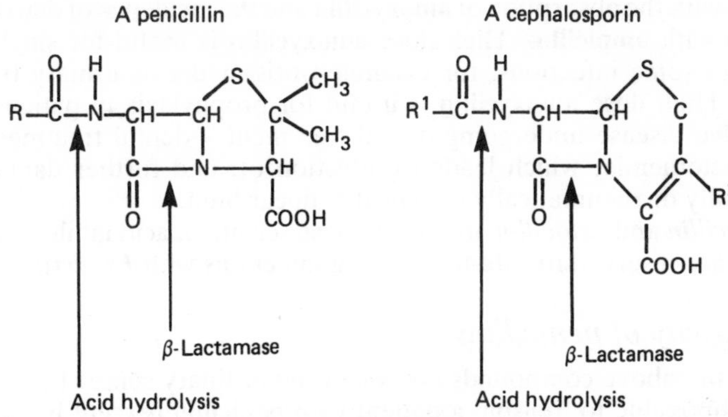

A penicillin   A cephalosporin

Figure 6.12 The penicillin and cephalosporin nuclei: the bonds susceptible to acid hydrolysis and β-lactamases

flamed). There is no significant metabolism. Elimination is by tubular secretion – 60–90% of the administered dose is eliminated in 1 hour. Excretion can be delayed and serum (and CSF) concentrations increased by *probenecid*, which competes for the choroid plexus and renal tubular active secretion mechanisms for organic acids.

Spectrum of activity – bactericidal at very low mic against Gram-positive and negative cocci and Gram-positive bacilli (*Table 6.3*): sensitivities vary. β-Lactamase opens the β-lactam ring and renders the drug inactive.

Procaine penicillin combines equimolar amounts of benzylpenicillin and procaine. Peak blood concentrations are reached in 4 h and drug is still detectable 24 h later. It is used in accident units prophylactically, to prevent gas-gangrene following trauma, with **benzylpenicillin** and *benethamine penicillin* as 'Triplopen'.

Phenoxymethylpenicillin (penicillin V) is acid stable. Chemical variants are available in tablet or elixir form. It is very effective in the treatment of streptococcal infections. It is useful prophylactically, to prevent streptococcal infections that would cause recurrence, in patients who have suffered rheumatic fever or glomerulonephritis.

Flucloxacillin is resistant to both β-lactamase and gastric acid. Food interferes with its absorption but even in the fasting state this is incomplete and a higher serum concentration is obtained by the im route, which is preferred in the acutely ill patient.

It should be reserved for infections with staphylococci and never be prescribed for infections due to an organism sensitive to **benzylpenicillin** or **ampicillin** because it is much less potent than either (*Table 6.4*).

Ampicillin has a wider spectrum of activity than **benzylpenicillin.** It is acid-stable and adequate serum concentrations are obtained after oral administration. It is, however, susceptible to β-lactamase and, like **benzylpenicillin,** it is rapidly eliminated by renal tubular secretion. Therapeutic concentrations are found in bile so it is useful for biliary tract infections and to eliminate the carrier state in typhoid fever. It may be given parenterally if required. Oral absorption is not complete and **amoxycillin** achieves a peak blood concentration about twice that of **ampicillin.** Comparative studies have shown little advantage of one drug or the other. Food does not interfere with the absorption of **amoxycillin** and the incidence of diarrhoea is less than with **ampicillin.** High dose **amoxycillin** is useful for single dose therapy in some infections, for example otitis media or urinary tract infections. High dose **amoxycillin** is useful for prophylaxis in patients with heart valve disease undergoing dental treatment – dental treatment produces bacteraemia, which leads to infection of, and further damage to, congenitally or rheumatically damaged endocardium.

Piperacillin and *azlocillin* are β-lactamase sensitive, acid labile and given iv. They are reserved for life-threatening infections with *Ps. aeruginosa.*

Host toxicity of penicillins

None of the above compounds is toxic in the ordinary sense. Indeed, it is almost impossible to 'poison' a patient with penicillin (except by administering it into the CSF where it is irritant). The predilection of this group lies in the production of hypersensitivity reactions (*see* page 25). This is most marked with **ampicillin** or **amoxycillin.** Reactions are of two kinds:

(1) immediate, for example, shock, collapse and death;
(2) delayed, for example, rash, urticaria, oedema, fever and serum sickness syndrome.

A rash with **ampicillin/amoxycillin** is more common at a dose of 2 than 1 g/day. It usually occurs when the antibiotic is prescribed irrationally for a viral infection, typically a sore throat, for example, infectious mononucleosis (*phenoxymethylpenicillin* is the treatment of choice for a streptococcal tonsillitis). It does not always signify allergy to all the penicillins.

There is a gradation in reactions produced – the first reaction is usually mild. Always ask a patient if he is sensitive to penicillin before prescribing any of the above drugs. Treatment consists of *adrenaline* im, **chlorpheniramine** slowly iv and *hydrocortisone sodium succinate* iv (page 27).

Other adverse reactions – nephritis and haemolytic anaemia – may occur usually in patients on long-term therapy, for example, for subacute bacterial endocarditis.

Cephalosporins and cephamycins

A family of antibiotics showing a common chemical nucleus (*Figure 6.12*) with substituents that condition the significant differences in properties between members.

There is a strong relationship to the penicillin family based on similarity of β-lactam and peptide parts of their nuclei. Thus the basis of cytotoxicity and selectivity is the same. Also members susceptible to and resistant to acid hydrolysis exist.

Most members show an antibacterial spectrum similar to **amoxycillin** combined with insusceptibility to β-lactamase.

The main adverse effects have hypersensitivity as their basis and about 10% of penicillin-hypersensitive patients are cephalosporin-hypersensitive too; therefore avoid these if there is a history of penicillin anaphylaxis.

Resistance (natural or acquired) can have drug destruction as its basis – a β-lactamase being produced (by *Kl., Ps.*) or drug insusceptibility.

Pharmacokinetically several show a rapid renal clearance by active tubular secretion (therefore $t_{\frac{1}{2}}$ about 45 min). One member is partially inactivated by metabolism rather than renal excretion – it would be preferable in renal insufficiency.

They are expensive; because valuable for their wide spectrum including many resistant hospital Gram-negative bacilli avoid use where a narrower spectrum agent will suffice.

Cephradine can be given orally or parenterally as an alternative to **ampicillin/amoxycillin**. It is less toxic than earlier cephalosporins. *Cefuroxime* and *ceftazadime* are less susceptible to β-lactamase than *cephradine* and are preferred in serious Gram-negative septicaemia.

Erythromycin

For mechanisms of **erythromycin** toxicity and selectivity *see* page 262. Absorption of the base from the gut is delayed by food. The drug is widely distributed throughout the body with the exception of the CSF. Significant metabolism occurs and elimination is via the bile and urine. Low doses are bacteriostatic but high doses are bactericidal. The spectrum of activity is similar to **benzylpenicillin** but it is also active against β-lactamase-producing staphylococci and *Legionella*, *Mycoplasma* and *Campylobacter*. Host toxicity is minimal and allergy rare. The estolate derivative should not be prescribed for more than 2 weeks because it may produce an intrahepatic obstructive jaundice.

Aminoglycoside antibiotics

For mechanisms of toxicity and selectivity *see* page 261. This group has several members with similar pharmacological characteristics. They are all soluble in water and strongly basic – absorption from the gut is therefore negligible. Distribution is predominantly extracellular; there is little penetration into tissues and no passage across the blood brain barrier. There is no significant metabolism and elimination is by glomerular filtration; no tubular secretion or reabsorption occurs. Renal clearance correlates well with the creatinine clearance.

Persistent high serum concentrations will produce high tone deafness by damaging the organ of Corti, as well as producing some vestibular damage and also result in renal tubular damage. This situation can be avoided by modifying the dose (*see* page 347).

Gentamicin is the most therapeutically useful member of the group. It has a wide spectrum of activity particularly against Gram-negative bacilli (including *Pseudomonas*). It is also useful prophylactically, to prevent infection in large bowel resection.

Streptomycin is a second line in the treatment of tuberculosis. It is a frequent cause of skin allergy and has caused congenital deafness when administered in pregnancy.

Neomycin is the most ototoxic member of the group and is given by mouth for 'sterilization' of the gut in the management of liver failure (page 266). It and *framycetin* are also useful topically (danger of skin sensitization, page 436) but note that some systemic absorption can occur with toxicity as a result. Topical preparations for the external ear are contraindicated if the eardrum is not intact.

Vancomycin

Vancomycin is a toxic bactericidal glycopeptide. It is used in the treatment of pseudomembranous colitis (given orally) and serious **flucloxacillin**-resistant staphylococcal infections (for example, septicaemia, endocarditis (given iv)). It is given intraperitoneally to treat peritonitis (*Staph. epidermidis*) in patients on continuous ambulatory peritoneal dialysis (CAPD).

Tetracyclines

This group contains several members with a wide spectrum of bacteriostatic activity, which includes most Gram-positive and Gram-negative cocci and bacilli as well as *Mycoplasma*, *Rickettsia* and *Chlamydia*. For mechanisms of toxicity and selectivity of tetracyclines *see* page 264. Absorption from the gut is incomplete but adequate. Two factors account for variability in absorption:

(1) the hydrochloride derivatives are soluble in water giving an acid solution; in a neutral or alkaline medium (the intestine) they tend to precipitate out or do not dissolve;
(2) they are chelating agents and will complex with the multivalent ions, Ca^{2+}, Al^{3+}, Mg^{2+} (milk, antacid mixtures) and **ferrous sulphate** significantly reducing bioavailability.

Disposition varies according to the degree of protein binding, biliary excretion and reabsorption (enterohepatic circulation) and tetracyclines are widely distributed throughout the body, including the CSF (concentration 10% that of serum). They complex with calcium in growing long bones and the enamel of developing teeth and should never be prescribed in pregnancy or in children under 7 years. Elimination occurs in both urine (glomerular filtration and tubular secretion) and faeces (biliary excretion).

Doxycycline is completely absorbed, need only be administered once daily and may be given if renal function is impaired and there is no alternative. It is expensive.

Host toxicity

Antibiotic-associated colitis (*see* page 292).
Tetracyclines (with the exception of *doxycycline*) and their metabolites

accumulate when renal function is impaired. Uraemia may be aggravated. Other adverse effects include photosensitization and rashes.

Chloramphenicol

Chloramphenicol is bacteriostatic and well absorbed when administered by mouth. Its wide distribution includes the CSF. It is metabolized and little unchanged drug is eliminated in the urine. Its conjugation mechanism in the liver is immature in the newborn, therefore it easily accumulates to toxic concentrations. It acts by inhibiting protein synthesis (page 262) and this is responsible for its major adverse effect – depression of the bone marrow. Therefore, monitor the full blood count (including platelets) every 48 h in patients receiving the drug. In sensitive subjects unpredictable development of complete marrow aplasia may occur that is ultimately fatal. This has restricted its use to infections with *Salmonella* (*S.*) *typhi* and to meningitis due to *H. influenzae*.

Ciprofloxacin

Ciprofloxacin is a recently developed member of the 4-quinolone family derived from the urinary antiseptic *nalidixic acid* (*see* page 266 for mechanism of action). A wide spectrum of bactericidal activity is demonstrated against many Gram-positive and negative organisms. It is particularly helpful against *S. typhi*, *N. gonorrhoeae* and *Chlamydia*. Widespread use of quinolones should be avoided as only small increments in bacterial resistance will result in therapeutic failure. Adverse effects include rashes, diarrhoea and CNS disturbance. Since these compounds inhibit DNA synthesis they must be avoided during pregnancy and childhood.

Metronidazole

Metronidazole (page 263) is well absorbed after oral or rectal administration. Active against strict anaerobes and some protozoa, it is very widely distributed throughout the body with good penetration into the brain and the interior of abscesses. It is useful in surgical prophylaxis, to prevent infection in pelvic surgery, and provides an alternative to *vancomycin* in the treatment of pseudomembranous colitis.

Host toxicity

Metronidazole resistance is rare. Nausea and other mild gastrointestinal effects are rare. In some patients taking ethanol a disulfiram-like (*see* page

249) effect can occur. Peripheral neuropathy is seen in patients on long-term therapy.

Sulphonamides

For mechanisms of toxicity and selectivity *see* page 256.

Drugs of this group are absorbed by mouth and are variably bound to plasma albumin, competing with other acidic drugs (anticoagulants, **tolbutamide**). Many undergo acetylation in the liver to a less soluble metabolite, which, together with the parent compound, is eliminated by glomerular filtration and tubular secretion. The proportion eliminated is increased if the urine is alkaline. Because of a relatively high incidence of adverse effects, they are much less frequently used than in the past.

Renal toxicity depends upon crystalluria – limited solubility of the sulphonamide or its metabolite.

Sulphamethoxazole was selected for combination with **trimethoprim** as *co-trimoxazole* because it possesses similar pharmacokinetic characteristics. The few toxic effects are attributable to the sulphonamide but folate metabolism can be disturbed in the elderly by the **trimethoprim. Trimethoprim** alone is sufficient for treatment of sensitive chest and urinary tract infections. *Co-trimoxazole* is useful mainly for the treatment of *Pneumocystis carinii* infections.

Sulphasalazine (an addition compound of sulphapyridine and 5-aminosalicylic acid) has been extensively use in the management of ulcerative colitis and Crohn's disease as a means of delivering the salicylate to the desired site of action in the colon where it is released by bacterial hydrolysis.

Sulphasalazine is also used as second line therapy in rheumatoid arthritis.

Superinfection

Any antibacterial drug with a wide bacterial spectrum and either incomplete absorption or partial gut elimination may reduce commensal organisms in the bowel, allowing the overgrowth of organisms naturally resistant to them (*Cl. difficile, Candida albicans*, resistant *Staphylococcus, Pseudomonas*). An extreme form of superinfection with *Cl. difficile* can lead to pseudomembranous colitis. Oral *vancomycin* effectively eliminates this organism; **metronidazole** is a less effective alternative.

Tuberculosis

Eradication of *Mycobacterium* (*M.*) *tuberculosis* from patients is now almost always achieved provided the patient takes the right drugs for the prescribed course. Antituberculous drugs have three kinds of action:

(1) slowly killing semidormant bacilli – **rifampicin** and *pyrazinamide* are most effective with **isoniazid** moderately effective;
(2) rapidly killing actively growing bacilli – **isoniazid** is the most effective;

(3) prevention of development of resistance to other sterilizing drugs – **isoniazid** and **rifampicin** have greatest activity in this regard.

Current antituberculosis chemotherapy involves quadruple therapy with **rifampicin, isoniazid,** *pyrazinamide* and *ethambutol* for 1–2 months (longer if *M. tuberculosis* can still be isolated from the sputum) with administration of the first two drugs being maintained for a further 3–6 months.

In countries outside Western Europe and North America **rifampicin,** because of its great expense, is used more economically. Very low rates of relapse have been found using a thrice weekly regimen for 8 months with *streptomycin,* **isoniazid,** *pyrazinamide* and **rifampicin** (thrice weekly for 4 months).

Isoniazid is bacteriostatic to dormant, but bactericidal to rapidly growing, mycobacteria. It penetrates cells to reach intracellular bacilli.

The mechanism of the antituberculous activity of **isoniazid** is unclear. It is well absorbed and crosses the blood brain barrier (may elevate mood). It is acetylated in the liver at a rate that is genetically determined (page 29) and toxic effects are more likely in slow acetylators. Polyneuropathy is corrected by *pyridoxine.* Liver damage (hepatitis-like) can be very severe.

Rifampicin has a wider spectrum of bactericidal activity (page 260) but is used mainly for tuberculosis because resistance readily develops and allergic reactions are common if interrupted therapy is practised. It can cause anorexia and nausea early in the course of treatment. Liver function should be monitored before and during therapy in an attempt to detect early signs of liver damage. Abnormal liver function tests are common but usually transient. Hepatic MFO enzyme induction results in a reduction of the efficacy of the low dose oestrogen oral contraceptives, corticosteroids, sulphonylureas, **warfarin** and anticonvulsants. Secretions including urine and tears are coloured pink.

Pyrazinamide is bactericidal in slightly acidic conditions, even against semidormant bacilli. It may cause arthralgia associated with hyperuricaemia or hepatic dysfunction.

Ethambutol is tuberculostatic. It is prescribed on a weight basis as high doses may damage visual acuity. Patients should be warned to report this early as continued exposure to the drug produces further optic neuritis. About 90% is excreted unchanged in the urine so dosage adjustment is necessary if renal function is impaired.

Chemotherapy of viral infections

Viruses are obligatory intracellular parasites having the genetic information for reproduction but no mechanism for carrying it out. The simplest comprises a single piece of nucleic acid containing just enough codons to reproduce itself. The large majority, including most human pathogens, also contain coding for a simple protein coating. The protein coat is worn when the virus particle is extracellular and confers antigenicity and affinity for specific cells.

Chlamydiae have properties intermediate between those of bacteria and viruses. They possess rigid cell walls, contain both DNA and RNA but can only reproduce inside other cells. Chlamydiae are susceptible to tetracyclines but diseases caused by them (trachoma, psittacosis and nonspecific urethritis) are infrequent in the UK.

True viruses contain only one type of nucleic acid and hence may be classified into:

(1) DNA viruses – herpes simplex (cold sores), herpes varicella/zoster (chicken pox, shingles), variola major (smallpox);
(2) RNA viruses – poliovirus (poliomyelitis), influenza virus, human immunodeficiency virus (AIDS), hepatitis viruses.

The viral replication process

(1) Virus particles exist free in the environment or host ECF.
(2) Adsorption onto specific cell surfaces.
(3) Penetration into susceptible cells.
(4) Lysozymal digestion of the protein coat. The liberated nucleic acid by-passes or takes over genetic control of the infected cell.
(5) Synthesis of early proteins (nucleic acid polymerases).
(6) Synthesis of RNA or DNA (multiple replicates of virus nucleic acid).
(7) Synthesis of proteins for coat.
(8) Assembly of virus particles.
(9) Release from the host cell with cell damage or death, induction of release of interferon and inflammation (gives localizing symptoms) and repair.

Thus the peak of viral multiplication has usually passed when illness becomes clinically obvious and there is little that an antiviral drug can be expected to do therapeutically.

Antiviral therapy

Immunization

The mainstay of antiviral therapy is prophylaxis provided by immunization. Immunological attack is directed against the protein coat of the virion. Viral vaccines provide active immunity. They may contain live attenuated virions (vaccines for poliomyelitis (Sabin), smallpox (vaccinia), German measles (rubella), measles and mumps) or suspensions of killed virions (vaccines for poliomyelitis (Salk), hepatitis B and influenza).

Immunoglobulins provide passive immunity. *Normal immunoglobulin* is prepared from pools of at least 1000 donations of human plasma. It is used to protect patients at risk from infectious hepatitis, measles and rubella. Specific immunoglobulins include *hepatitis B*, *varicella-zoster* and *rabies immunoglobulins*. They are prepared by pooling the blood of convalescent or immunized donors.

Antiviral drugs

Antiviral drugs have a very limited role in the prophylaxis or treatment of viral infections. They may be classified according to the mechanism of antiviral action.

Inhibition of adsorption to or penetration of host cells

Since the virion is prevented from moving into the intracellular compartment it remains susceptible to the host's immunological defences. *Amantadine* inhibits cell penetration by certain RNA- or DNA-containing virions. It reduces the incidence of influenza 'A' strain infections if administered continuously during epidemics and it may reduce the duration of illness if taken after the onset of symptoms. *Amantadine* is also effective in the treatment of herpes zoster infections (shingles).

A beneficial effect of *amantadine* in parkinsonism (page 221) was discovered as a side-effect during tests of the antiviral action. Unwanted effects (nervousness, insomnia, gastrointestinal disturbances) are rarely troublesome but may be attributable to the dopamine-like activity of the drug.

Inhibition of viral nucleic acid synthesis

Drug or prodrug analogues of deoxyribonucleoside can interfere with the synthesis of viral DNA.

Idoxuridine is an analogue of thymidine, competing with it for nonselective incorporation into DNA and yielding a functionally deficient DNA analogue. Therefore *idoxuridine* is lethal to all cells actively synthesizing DNA (page 268) and is so toxic that it cannot be used systemically.

Idoxuridine is used topically to treat infections with herpes simplex or zoster, and since herpes-infected cells synthesize DNA some 1000 times faster than normal cells, the drug exhibits some biochemical selectivity. In topical use this is reinforced by distributional selectivity (selective administration).

Acyclovir is a prodrug that is activated only in herpes-infected cells. A virally coded kinase (not present in healthy cells) catalyses its conversion to a monophosphate derivative. Host cell-coded kinases subsequently convert the monophosphate to a triphosphate, which is the active drug. The triphosphate derivative of **acyclovir** inhibits the replication of viral DNA more readily than the replication of host cell DNA. Hence the high selectivity of **acyclovir** has both a distributional (activation only in infected cells) and a quantitative biochemical basis. It is the available antiviral agent that exhibits the most selective toxicity.

Acyclovir is useful topically in the treatment of herpes simplex infection of the cornea and orally or by iv infusion in the treatment of herpes encephalitis. It is also useful prophylactically for those at risk from developing severe herpes virus infection. Treatment is not completely curative as the virus is not eliminated.

Ganciclovir is related to **acyclovir** but is much more active against cytomegalovirus. It is, however, much more toxic than **acyclovir,** possibly because it can more easily be phosphorylated by cellular thymidine kinase. Consequently its use is restricted to life threatening cytomegalovirus infections in immunocompromised patients.

Zidovudine (AZT) is a nucleoside analogue activated by cellular thymidine kinase, and is used in the treatment of human immunodeficiency virus (HIV), the agent responsible for the development of AIDS. *Zidovudine* inhibits the reverse transcriptase activity of retroviruses (HIV) at concentrations lower than those required to interfere with host cell DNA synthesis. *Zidovudine* therapy improves (partially) immune function, reduces the incidence of opportunistic infections (for example, pneumocystis, cytomegalovirus) and increases survival in patients with AIDS. It may also be helpful in prolonging survival in patients who have positive antigenic plasma tests for HIV infection but who have not yet developed AIDS (preAIDS). It is, however, very toxic against the bone marrow.

Chemotherapy of malignant neoplasms

Next to heart disease, cancer (malignant neoplastic disease) is the major cause of death. Cancer can arise in all tissues. Although new tissue growth can be regarded as a common factor, each type of tumour must be considered as a disease on its own. The biology of the tumour, the clinical symptoms and treatment are diverse. Some tumours may be cured but treatment of others hardly affects tumour growth and dissemination. Colonic and lung cancers grow slowly and are only terminally associated with gross bodily changes. In contrast, pancreatic tumours grow quickly and secrete hormones that produce early and dramatic secondary changes. The incidence of the different cancers also varies and may have a biological basis (sex organ and breast cancers) or may be related to social and industrial conditions (cigarette smoking and lung cancer, aniline dyes and bladder cancer). In general the incidence of cancer is decreasing; however the incidence of malignant melanoma, breast and cervical cancers is increasing.

In the past, due to poor therapeutic responses and a high incidence of adverse effects, chemotherapy was considered only as a last resort, after the apparently more successful treatments, surgery and radiotherapy, had failed. Recent progress (particularly with intermittent combination chemotherapeutic schedules) holds considerable promise and chemotherapy is now the preferred form of treatment of the leukaemias, lymphomas, choriocarcinomas and certain other tumours.

The greater proportion of tumours is resistant to chemotherapy (for example, those of the lung and colon).

Metastasis of the tumour via the blood and lymph gives rise to secondary tumours throughout the body. When this has occurred radiation and surgery are impractical and chemotherapy must be used.

The main problem in cancer chemotherapy is the lack of highly selectively toxic agents. With those currently used, many rapidly dividing normal cells (bone marrow, gut epithelium, spermatogenic cells, lymphoid tissue, hair follicles, fetus) are also killed.

As the therapeutic index of these drugs is low, doses should be optimized for each patient. Drugs may be given per kg body weight or per m^2 of body surface area, the latter being computed from the height and weight of the patient.

Chemotherapy may cure a minority of cancers (for example, Hodgkin's disease, testicular cancer). However for the majority of patients palliation of the symptoms or modest prolongation of survival is usually achieved.

The limited success (enhanced tumour regression, longer remission periods, decreased adverse effects) of intermittent combination therapy has been obtained by rather empirical clinical methods. Developments in knowledge of cell-cycle kinetics (and pharmacokinetics) provide some understanding of the mechanisms involved.

Cell kinetics and dose strategy

Transformation of a normal cell to a neoplastic cell that produces a tumour is associated with changes in the expression of oncogenes. Oncogenes promote uncontrolled cell division and dedifferentiation to a more primitive type.

Cellular replication involves passage through a cell-cycle (*Figure 6.13*).

In general, anticancer drugs may be described as being either cell-cycle phase-dependent or phase-independent.

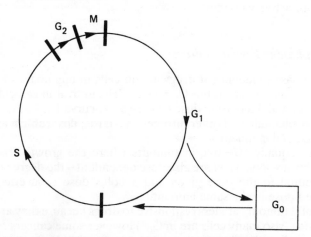

Figure 6.13 G_0 = nonproliferating cells which can reenter the cell cycle; G_1 = variable (usually long) interphase period prior to DNA synthesis (cells grow in size); S = period (6–8 h) of DNA synthesis; G_2 = period (about 2 h) prior to mitosis (tetraploid); M = mitosis

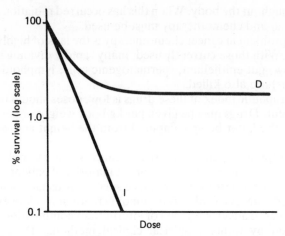

Figure 6.14 Tumour colony-forming cells in culture: D = cell-cycle phase-dependent drug; I = cell-cycle phase-independent drug

Cell-cycle phase-dependent drugs

Cell-cycle phase-dependent drugs act chiefly on cells in certain phases of the cell-cycle (but not G_0). When a cell culture is treated with drugs in this group the percentage of colony-forming cells surviving falls rapidly at first with increasing dose but reaches a plateau where further increase in dose produces no further increase in cell death (*Figure 6.14*, curve D). **Methotrexate,** *mercaptopurine*, *fluorouracil* (S) and vinca alkaloids (M) are phase-dependent drugs.

The cell kill is greater if the drug is given in repeated fractions rather than as the summated single dose.

Most are antimetabolites each producing a particular biochemical blockade. They are most effective in those tumours with a large proportion of the cells that are actively dividing.

Cell-cycle phase-independent drugs

Cell-cycle phase-independent drugs act on cells in any phase of the cycle including a slight effect on the G_0 phase. Cell survival in cell culture falls progressively with increasing dose (*Figure 6.14*, curve I).

Cyclophosphamide and other nitrogen mustards, **doxorubicin** and *cisplatin* are phase-independent.

They are equally effective in tumours where the growth fraction and mitotic index are low. They are also dose dependent – the degree of cell-kill is proportional to the dose given and a bolus dose is as effective as a fractionated dose of the same amount.

Large solid tumours are less responsive to drugs because they are not well vascularized. Also many cells are in G_0. However some cancers respond to the use of cell-cycle phase-independent drugs first, both to reduce cell numbers and promote recruitment of cells into the growth phase of the cell-cycle, thus rendering them susceptible to cell-cycle phase-dependent drugs. If exposure to cell-cycle phase-independent drugs is prolonged (say more than two cell-cycles, about 48 h in man) many normal cells will also be drawn out of G_0 and killed.

Cell kinetic studies have provided a logical basis for the fact that high dosage intermittent combination therapy is the most effective treatment mode. Drugs and timings are selected that allow maximal tumour cell killing, recovery of normal tissue during the drug-free interval and minimal emergence of drug resistance.

Cell-cycle nomenclature

Cell-cycle time: the time for a proliferating cell to pass through the cell-cycle to produce a daughter cell. It is very variable between tumours but fairly constant for a particular tumour type.

Doubling time: the time required for the cell population to double (acute leukaemia – 2 days; breast cancer – 200 days).

Growth fraction: the overall proportion of proliferating tumour cells.

Mitotic index: the fraction of cells in mitosis in a steady state situation.

Principal adverse effects of cancer chemotherapy

When compared with other drug therapy, adverse effects are severe and may necessitate supportive drug therapy and intensive nursing care. Their appearance may be life threatening and may limit the further use of the drugs.

Immediate

(1) Nausea and vomiting are relieved by *metoclopramide* and other anti-emetics, especially ondansetron, a highly selective antagonist at 5-HT$_3$ receptors, acting on the area postrema and possibly on vagal efferent fibres in the gastrointestinal tract. It is usually delayed after bolus injection: the maximum effect occurs 8–10 h after treatment. It is a central action exerted on the CTZ.

(2) Irritancy. Extravasation at the injection site leads to pain and inflammation.

Delayed

(1) Bone marrow depression occurs 7–10 days after a single dose. Neutrophils are most susceptible. Myelosuppression is indicated by decrease in platelet and leucocyte counts and may be used as an indicator of the efficacy of treatment (may lead to bleeding disorders, increased susceptibility to infection and even marrow aplasia). Severe myelosuppression and septicaemia can be reduced by the concurrent administration of granulocyte colony stimulating factor (G-CSF).

(2) Immune suppression is related to marrow depression and to a direct effect on lymphocytes and other 'immunocytes'. There is a low resistance to infection and may be a reduced immunological response against the neoplasia itself.

(3) Gastrointestinal tract disturbances – mucosal ulceration (inspect the mouth), bleeding and diarrhoea.

(4) Epilation (hair loss) is often complete but reversible.

(5) Neurotoxicity (commonly with vinca alkaloids) is seen as peripheral neuropathy that leads to constipation and ileus.

(6) Hepatic damage may be due to toxic metabolites.

(7) During pregnancy, cancer chemotherapeutic drugs must be avoided as animal studies have shown them to be teratogenic.

(8) Impaired growth in children.

(9) Infertility, often irreversible, associated with premature menopause in women and azoospermia in men.

(10) Mutagenesis – alkylating agents are associated with an increased incidence of secondary malignancies, for example, acute myeloid leukaemia after combination therapy and bladder cancer after treatment with **cyclophosphamide.**

Many of the anticancer drugs (*azathioprine*, **cyclophosphamide**) are also immunosuppressive agents, useful alone and in relatively low doses for longer periods after organ transplantation and for the treatment of certain autoimmune diseases (systemic lupus erythematosus).

Antimetabolites

Drugs in this category interfere by competitive inhibition or substrate competition with the synthetic metabolism of nucleic acids (for example replacing —OH and —H in folic acid with —NH_2 and —CH_3 respectively produces **methotrexate**) (purines and pyrimidines).

Methotrexate inhibits DHF hydrogenase (page 257) (affinity for this enzyme is 100 000 times that of folate). It is effective against a wide variety of solid and blood tumours but is particularly prone to produce gastrointestinal lesions. Its toxicity to normal cells can be overcome by the concurrent administration of folinic acid.

Fluorouracil and *cytarabine* – (page 259)

Mercaptopurine (page 258) is metabolized in the liver by xanthine oxidase; this can be prevented by **allopurinol,** which is occasionally used to increase the cytotoxic action.

Azathioprine is a prodrug of mercaptopurine (page 258); its main effect is depression of the immune response and it is reserved for this purpose.

Drugs affecting DNA

Hydroxyurea is a specific inhibitor of DNA synthesis that blocks the cell-cycle at G_1. It is well absorbed. Clinical use is restricted to the treatment of the chronic leukaemias, generally resistant to alkylating agents.

Doxorubicin is an anthracycline antibiotic and has a planar ring structure that is intercalated into the DNA helix and inhibits DNA replication. It has potent effects on bone marrow and is effective in acute myeloid leukaemia and a variety of solid tumours. It is highly toxic to normal tissue and is administered iv in a fast running infusion. Cardiac muscle is particularly susceptible and latent cardiomyopathy may be produced. Related drugs are *mitozantrone* and *epirubicin*, both with a similar spectrum of activity but less cardiotoxic.

Procarbazine binds to DNA and promotes single strand breaks. It is a first line drug in Hodgkin's disease. A disulfiram-like effect is produced if ethanol is ingested.

Actinomycin D [dactinomycin] is the most potent cytotoxic drug on a molar basis. It combines with DNA and prevents transcription to RNA. It is reserved for certain paediatric tumours.

Bleomycin is a generic name for a group of anticancer antibiotics. It inhibits cell proliferation and prevents DNA replication by selective DNA inhibition so that progression of cells through the S-phase of the cycle is inhibited. It is active against squamous cell carcinoma, particularly of head and neck, cervix and lung. It is also used in the lymphomas and testicular cancer. Its main advantage is that it does not produce myelosuppression and therefore can be given in patients whose bone marrow function is compromised. However, it has a propensity to cause pulmonary fibrosis and therefore the total dose must be restricted to 300 mg.

Alkylating agents

Nitrogen mustards are all derivatives (different R-groups) of the basic structure given in *Figure 6.4*.

Mechanism of action – form ethyleniminium ions (page 259) and replace hydrogen in the DNA molecule by an alkyl group. Breaking and cross-linking of DNA chains disrupts cell replication.

Mustine (R = CH_3) is given by iv injection only. It is the most highly reactive and effective member of the group but also the most toxic – used in combination with other agents for the treatment of Hodgkin's disease.

Cyclophosphamide is a 'wide spectrum' antitumour drug given either by mouth or injection. It is a prodrug that requires activation by liver (MFO, page 326) enzymes. A metabolite (acrolein) is irritant to the bladder causing haemorrhagic cystitis that is avoided by hydration and simultaneous administration of the antagonist (by neutralization) *mesna*. One of its active metabolites may denature cytochrome P_{450} thus impairing the biotransformation of various drugs including **cyclophosphamide** itself.

Ifosfamide is structurally similar but has different pharmacological and toxicological properties. The dose-limiting toxicity is damage to the bladder and therefore the uroprotector *mesna* must be given concurrently.

Lomustine is a fat soluble nitrosourea, useful in the treatment of brain tumours.

Chlorambucil is the slowest-acting nitrogen mustard and the treatment of choice in chronic lymphatic leukaemia. Orally active, it is considered by many to be a 'mild' agent but in the correct dosage is as toxic as **cyclophosphamide** – particularly prone to produce thrombocytopenia when given continuously.

Melphalan (R = *l*-phenylalanine) is usually reserved for myeloma and occasionally breast and ovarian carcinoma.

Busulphan (a dimethanesulphonate derivative, not an N mustard) is the least toxic of the alkylating agents (page 260). Platelet depression is unusual but it may produce marrow aplasia so frequent monitoring of the blood count is necessary. It is the treatment of choice for chronic myeloid leukaemia: active orally. Fibrosing alveolitis is an adverse effect (*'busulphan* lung') peculiar to this agent.

Tumour cells may become resistant to alkylating agents with time, perhaps as a result of enhanced DNA repair mechanisms (animal studies indicate that agents that inhibit DNA repair processes, *caffeine* and **chloroquine,** tend to lessen this resistance when given concurrently).

Cisplatin (*cis*-diamminedichloroplatinum) is an organometal compound. The mechanism of action is unknown but is thought to be one of alkylation, which causes damage to DNA by producing cross-links. It has a wide spectrum of clinical activity including ovarian and testicular cancer, head and neck cancer, lung cancer. The main problem is nephrotoxicity and therefore it must be given with hydration. It causes considerable emesis, which can be controlled with ondansetron. Should sepsis result from therapy, aminoglycosides must not be given as their interaction may precipitate acute renal failure.

Carboplatin is an expensive organic analogue of *cisplatin* that is less emetic, not nephrotoxic and has the same spectrum of activity. Dose is directly related to renal clearance.

Vinca alkaloids

These consist of two plant alkaloids with only a small difference in structure but different chemical and physical properties. Administration is by iv injection only.

Vinblastine – effective against Hodgkin's disease, sarcomas, testicular cancer and non-Hodgkin's lymphoma.

Vincristine – effective against acute lymphatic leukaemia, Hodgkin's disease and non-Hodgkin's lymphoma.

Cells accumulate the vinca alkaloids, probably due to their capacity to bind to tubulin and interfere with microtubule assembly within the cell. Microtubules are associated with spindle formation before mitosis and axoplasmic flow; the latter may account for the neurotoxic adverse effects.

Etoposide is a semisynthetic derivative of podophyllotoxin. It is a mitotic inhibitor acting in the cell-cycle at or before the initiation of mitosis but by a mechanism of action different from the classic mitotic inhibitors the vinca alkaloids. It is both cell-cycle dependent and phase specific. It has a wide spectrum of activity, particularly in lung, testes, lymphoreticular disorders and Hodgkin's disease. It may be given both by mouth or by injection but the oral route has erratic absorption and the iv route is to be preferred. After repetitive treatments peripheral neuropathy may develop.

Hormones

Prednisolone is widely used in combination chemotherapy. The lymphosuppressive action of glucocorticoids is exploited in the treatment of leukaemias and lymphomas; there is also antitumour activity against some solid tumours. They promote a sense of well being. Immunosuppression does not appear to compromise treatment.

Specific hormonal therapy started in 1939 with the treatment of prostate cancer with oestrogens. The tumours that respond are generally less ana-plastic (more highly differentiated) than those that do not. Hormones are often used in preference to other drugs because of the latter's undesirable effects on the immune response.

Androgen dependent prostate cancer regresses in response to pharmaco-logical manipulation of androgenic activity (oestrogens, androgen antag-onists, *goserelin*).

Advanced breast cancers are routinely screened for oestrogen receptors. Receptor negative tumours are only treated by chemotherapy. Two-thirds of tumours possess receptors and half of these respond to hormonal manipu-lation – removal of ovaries, **tamoxifen** (page 164), *gonadorelin, aminoglu-tethimide*, removal of adrenals or, paradoxically, large doses of oestrogens or androgens. **Tamoxifen** is relatively free of adverse effects. It has become the hormonal agent of first choice in postmenopausal women with metastatic breast cancer and if often chosen as the initial treatment in premenopausal women.

Progestogens are used for endometrial and renal tumours.

Radiotherapy

Radiotherapy (X-rays, neutrons) is an extremely effective way of treating localized tumours by the generation of highly reactive free radicals that react with DNA: a second course of radical treatment cannot be given as this would damage normal tissues. It is often used in combination with cytotoxic drugs.

^{32}P is as effective as *busulphan* in chronic myeloid leukaemia. ^{131}I is the treatment of choice for elderly patients with thyrotoxicosis. It is selectively concentrated in the thyroid tissue (page 176) and therefore useful in the treatment of differentiated tumours of the thyroid gland.

Manipulation of immunity

The interleukins (including interferons) (page 203) act as immunomod-ulators and may also have therapeutic potential as anticancer agents.

7

Drug disposition

Aims

- To explain the entry of drug molecules into body tissues and their subsequent removal in terms of familiar physical, chemical and biological processes.
- To introduce the concepts underlying the quantitative description of drug handling.
- To focus attention on the entry and removal of particular drugs which serve as type substances for broad groups with similar physicochemical properties.
- To provide the scientific basis underlying the therapeutic choices of routes of administration and dosage regimens of drugs.

Introduction

The relationship between drug concentration and tissue response and the nature of that response are studied in the science of pharmacodynamics. Several processes collectively determine the concentration of drug at its site of action and how the concentration alters with time (*Figure 7.1*). These dispositional processes are studied quantitatively in the science of pharmacokinetics.

Disposition is a comprehensive term that includes the processes of absorption, distribution and elimination.

Absorption is the entry of drug molecules into the systemic blood via the mucous membranes (for example, the alimentary or respiratory tracts), via the skin or from the site of an injection.

Distribution is the movement of drug molecules between the water, lipid and protein constituents of the body.

Elimination is the removal of the original drug molecule from the body by excretion or by metabolism (alteration of the structure of the molecule).

Clearly an understanding of the pharmacokinetic properties of a drug can

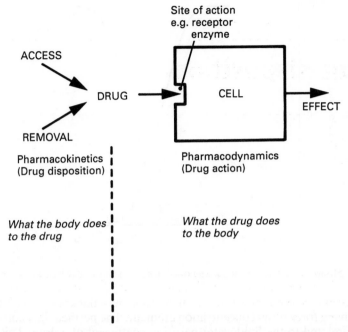

Figure 7.1 The distinction between drug disposition and pharmacodynamics

aid the definition of its dosage regimen to optimize therapy and minimize toxicity. Also, variability in drug response and selectivity of a drug between tissues can have dispositional as well as pharmacodynamic causes.

Drug movement through membranes

Plasma membranes typically consist of a bimolecular lipid sheet (10 nm thick) with polar (hydrophilic) groups outside and nonpolar (hydrophobic) groups inside. Most membranes behave as if they have very small water-filled pores (1 nm diameter). Drugs can pass through membranes by passive processes involving lipid or aqueous diffusion or by utilizing specific carrier systems.

Therefore, the major determinants of the disposition of drugs are the physical properties of membranes and the physicochemical properties of drugs.

Lipid diffusion

Most drugs move through the lipid part of the membrane by passive diffusion. The rate can be expressed by Fick's law:

$$dQ/dt = P_k A (C_1 - C_2) / w$$

where: dQ = amount of drug diffusing within the time interval dt; P_k = permeability constant; A = membrane area; C_1 and C_2 are the drug

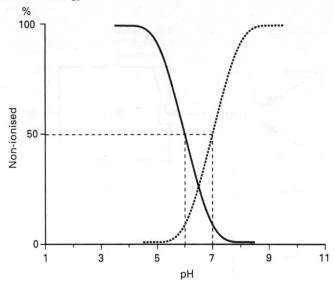

Figure 7.2 Ionization curve for a weak acid (——, $pK_a = 6$) and a weak base (----, $pK_a = 7$)

concentrations on either side of the membrane; w = thickness of membrane. The driving force is the concentration gradient. The permeability constant is closely related to the lipid/water partition coefficient of a drug. This physicochemical property can be measured by the extent to which the drug partitions into an organic solvent (*n*-octanol) relative to an aqueous phase. Therefore, lipid-soluble drug molecules or species penetrate rapidly across membranes while water-soluble drugs or species do not.

Many drugs can be ionized in aqueous solution but only the nonionized species is lipid-soluble. The proportions of ionized and nonionized species are determined by the pH of the medium (*Figure 7.2*) and the ionization constant of the drug (the pK_a = the pH at which half the drug molecules are ionized). This relationship is expressed in the Henderson–Hasselbach equation:

Acid form: $HA = A^- + H^+$
$$pH = pK_a + \log([A^-]/[HA]) \tag{7.1}$$
Basic form: $BH^+ = B + H^+$
$$pH = pK_a + \log([B]/[BH^+]) \tag{7.2}$$

The rate of drug movement is thus proportional to the concentration gradient and lipid solubility of the nonionized, readily diffusible species where permeability is rate limiting.

Aqueous diffusion

Water-filled pores can be penetrated by water-soluble drugs if the molecules are small enough (MW less than 100 Da); examples: ethanol (MW = 46) and urea (MW = 60). Aqueous diffusion is not an applicable mechanism of transport for most drugs as they have MW between 100 and 400 Da.

Specific carrier systems

Some membranes possess active transport or passive facilitated diffusion systems, which exhibit substrate specificity, stereospecificity, saturability and competition between analogues; for example, *l*-amino acids and analogues (**levodopa** and *methyldopa*), *thyroxine*, antimetabolites (purine and pyrimidine analogues). Few drugs meet the structural requirements for carrier transport.

Diffusion across a membrane is rarely rate limiting for highly lipid-soluble drugs and those moving by aqueous diffusion. For these compounds the rate of blood flow is usually limiting – that is they exhibit perfusion rate limitation. Ethanol absorption from stomach, for example, is limited by intestinal blood flow.

Some membranes (for example, endothelia of capillaries, glomeruli) effectively have large water-filled pores (10 nm) that allow the permeation of most drugs.

Absorption

Formulations and routes of administration

Most drugs are administered as a medicine, formulated along with other materials known as excipients, which are pharmacologically inactive. The formulation serves some or all of the following purposes:

(1) an accurately measured dose can be administered;
(2) drug stability is improved;
(3) the drug is presented in a convenient form for administration;
(4) the rate of disintegration and/or solution of the medicine is regulated.

Oral formulations

Disintegration and dissolution

These two processes precede absorption for most oral formulations. Tablets often contain excipients that cause them to swell on contact with water and disintegrate into fine particles. Dissolution then occurs from the surface of the particles. For many medicines the rate of dissolution is faster the smaller the particles because of the larger surface area/mass ratio of the particles.

Many drugs are weak acids or bases and so exhibit pH-dependent dissolution. They can be formulated with a buffering agent (**aspirin** with sodium bicarbonate) to aid dissolution of the acid. On mixing with the environment of the gastrointestinal lumen the drug reprecipitates but as a micronized form that dissolves more readily.

Rate of absorption

The rate of absorption from the gut can be influenced by many factors.

Drug absorption can occur from the stomach but the small intestine is quantitatively much more important because of its vastly greater area and blood flow. If the time to gastric emptying is increased (for example, by taking a drug with food) then the rate of absorption is usually decreased.

If dissolution from the formulation is slower than the rate of drug absorption then absorption is described as dissolution rate limited. However, if dissolution is rapid the permeability characteristics of the drug dictate the rate of absorption.

Sustained and delayed release oral formulations

Rapid dissolution of drugs may cause local damage to the gut mucosa (**aspirin,** potassium chloride, iron salts), or systemic adverse effects due to a brief, high peak of concentration in the blood (*aminophylline* – CNS stimulation). Alternatively the duration of drug response may be too short for practical day-to-day treatment (*quinidine*). These problems are sometimes solved by producing pharmaceutical formulations that release drug slowly or after a delay. Not all these formulations are justified but all are more expensive than the standard drug. A variety of techniques is employed.

Enteric coated tablets

The coating dissolves on reaching a nonacid medium. It is used to protect the drug from acid or to protect the stomach from the drug (**aspirin, prednisolone**). The thicker the coating the slower the solution.

Capsules

Smoothly sustained release may be obtained by filling capsules with mixed granules having different solution rates (*aminophylline*). A thin or soluble coating to the granules gives immediate release. A thick or insoluble coating gives delayed release.

Mucous membranes other than stomach and small intestine

These routes can be used for drugs that are required to provide a local effect or for systemic absorption for drugs that are susceptible to intestinal or liver metabolism. Since the venous drainage of these membranes occurs into the systemic circulation, gut and liver enzymes are avoided. The rate of systemic absorption is dictated by surface area and/or blood flow.

Buccal mucosa

Buccal mucosa provides a convenient site for highly lipid-soluble compounds (**glyceryl trinitrate** in the prophylaxis of effort angina and the treatment of heart failure – there are short acting sublingual and sustained release tablets available).

Respiratory mucosa

Bronchial mucosa and alveoli provide the largest surface area of any mucous membrane and are accessible to vapours and ultrafine droplets (aerosols). Particle size of droplets is of critical importance to achieve drug deposition in the smallest airways.

Examples	*Uses*
Halothane, nitrous oxide	Anaesthesia
Salbutamol	Relief of bronchial asthma

Nasal mucosa

Nasal mucosa provides an inefficient (high proportion of dose is wasted) but convenient route of entry for relatively low MW peptides. They can be administered as a nasal spray.

Examples	*Uses*
Lypressin	Diabetes insipidus
Sodium cromoglycate	Allergic rhinitis

Rectal mucosa

Rectal mucosa provides a useful absorptive surface when the patient is unconscious, vomiting or suffering local gastric adverse effects. The absorption of lipid-soluble drugs can be delayed by presentation in a fatty suppository, into which the drug partitions preferentially.

Examples	*Uses*
Rectal **diazepam** solution	Serial seizures
Sulphasalazine suppositories	Ulcerative colitis
Prednisolone foam	Ulcerative colitis
Metronidazole suppository	Prophylaxis of surgical wound infection

Skin

Healthy skin

Healthy skin is a highly specialized protective envelope that prevents uncontrolled water loss. Skin is several mm thick and normally has a low blood flow. Thus, the entry of water-soluble compounds is limited. However, many lipid-soluble drugs can enter and produce therapeutic or unwanted effects.

Examples	*Uses/Effect*
Glyceryl trinitrate skin patch	Prophylaxis of effort angina
Glucocorticoid esters	ACTH suppression

Infants and toddlers are specially vulnerable to the undesired effects of substances absorbed through the skin because of their high surface area/mass ratio (*Table 7.1*).

Table 7.1 Changing average surface/mass ratio with age

	Child (1 month)	Child (5 years)	Adult
Height (m)	0.50	0.90	1.8
Surface area (m²)	0.25	0.67	1.9
Weight (kg)	5.00	20.00	70.0
m²/kg x 100	5.00	3.40	2.7

Diseased skin

In diseased skin, due to extensive burns, wounds or dermatitis, the water barrier is lost; even water-soluble drugs can enter and fatal accidents have resulted. Occlusive dressings, by increasing the hydration of the skin, augment transdermal absorption.

Examples	*Effects*
Sulphonamides	Crystalluria
Neomycin	Deafness

Parenteral routes

The parenteral (injection) route is necessary when the proportion of the orally administered drug that is absorbed is low. Absorption rate is dictated by blood flow at the site of injection unless sustained release formulations are used.

Intravenous

Absorption is complete when injection is complete unless part of the dose was spilled accidentally outside the blood vessel. The intravenous (iv) route is used when a rapid effect is required, the drug is too irritant by other routes or when abdominal surgery prevents the use of the oral route.

Intramuscular

Skeletal muscle has a rich capillary plexus. The capillary endothelium has large water-filled pores that are freely permeable even to water-soluble drugs of high MW. The intramuscular (im) route is the standard one for injections by nurses. Many emergency drugs (analgesics, antiemetics, oxytocics) are given by this route (deltoid, gluteal and quadriceps muscles). The rate of absorption is proportional to the dose, the extent of dispersion through the muscle and the rate of tissue blood flow – exercise promotes absorption.

Subcutaneous

Subcutaneous tissues are poorly perfused especially in low cardiac output states (haemorrhagic shock, acute diabetic ketoacidosis). The subcutaneous (sc) route is the standard one for self-injection (diabetes) – convenient sites are the upper arm, thigh and abdomen. Absorption is relatively slow even in healthy subjects and may be deliberately delayed by administration of sustained release formulations (depot insulins) or by co-administration of a vasoconstrictor (*adrenaline* with **lignocaine**).

Sustained and delayed release parenteral formulations

Solution in oil

An ester of drug and long chain fatty acid (*fluphenazine decanoate*) is dissolved in nontoxic oil. Drug very slowly diffuses out from an injection site over a period of weeks. The rate-limiting step is hydrolysis to fluphenazine at the surface of the oil. This formulation is used for maintenance dosage in psychotic patients who otherwise fail to take prescribed treatment.

Soluble colloid complex in water

A drug is held in a micelle by weak hydrogen bonds. Release from the complex occurs slowly in the circulation after absorption (*iron dextran* given iv or im).

Suspension of insoluble complex

A complex between soluble drug and a relatively inert molecule is almost insoluble. Soluble drug is slowly released from suspension at the site of im or sc injection. This extends the duration of action of **benzylpenicillin** (*procaine penicillin*) or insulin (*isophane insulin*).

Suspension of crystals

Notably *insulin zinc suspension* – the smallest particles (*amorphous*) give most rapid absorption. The largest crystals (*crystalline*) give the slowest absorption and longest duration of action. A mixture of *amorphous:crystalline* in the ratio of 3:7 spans 4–24 h.

Systemic bioavailability

Systemic bioavailability can be defined as the fraction (F) of the dose of drug administered that reaches the systemic circulation. For iv injection F equals 1 but by other routes, particularly after oral administration, F may be less than 1 (*Table 7.2*). Some drugs may be extensively metabolized on their 'first pass' through the liver.

Table 7.2 Reasons for low systemic bioavailability of drugs after oral administration

Mechanism	Examples
Incomplete solution	**Aspirin** in enteric-coated tablets
Breakdown in gut lumen	**Benzylpenicillin**
Binding in gut lumen	Tetracyclines with divalent cations
Negligible absorption	**Gentamicin**
Metabolism by gut wall	*Isoprenaline*, **levodopa**
Metabolism by liver	**Glyceryl trinitrate**

Where systemic bioavailability after oral administration is low, drugs may need to be given via other mucous membranes or parenterally. The oral route may still be suitable, despite extensive metabolism, if the metabolites are pharmacologically active (**aspirin** is converted to salicylic acid).

Distribution

Distribution involves the movement of drug molecules from the circulating blood to other areas of the body, including the sites of action, of binding and of elimination. Drug action at one site and not another may be due to selective access of drug (pharmacokinetic selectivity) rather than differences in the sites of action (pharmacodynamic selectivity). For drugs applied to the site of action (for example, local anaesthetics injected for nerve block) absorption and distribution reduce drug effects.

Once a drug has entered the blood it mixes rapidly (circulation time = 20 s). The rate and extent of distribution depend upon the relative arterial blood perfusion rates of different organs and the permeability characteristics of cell membranes towards different drug molecules. The initial driving force is the concentration gradient between plasma and the site to which distribution is occurring.

Haemodynamic (perfusion) factors

The whole of the right heart output (and therefore the 'absorbed' dose) is passed through the lungs to the left heart. The bulk of the absorbed dose is then carried rapidly to the 'vessel-rich' group of organs (brain, myocardium, liver, kidneys, adrenals and thyroid), which receive about 80% of the cardiac output at rest. During late pregnancy the uterus and placenta are included.

A few minutes after a drug is injected as an iv bolus it is relatively concentrated in these organs. Drug is more slowly distributed to skeletal muscle, which has a relatively low blood flow at rest. More slowly still it reaches skin and adipose tissue and only very slowly indeed does it reach avascular structures (tendon, cartilage).

Permeability factors

Arterial blood flow determines the rate at which drug reaches the interstitial fluid of a given organ or tissue. The capillary endothelia of most tissues contain large pores (50–100 nm diameter) and therefore present no diffusional barrier to even water-soluble drugs/ionized species (*Figure 7.3*). Particularly the nonprotein-bound drug readily diffuses into interstitial fluid. Therefore, virtually all drugs can gain access to interstitial fluid/cell surface. This may be their site of action (**tubocurarine**).

The rate of penetration into cells and across special tissue barriers is, however, dependent on the physicochemical properties of the drug molecule as the boundary is a lipid membrane (*Figure 7.3*). Highly water-soluble drugs (**gentamicin**) behave like inulin; that is they penetrate into cells slowly or not at all. Conversely highly lipid-soluble drugs (**thiopentone** and inhalational anaesthetics) penetrate very rapidly.

Rate and extent of distribution

For any one drug and one organ the rate of distribution can be perfusion or permeability rate limited.

Perfusion limits the rate of distribution for highly lipid soluble drugs traversing most membranes and for most drugs crossing membranes with large pores. For example, **thiopentone sodium** is so lipid soluble that its rate of entry into the CNS is dictated solely by cerebral blood flow (*Table 7.3*). If a drug has a high affinity for the tissue (high tissue/plasma partition coefficient) then much drug needs to be delivered before equilibrium is reached.

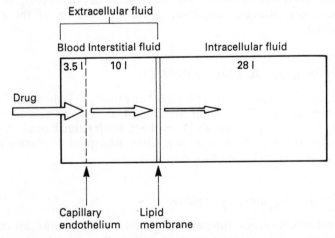

Figure 7.3 The physiological fluid spaces in man and the distribution of drug molecules across these membranes

Therefore, the time to equilibrium is long with low tissue perfusion and a high partition coefficient.

Permeability limits the rate of distribution for water soluble drugs crossing membranes with small pores. Here the time to equilibrium is longer the less permeable the drug and the greater the proportion of drug present as the ionized, nondiffusible species. The factors dictating removal of drug from an organ are the same as those regulating its access.

The differences between drugs in their time to onset of effect after iv administration due to their different physicochemical properties are illustrated in *Table 7.3*.

Table 7.3 Effect of physicochemical property of a drug on the time to the onset of action

Drug	Physico-chemical property	Effect	Time to onset	Rate-limiting process
Thiopentone	Lipid soluble	Anaesthesia	15 s	Circulation time CNS perfusion
Morphine	Weak base	Analgesia	10 min	Diffusion into CNS
Digoxin	Intermediate solubility	Increased ventricular force	30 min	Diffusion into cardiac cell

Binding of drugs by proteins (and other macromolecules)

Virtually all drugs are adsorbed to macromolecules in tissues and in plasma in a readily reversible manner involving noncovalent bonds. The drug/macromolecule complexes associate and dissociate with a half-life $(t_{\frac{1}{2}})$ measured in milliseconds. Rarely, therefore, is the dissociation of the complex rate-limiting.

Binding of drugs to plasma proteins

The total drug concentration in plasma at any time (C) is the sum of the free drug concentration $(C \times f_u)$ and that bound $(C \times f_b)$ to plasma proteins; where: f_u = fraction unbound and $f_b = (1 - f_u)$ = fraction bound. Few drugs exist in plasma solely in the free form. Drug adsorption to plasma proteins can be considered to be of two kinds.

Simple partitioning into a lipid phase

Many lipid-soluble drugs (**thiopentone**) preferentially partition into the non-aqueous phase of plasma. f_u is constant over the therapeutic range of plasma concentrations (*Figure 7.4*).

Association with specific ionic binding sites

Many acidic drugs (salicylic acid, sulphonamides, **warfarin**) bind to one (the same) specific site on each albumin molecule and some basic drugs (**diazepam, propranolol**) bind to α_1-acid glycoprotein and lipoproteins. Usually the number of binding sites considerably exceeds the number of drug molecules, therefore, f_b is constant over a wide range of total drug concentrations.

For just a few drugs, such as those with a high affinity for specific binding sites (salicylic acid, **sodium valproate**), as the total drug concentration in plasma rises within the clinically encountered range, the binding sites become saturated, f_b falls (*Figure 7.4*) and, therefore, the concentration of unbound drug rises out of proportion to the total plasma concentration.

Binding of drugs to tissue macromolecules

Most drugs equilibrate at a higher concentration in tissues than in plasma. Such drug adsorption is reversible. For **digoxin** (page 349) this binding dominates its pharmacokinetics.

Nonreversible binding can occur.

Examples:

Drug	Site	Mechanism
Tetracyclines	Bones, teeth	Binds when blood flow moderate associated with growth Later blood flow very low Also chelation to Ca^{2+}
Cyclophosphamide	Nuclei	Covalent bonding to purine and pyrimidine bases

Dispositional significance of protein binding

(1) The plasma protein/drug complex is a pharmacologically inactive mass transit system, carrying drugs to tissues. Often the total plasma concentration of a drug exceeds its aqueous solubility due to protein binding (**phenytoin, propranolol, benzylpenicillin**) so distribution is more rapid.

(2) Drug/protein complex (plasma/tissue) acts as a reservoir, which smooths fluctuations in the concentration of free drug in plasma water and at the site of action and prolongs its action. If albumin concentration is low (nephrotic syndrome, liver failure, malabsorption, starvation) this effect is reduced.

(3) Two acidic drugs can compete for specific binding sites on plasma albumin. An interacting drug can exaggerate the effects of the target drug (page 40).

Special compartments and special barriers

The rate and extent of distribution of a drug to and from these tissues can be limited either by perfusion or permeability factors. For tissues with a lipid membrane between plasma and the site of drug action and a high blood flow (for example, brain, placenta) drug permeability across the membrane is usually limiting. Only for the most lipid-soluble drugs (**thiopentone sodium**) is blood flow limiting. For tissues with a low blood flow, distribution is usually perfusion limited.

Brain

Thin astrocyte processes envelop the capillary endothelium and provide a lipid membrane between blood and CSF.

Highly polar, water-soluble drugs (**gentamicin**) penetrate slowly, if at all. Nonpolar, lipid-soluble drugs (**thiopentone** and inhalational anaesthetics) penetrate rapidly and drugs with intermediate solubility (tetracyclines) penetrate at an intermediate rate.

The stronger an acidic drug (the lower the pK_a) the smaller the concentration of unionized molecules at pH 7.4 and the slower the rate of penetration into brain – salicylic acid (pK_a 3) penetrates slowly. Similarly, the stronger a basic drug (the higher the pK_a) the smaller the concentration of unionized molecules and the slower the rate of penetration into brain – **morphine** (pK_a 8) penetrates slowly. The penetration of acidic and basic drugs depends also on the lipid solubility of the unionized molecules – *adrenaline* has few CNS effects but the less polar amphetamine (no —OH groups) has marked CNS effects.

Several drugs are transferred from the CSF to the plasma across the choroid plexus against a concentration gradient. This mechanism resembles the transport system in the renal tubule.

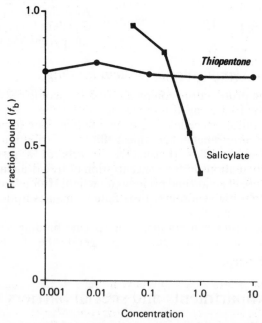

Figure 7.4 Relationship between fraction of drug bound in plasma and total plasma concentration of drug (on a log scale) for **thiopentone** and salicylate. ■ salicylate (mg/ml); ● **thiopentone** (µg/ml)

Examples:

Anions	*Cations*
Benzylpenicillin	**Tubocurarine**
Probenecid	

This process reduces the concentration of penicillins in the CSF and, there-fore, impairs their effectiveness against bacterial infections within the CNS. As a consequence very large doses of these antibiotics are required.

Essential nutrients (amino acids, glucose, purines, pyrimidines) are actively transported into the CSF and brain. *Methyldopa* and **levodopa** also enter by this means.

Placenta

Lipid-soluble drugs (general anaesthetics) penetrate readily and can inter-fere with respiration in the newborn child. **Morphine** and related analgesics cause the same problem. All drugs penetrate into the fetal circulation at some rate. Even highly polar water-soluble drugs (**gentamicin**) penetrate to the fetus slowly. Slow penetration only protects the fetus if delivery is imminent.

Breast

The breast is an example of a pharmacokinetic 'deep' compartment with a moderate blood supply. Most drugs enter breast milk by passive lipid diffusion. Compounds with MW less than 100 Da (ethanol) enter by passive aqueous diffusion. Iodine is actively transported and, therefore, adminis-tration of radioactive iodide to the mother is an absolute contraindication to breast feeding. For most drugs concentrations in milk are similar to those in plasma at equilibrium. However, as the amount of drug in plasma is usually small in relation to the total amount in the body, so the total amount of drug delivered to the infant during breast feeding is small in relation to doses recommended for therapeutic purposes in infants. Hence breast feeding can be continued when the mother is taking **digoxin,** tricyclic antidepressive drugs, **paracetamol, phenytoin,** diuretics and even **warfarin.**

Breast feeding should be discouraged where the mother is taking drugs for prolonged periods and where the drugs could have serious adverse effects on the infant (radioactive iodide, cytotoxic drugs, **carbimazole,** theophylline, sulphonylurea oral hypoglycaemic drugs).

Eye

Anterior compartment

The conjunctiva, sclera, iris and ciliary muscle receive a moderate blood supply but the cornea and lens are avascular. Drugs can penetrate to these structures and the aqueous humour from the conjunctival sac (*chloramphen-icol*). As there is little perfusion of either side of the membranes, the rate of drug movement is mainly proportional to the lipid solubility of the drug and the proportion that is nonionized. As the stroma of the cornea has a high water content, relatively water-soluble drugs (*pilocarpine*) can penetrate into aqueous humour.

Note: **benzylpenicillin** is extruded from the aqueous humour as it is from the CSF.

Posterior compartment

The sclera, choroid and retina are moderately vascular but the vitreous humour is avascular. These structures are not penetrated from the conjunctival sac as the diffusion distance is too great but are reached from the systemic circulation.

Serous cavities

In general, all drugs enter and leave serous cavities (pleural, pericardial, peritoneal sacs, joint spaces) slowly. Water-soluble drugs penetrate slowly and lipid-soluble drugs more rapidly. Acute inflammation facilitates the penetration of drugs but chronic inflammation with fibrosis impedes it.

Bones and teeth

Drug access is proportional to the local blood flow. Infection produces oedema, ischaemia and avascular necrosis so that only prompt treatment is effective. The growth region of bone is moderately well perfused. Blood flow becomes very low when growth ceases. Certain drugs and ions complex with bone salt especially in growing bone (lead, fluoride and tetracyclines).

Skin and nails

These are avascular and thus penetration of drugs from the systemic circulation is very slow. **Griseofulvin,** an antifungal agent, has an affinity for keratin and so achieves selective concentration in skin.

Abscess cavities

Acute abscesses are thin walled, local blood flow is increased and antibiotics penetrate readily. Chronic abscesses have thick avascular walls and drugs do not penetrate. Similarly penetration into sputum is slow. In acute otitis media the organisms are accessible but not in chronic otitis media.

Extent of distribution – apparent volume of distribution

After a dose of drug is administered eventually distribution equilibrium will be reached. The extent of distribution can be defined as the apparent volume of distribution (V).

$$V = \frac{\text{Amount of drug in body at equilibrium}}{\text{Plasma drug concentration}}$$

The concept can be illustrated with a dye model (*Figure 7.5*). A known dose (*D*) of dye is injected into a beaker of water, the compartment well stirred and a sample taken. Measurement of dye concentration enables calculation of compartment volume (*Figure 7.5a*), which is the same as the actual volume. This is the situation for a few drugs, which are either restricted to plasma (very large molecules or plasma protein bound) or restricted to ECF (highly water-soluble) or distribute evenly throughout the body (*Table 7.4*). Most drugs have a tissue/plasma partition coefficient much greater than 1, that is, they exhibit some tissue binding. These drugs therefore 'appear' to have a *V* greater than total body volume (*Figure 7.5b*).

Table 7.4 Examples of apparent volumes of distribution (V)

Substance	V (l)	Equivalent physiological space
Evans blue, **heparin**	3.5	Plasma water
Inulin, **gentamicin**	13.5	ECF
Tritiated water, ethanol	41.5	Total body water
Digoxin	350	None

Elimination

Elimination is achieved by excretion of the unchanged drug or its metabolism. Excretion of drugs is mainly by the kidney but also by other organs that communicate with the exterior. Excretion is important for water-soluble drugs and water-soluble metabolites of the more lipid-soluble drugs.

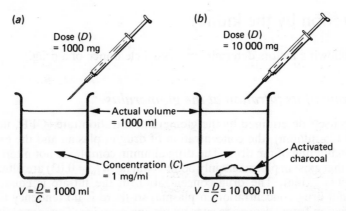

Figure 7.5 Dye model to illustrate apparent volume of distribution: (a) with no 'tissue binding' and homogeneous concentration; (b) with 'tissue binding' simulated by activated charcoal

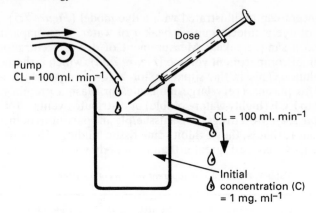

Figure 7.6 Dye model to illustrate clearance

Clearance is used as a measure of elimination. The concept of clearance can be illustrated with a dye model (*Figure 7.6*). Dye solution is pumped from a beaker and clean water is replaced at the same rate to keep the volume of distribution constant.

$$\text{Rate of elimination of dye} = \text{CL} \times C$$
$$= 100 \text{ ml/min} \times 1 \text{ mg/ml}$$
$$= 100 \text{ mg/min}$$

Clearance (CL) is the proportionality constant between the rate of elimination and concentration. As the concentration falls so the rate of elimination decreases in direct proportion.

Renal plasma clearance is the volume of plasma effectively stripped of drug by the kidney per unit time. The total drug clearance is the sum of the renal plasma clearance and clearance by metabolism or by excretion through other organs notably the liver.

Excretion by the kidney

The following factors determine the renal clearance of a drug.

The rate of its filtration at the glomerulus

This is itself determined by the glomerular filtration rate (GFR, normally about 125 ml/min), the concentration of drug in plasma and the extent of protein binding of the drug. The drug/albumin complex is not filtered, thus drugs that exist in plasma mainly bound (**warfarin** $f_u = 0.03$) are filtered to a negligible extent. The drug concentration in the filtrate is equal to the unbound drug concentration in plasma, so there is no tendency for drug dissociation from adsorption sites on plasma proteins. The rate of filtration is not directly affected by the lipid solubility or by the degree of ionization of the drug.

Tubular reabsorption

Passive

Water and salt are removed from the filtrate in the renal tubules and drug molecules diffuse back into the peritubular plasma down a concentration gradient. The rate of reabsorption depends on the same physicochemical properties of a drug that govern its absorption.

Highly polar water-soluble drugs (**gentamicin,** oxidized drug metabolites and conjugates) are too large to penetrate the water pores of cells and have negligible solubility in the membrane lipids. There is little reabsorption and the renal clearance is a high proportion of the GFR. Drugs with intermediate polarity (**digoxin**) resemble the water-soluble drugs. Nonpolar, lipid-soluble drugs (**thiopentone, phenytoin,** inhalational anaesthetics) are reabsorbed from the tubular urine almost completely. Their renal clearance is negligible.

Acidic drugs (pK_a 2–7.4) (salicylic acid) show pH-dependent excretion. The lipid-soluble species (nonionized form) is reabsorbed but the charged, polar species (anion) is not. The maximum renal clearance is obtained at the maximum attainable urine pH, usually 8 (*Table 7.13*). Basic drugs (pK_a 6–12) (**lignocaine**) also show pH-dependent excretion. The lipid-soluble species (nonionized form) is reabsorbed but the charged, polar species (cation) is not. The maximum renal clearance is obtained at the minimum attainable urine pH, usually 5 (*Table 7.16*).

Active

This occurs for drugs that resemble essential metabolites (*l*-amino acids, *thyroxine, methyldopa*). The active reabsorption of uric acid is inhibited by another acid, *probenecid*.

Tubular secretion

Secretion implies active transport into the renal tubules against a concentration gradient. There are two distinct systems each with a low specificity. Each system shows competition and saturation kinetics. Compounds with a low rate of transport can act as inhibitors. The transport is often bidirectional. Examples of anions actively secreted are penicillins, thiazides and loop diuretics, salicylates and drug conjugates. Cations actively secreted include **neostigmine** and **morphine.**

Renal clearance usually exceeds GFR and can be as large as the renal plasma flow. Clearance can exceed renal plasma flow if drug concentrated in red cells is available for secretion (*prilocaine* in highly acid urine). The drug/albumin complex dissociates very rapidly as free drug is secreted, so that renal clearance is not reduced by the protein binding. Thus, although **benzylpenicillin** is about 50% bound the renal clearance approximates to renal plasma flow.

Drug disposition in renal insufficiency

There is accumulation of unchanged drug or metabolites in plasma until the clearance of a small volume of plasma with a high drug concentration equals the rate of intake. Nonrenal elimination mechanisms may become more important.

Water-soluble and intermediate solubility drugs accumulate – **gentamicin** (toxic effects on inner ear and kidney) and **digoxin** (toxic effects on the heart).

Lipid-soluble drugs (**phenytoin**) do not accumulate but the water-soluble hydroxylated metabolites do, and their effects may be clinically detectable.

Actively transported drugs show intermediate accumulation. Large doses of the diuretic **frusemide,** which is actively secreted, can be given without evidence of systemic toxicity.

Creatinine clearance

The clearance of creatinine is widely used to measure GFR when assessing renal impairment. Creatinine is a catabolic product of amino acid metabolism derived from muscle. Its rate of production is proportional to muscle mass and is fairly constant for an individual. Creatinine (MW 113 Da) is water-soluble, distributes through ECF, exhibits limited binding to proteins and is eliminated by renal filtration at a rate equal to GFR. There is some passive reabsorption of creatinine, which is matched by active secretion. Creatinine clearance can be determined in two ways:

(1) by collection of a 24-h urine sample, a blood sample at the midpoint of the 24-h period and assay of their creatinine contents;

$$\text{CL}_{\text{CR}} \text{ (ml/min)} = \frac{\text{Creatinine content of 24-h urine sample (mg/24 h)}}{\text{Serum creatinine content (mg/ml)} \times 60 \times 24}$$

(2) more commonly by collection and assay of a blood sample and by calculation of creatinine production from an estimation of muscle mass using easily measured physical characteristics (height, weight, sex). At a steady state, the rate of elimination of creatinine equals its rate of production.

CL_{CR} in a young adult is about 125 ml/min. Serum creatinine concentration is relatively constant within an individual as both creatinine production and CL_{CR} fall with age. Renal clearance of a drug at a rate greater than 125 ml/min implies some active secretion while renal clearance at less than the CL_{CR} implies some reabsorption or plasma protein binding. As urine flow is normally about 1 ml/min it can be deduced that more than 99% of water filtered at the glomerulus is reabsorbed.

Where glomerular filtration is the predominant mechanism of drug elimination, there is a close correlation between drug clearance and CL_{CR}. In renal insufficiency the loading dose required will be similar to that of a healthy individual (V is unchanged) but the reduced maintenance dose rate can be calculated using nomograms (graphical representations between the variables dose rate and CL_{CR}).

Excretion – other routes

Liver

Bile flow is low, about 0.5 ml/min. Therefore, biliary clearance of unmetabolized drugs, which enter bile by simple diffusion, is negligible. Biliary excretion is significant for drug metabolites. Active transport systems exist for polar compounds with MW greater than 250 Da. These mechanisms are applicable for carbohydrates (dextran, inulin, sucrose, *mannitol*) and acidic compounds (bile acids, bilirubin, iodine contrast media, glucuronide, glycine and sulphate conjugates and penicillins).

Excreted compounds are often reabsorbed from the gut; they may be re-excreted by the liver to produce 'enterohepatic recycling' (contraceptive steroids, phenothiazines, *Figure 7.7*). The reabsorbed drug, metabolite or conjugate is often finally excreted by the kidney.

Biliary obstruction and hepatocellular failure produce impairment of biliary excretion.

Lungs

Drug molecules may diffuse across alveolar membrane. The lungs are the major organ of elimination of volatile anaesthetics. Excretion in expired air may be obvious to smell but quantitatively insignificant (ethanol, *paraldehyde*, thiols).

Saliva, milk, sweat, sebum

The amounts of drug excreted are small but relevant to the breast-fed infant and to the treatment of acne with antibacterial drugs that partition into sebum (*tetracycline*).

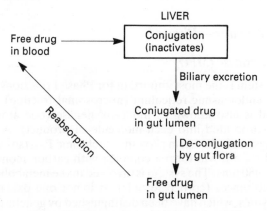

Figure 7.7 Enterohepatic circulation of steroids

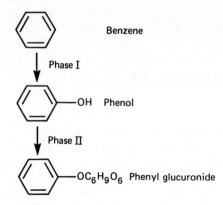

Figure 7.8 The phases of benzene biotransformation

Drug metabolism

Most lipid-soluble compounds are metabolized to more water-soluble products. Drugs must possess some degree of lipid solubility to be able to pass
through cell membranes to gain access to enzymes. The metabolism (biotransformation) of foreign compounds (xenobiotics) occurs mainly in liver,
although kidney, adrenal cortex, lungs, placenta, skin and even lymphocytes may be involved to a small extent.

Atracurium (page 77) is an unusual drug in that it undergoes spontaneous
hydrolysis in blood (at pH 7.4, 37°C) to inactive products so terminating its
neuromuscular blocking action.

The biotransformation of most drugs occurs in two phases (*Figure 7.8*).

Phase I – reactions that unmask or insert a hydrophilic functional group
(—OH). Phase I reactions generally produce a more water-soluble and less
active compound.

Phase II – conjugation reactions. The conjugation occurs at the site of a
reactive group (-OH, added perhaps by a Phase I reaction). A Phase II
reaction renders a compound much more water-soluble and totally inactive.

Metabolic pathways – Phase I

Mixed function oxidase (MFO)

This enzyme system is the most important for Phase I reactions. It is located
in the smooth endoplasmic reticulum (microsomal fraction), is relatively
nonspecific and is also known as mono-oxygenase (one atom of the O_2
molecule is incorporated into each molecule of product). A major component of the system is the haem protein cytochrome P_{450} (so called because
in the reduced state it will form a complex with carbon monoxide, which
absorbs light at 450 nm). The system is involved in the metabolism of several
endogenous substances (corticosteroids). It is not one oxidase but many
oxidase isoenzymes, which have been distinguished by genetic means and by
selectivity for particular substrates.

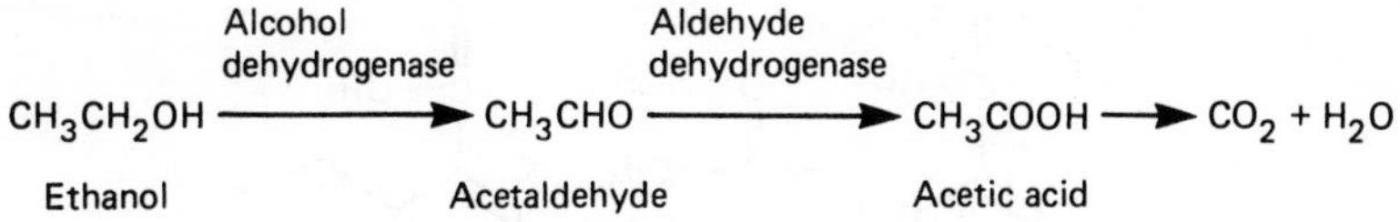

$$CH_3CH_2OH \xrightarrow[\text{dehydrogenase}]{\text{Alcohol}} CH_3CHO \xrightarrow[\text{dehydrogenase}]{\text{Aldehyde}} CH_3COOH \longrightarrow CO_2 + H_2O$$

Ethanol   Acetaldehyde   Acetic acid

Figure 7.9 Oxidation of ethanol

Examples:
Chemical reaction   *Example*
Hydroxylation of aromatic ring   Benzene → phenol
Hydroxylation of alkyl chain   Toluene → benzyl alcohol
Epoxidation   Benzopyrene → benzopyrene
                                                       epoxide
Oxidative deamination   Amphetamine → phenylace-
                                                       tone

Other oxidations

Some are cytoplasmic (ethanol metabolism, *Figure 7.9*), others are mitochondrial (MAO – substrates include NA, tyramine, page 101).

Reductions

Reductive metabolism of drugs (*Figure 7.10*) is less common that oxidation.

Hydrolysis

Ester bonds (in **aspirin, atropine,** *pethidine*) and amide bonds (in **lignocaine**) can be hydrolysed (*Figure 7.11*). Esterases are present in gut, liver, plasma and other tissues.

Metabolic pathways – Phase II

Glucuronide conjugates

Glucose is oxidized to glucuronic acid. This in turn is combined with alcoholic or phenolic hydroxy groups or amines to form glucuronide conjugates (*Figure 7.8*).

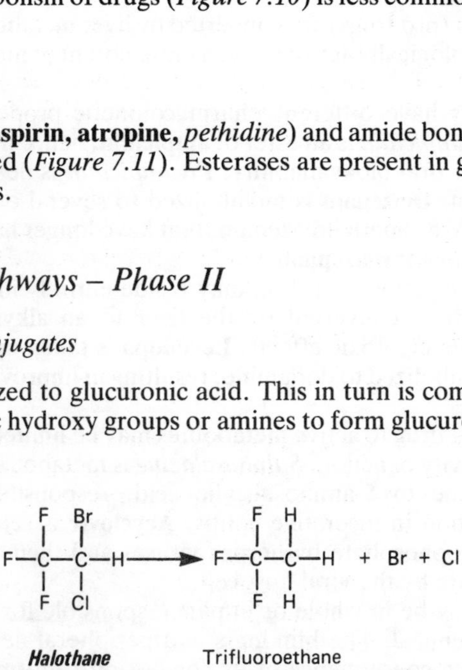

$$\begin{array}{ccc} F & Br & \\ | & | & \\ F-C-C-H & \longrightarrow & F-C-C-H + Br + Cl \\ | & | & \\ F & Cl & \end{array}$$

Halothane   Trifluoroethane

Figure 7.10 Reductive metabolism of **halothane**

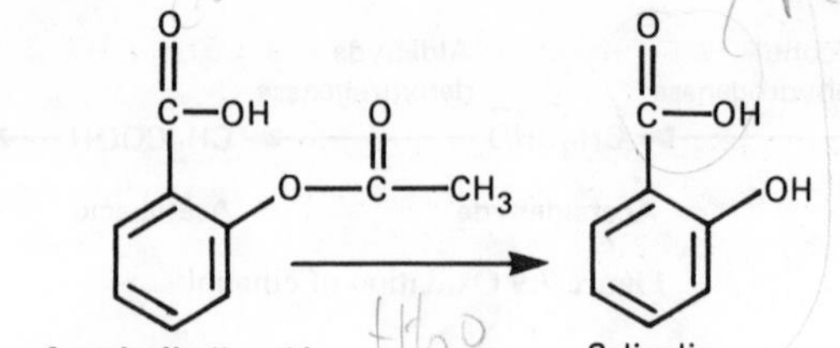

Figure 7.11 Hydrolysis of acetylsalicylic acid (**aspirin**)

Other conjugates

Products from Phase I metabolism or parent drugs can form addition compounds with sulphate (paracetamol sulphate), acetate (acetylisoniazid), glycine (salicyluric acid) and a methyl group (NA to adrenaline).

Pharmacological importance of drug metabolism

Usually liver metabolism involves the conversion of lipid-soluble to more water-soluble compounds. The high MW conjugates are actively transported into the bile duct or the metabolites diffuse into the blood and are excreted by the kidney. The majority of metabolites are less pharmacologically active (potent) than the parent drugs.

Prodrugs

Some compounds (prodrugs) are converted by liver metabolism to products that are pharmacologically active or even more potent or more toxic than the parent chemical.

Some prodrugs have different pharmacokinetic properties from their metabolites. *Pivampicillin* is an ester of **ampicillin,** hence more lipid soluble and with a higher oral bioavailability. *Pivampicillin* is de-esterified by the liver to ampicillin. **Diazepam** is metabolized to several other benzodiazepines, including *N*-desmethyldiazepam, that have longer half-lives and contribute to the action of **diazepam.**

The therapeutic action of a drug may reside entirely in its metabolites. **Cyclophosphamide** is converted by the liver to an alkylating derivative responsible for the cytotoxic effects. **Levodopa** is taken up by neurones in the CNS and metabolized to dopamine, resulting in improvement in Parkinson's disease.

Conversion of a drug to active metabolites may be limited to one organ so increasing selectivity of action. *Sulphasalazine* is metabolized by bacteria in the large intestine to 5-aminosalicylic acid, responsible for the anti-inflammatory action in ulcerative colitis. **Acyclovir** is selectively metabolized to the monophosphate by herpes viruses and then converted to the active triphosphate by the viral host cell.

Metabolites may be in whole or in part responsible for the toxic effects of the parent chemical. The blindness and peripheral neuropathy caused by methanol are a consequence of its conversion to formaldehyde. **Paracetamol** is mainly metabolized to inactive conjugates but a minor oxidized metabolite is a reactive quinone. Normally this derivative is conjugated with glutathione in the liver. In **paracetamol** overdosage the liver content of glutathione is soon consumed. The remaining reactive quinone covalently bonds to proteins resulting in hepatic necrosis. Early treatment with *acetylcysteine*, which is converted to glutathione, can prevent liver failure in **paracetamol** overdose.

Metabolic rate

The concept of clearance (page 320) can be equally applied to liver metabolism. An organ clearance can be defined in terms of drug removal across the eliminating organ. Hepatic clearance equals liver blood flow (normally about 1500 ml/min) multiplied by the extraction ratio (the proportion of drug presented to the liver at each pass that is metabolized by it). The extraction ratio can vary from one (virtually all drug presented is removed) to zero (no drug metabolized).

Examples:

Low extraction ratio	*High extraction ratio*
Phenytoin	**Lignocaine**
Salicylic acid	**Glyceryl trinitrate**
Warfarin	**Morphine**

For drugs with a high extraction ratio, the liver has such a high capacity for metabolism that the clearance is unaffected by changes in enzyme activity or fraction protein bound but is proportional to blood flow (changes in amount delivered). Shock (with reduced hepatic blood flow) decreases metabolism. **Lignocaine** and **morphine** are unusually persistent in patients with cardiogenic shock. This category of drug exhibits considerable 'first pass' metabolism (when absorbed from the gut all the drug is presented to the liver but on the first circulation only).

For drugs with a low extraction ratio, blood flow delivers them in amounts in excess of either drug diffusion into the liver or the liver's capacity to metabolize. Therefore, clearance is sensitive to changes in fraction of drug in plasma that is unbound and enzyme activity but not blood flow. The liver can still be the major route of elimination for drugs in this group.

Most drug metabolizing systems exhibit first order kinetics (rate of enzymatic elimination is proportional to C^1) within the therapeutic range of drug plasma concentrations; a few, specifically salicylic acid (page 362), **phenytoin** (page 354) and ethanol (page 356), exhibit saturation or zero order kinetics (rate of enzymatic elimination is proportional to C^0, that is, is independent of C).

There is a genetically determined variation in the rate of metabolism by some specific enzyme systems. The best studied examples are *N*-acetylation (page 29), plasma ChE (page 30) and drug hydroxylation by MFO (page 30).

Metabolism and drug interactions

The MFO system is inducible by a few drugs. As a result, there is an increased rate of elimination of the inducing drug itself and many other drug substrates (page 41).

A number of the enzyme systems can be inhibited by drugs, leading to decreased elimination of other drugs or endogenous substrates. This can lead to excessive drug effects although often the interaction is not of major clinical significance or can be taken into account by change in dosage (page 42).

Pharmacokinetics

Pharmacokinetic knowledge contributes in many ways to the practice of therapeutics. These include:

(1) distinguishing between pharmacokinetic and pharmacodynamic causes of an unusual degree of response to a drug;
(2) evolving concepts that are common to all drugs; thus information gained about one drug helps in anticipating the pharmacokinetics of another drug;
(3) often explaining the manner of a drug's use and occasionally suggesting a more convenient or an improved dosage regimen;
(4) often allowing anticipation of the likely outcome following a therapeutic manoeuvre.

One-compartment open model

A stirred beaker of water that is continuously emptied and replenished by a pump (*Figure 7.6*) simulates the major processes of drug disposition. The rate and completeness of absorption are under the control of the operator when injecting a dose of a dye into the beaker. Immediate injection is equivalent to bolus iv injection in a patient. This dose is then distributed throughout the volume of water in the beaker (or apparent volume of distribution, *Figure 7.5*) at a rate that is determined by the stirrer (equivalent to the heart). Elimination from the beaker (equivalent to the kidneys, liver and lungs) starts as soon as some dye has entered and is determined by the rate at which coloured water overflows and the pump replaces it by clean water; that is the rate at which the pump 'clears' the water in the beaker.

It is characteristic of this model that the dye does not disappear at a steady rate. The higher the concentration the more rapidly does it fall. In fact, the rate of elimination of dye (the slope in *Figure 7.12a*) is proportional to the concentration. This is the characteristic of an exponential process and a convenient statistic for describing an exponential process is the half-time $(t_{\frac{1}{2}})$.

This simple model adequately describes the handling of most drugs used in patients although it is sometimes necessary to postulate more than one distribution compartment and an elimination process that can be saturated at high concentration. In what follows, this simple model is used to illustrate the principles of pharmacokinetics.

Intravenous bolus dose

If a dose (D) of drug is injected slowly iv into an average patient he behaves towards the drug as though composed of a well stirred single open compartment of volume (V), see *Figure 7.5a*. The peak concentration that would have been reached at zero time, i.e. $C_0 = D/V$, can be deduced by assaying the plasma concentration (C) at various times (t) and extrapolating back to zero time – see *Figure 7.12a*.

The compartment, with apparent volume of distribution V, loses drug by a process of elimination to the outside world (hence 'open'). This loss results in the decay of the compartment's drug concentration in a time dependent (kinetic) fashion. The rate of decay (dC/dt) is proportional only to the concentration (i.e. is exponential) so the process is described as 'first order':

$$dC/dt = -k_{el}\, C \qquad \text{(differential form)}$$
$$C = C_0 e^{(-k_{el}t)} \qquad \text{(integral form)}$$

C is an exponential function of time and any of the three interrelated parameters can be used to describe the rate of the decay of C with time:

(1) half-life (or half-time) $t_{\frac{1}{2}}$;
(2) elimination rate constant k_{el};
(3) elimination clearance CL.

The time taken for the concentration to halve ($t_{\frac{1}{2}}$ – units = time) is constant irrespective of the concentration or the elapsed time. This is a

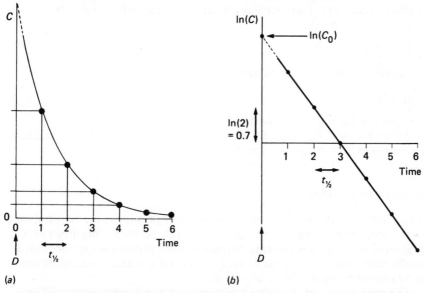

(a)   (b)

Figure 7.12 The exponential decay of concentration: (a) on an arithmetic scale; (b) on a logarithmic scale, with time after injection of a dose (D) into a one-compartment open model

characteristic feature of exponential processes. Another is that replotting the same data on the same abscissa but a logarithmic ordinate produces a straight line (*Figure 7.12b*). (This is how, by back extrapolation to $t = 0$, the peak concentration (C_0) and hence V could be deduced).

Using natural logarithms (ln) the negative slope of this semilogarithmic relationship is the elimination rate constant, k_{el} (units = time^{-1}). A k_{el} of 0.1 h^{-1} implies that 10% of the drug is eliminated per hour. k_{el} is closely related to $t_{\frac{1}{2}}$

$$k_{el} = 0.7/t_{\frac{1}{2}} \tag{7.3}$$

(the value of ln(2) is approximately 0.7)

The third parameter of rate of decay of plasma concentration is the elimination clearance CL (units = volume time^{-1}). This is the proportionality constant in the relationship between rate of drug elimination (units = mass time^{-1}) and its driving force, the plasma concentration. Clearance can also be defined as the volume of plasma that contains the mass of drug eliminated in unit time.

$$\text{Rate of elimination} = \frac{\text{mass of drug eliminated}}{\text{time}} = V \times dC/dt \tag{7.4}$$

For an exponential process, the rate of elimination is proportional to concentration:

$$V \times dC/dt \, \alpha \, C \tag{7.5}$$

$$V \times dC/dt = CL \times C \tag{7.6}$$

where CL is the proportionality constant, the clearance. From this equation it can be seen that clearance has the units of volume per unit time.

It can be shown that:

$$k_{el} = CL/V \tag{7.7}$$

Therefore, combining equations 7.7 and 7.3:

$$t_{\frac{1}{2}} = 0.7 \, V/CL \tag{7.8}$$

Equation 7.8 is an important one for you to understand.

Note (*Figure 7.13a and b*) that an empirically observed long $t_{\frac{1}{2}}$ can have two independent causes – a small CL or a large V!

Intravenous infusion

The iv infusion of a drug at a constant rate (D/T) results in the accumulation of the drug in the compartment to a steady state plateau concentration (C_{ss}) (*Figure 7.14a*). This is because the elimination process is exponential. Initially drug output is zero but as the concentration rises the output increases until output = input (the steady state).

The time course of the growth of concentration is asymptotic and its $t_{\frac{1}{2}}$ is identical with the elimination $t_{\frac{1}{2}}$. The time to reach the plateau depends only on $t_{\frac{1}{2}}$. The shorter the $t_{\frac{1}{2}}$ the quicker the plateau is attained (*Figure 7.14b*).

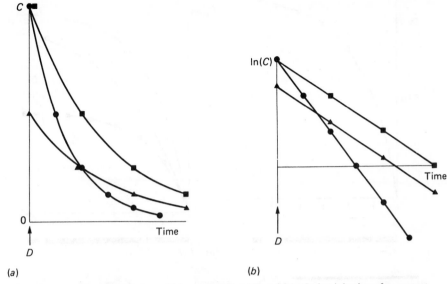

Figure 7.13 Change with time of (a) concentration (C) or (b) ln C after injection of a constant dose (D) into a one-compartment open model: the effect of altering volume of distribution (V) or elimination clearance (CL). ● = initial values of V and CL; ▲ = effect of doubling V and hence doubling $t_{\frac{1}{2}}$ or halving k_{el}; ■ = effect of halving CL and hence doubling $t_{\frac{1}{2}}$ or halving k_{el}

It is conventional and convenient to regard the steady state as effectively attained when more than 95% of the steady state concentration (C_{ss}) is reached. Five half-lives must elapse before more than 95% of C_{ss} is attained (*Table 7.5*).

Table 7.5 Time course of approach to steady state

Time (in multiples of $t_{\frac{1}{2}}$)	Plateau concentration (% of C_{ss})
1	50
2	75
3	87.5
3.3	90
4	93.75
5	96.87

The actual concentration at steady state (the plateau concentration) is determined by the rate of drug infusion and the clearance. Note that an increase in V will slow the rate of attainment of a steady state but will not affect C_{ss}.

At a steady state the concentration of drug in the compartment does not change. The rate of drug input to the compartment is the infusion rate (D/T), the rate of output is the rate of elimination ($CL \times C_{ss}$, from *Equation 7.6*). Hence

$$D/T = CL \times C_{ss} \tag{7.9}$$

Equation 7.9 is an important one for you to understand.

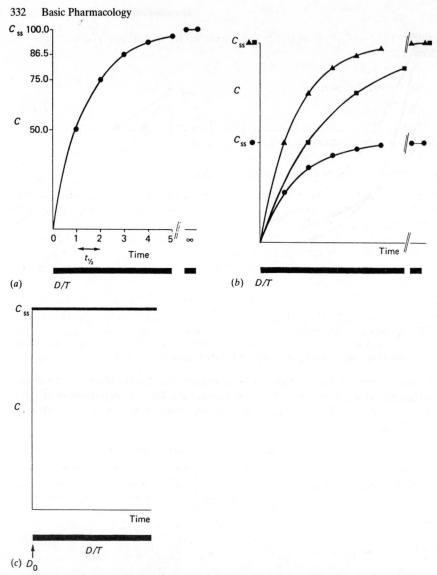

Figure 7.14 Change of concentration (*C*) with time after constant infusion (rate *D/T*) into a one-compartment open model: (a) accumulation asymptotic to C_{ss}; (b) the effect of altering infusion rate or elimination clearance (CL); ● = initial values of *D/T* and CL; ▲ = effect of doubling *D/T*; ■ = effect of halving CL and hence doubling $t_{\frac{1}{2}}$; (c) the effect of the loading dose D_0

Intravenous bolus dose and infusion

The delay in establishing the steady state inherent in iv infusion of a drug with a significant $t_{\frac{1}{2}}$ can be eliminated by injecting a suitable bolus dose (loading dose) as the infusion is begun. *Figure 7.14c* shows the algebraic sum of *Figure 7.13a* and *Figure 7.14a*.

The loading dose (D_0) that is needed is that which produces a peak concentration (C_0) equal to the C_{ss} produced by the infusion (maintenance dosing).

$$D_0/V = C_0 = C_{ss} = (D/T)/CL$$

Hence from *Equation 7.8*

$$D_0/(D/T) = t_{\frac{1}{2}}/0.7 \tag{7.10}$$

That is, the greater the $t_{\frac{1}{2}}$ of a drug the larger the bolus dose will need to be in relation to the maintenance dose rate.

Regularly repeated intravenous bolus doses

The smoothed average compartmental concentration (C_{av}) resulting from regular bolus dosing is no different from that resulting from infusion at the same drug input rate (D/T).

The rate of approach to steady state depends only on $t_{\frac{1}{2}}$. The steady state average concentration (C_{avss}) is determined by the dose rate and clearance. However each injection produces a spike increment of concentration over the previous trough of D/V (*Figure 7.15*).

Large trough to peak fluctuations are caused by large infrequent dosing and smaller fluctuations at the same dose rate are caused by smaller doses at more frequent intervals.

Intravenous bolus dose and repeated doses

As in the case of iv bolus dose and infusion (page 332) the time it takes to reach steady state can be reduced by starting the sequence with an

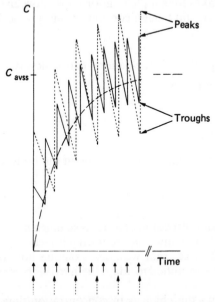

Figure 7.15 Change of concentration (C) with time after dosing a one compartment open model with a constant dose rate (D/T) but varying interdose intervals (T): --- = smoothed average C with T near 0 as with iv infusion: → = repeated bolus injections at significant dose intervals; ⇢ = repeated bolus injections at longer T

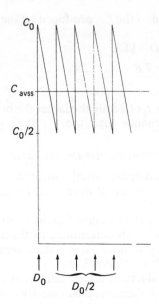

Figure 7.16 The early establishment of a steady state in discontinuous dosing by a loading dose

appropriately sized loading dose (*Equation 7.10* applies). When the dosing interval equals the $t_{\frac{1}{2}}$ the maintenance dose must be one-half the loading dose to make good the loss (*Figure 7.16*).

Note that this makes for simple relationships between both doses, volume of distribution, peak and trough concentrations and dosing interval:

$$C_{\text{avss}} = C_0/(2 \times 0.7)$$

For other dosing intervals the general expression is:

$$C_{\text{avss}}/(D/V) = t_{\frac{1}{2}}/(0.7\ \text{T}) \tag{7.11}$$

or in mass terms

$$A_{\text{avss}}/D = t_{\frac{1}{2}}/(0.7\ \text{T})$$

where A_{avss} is the average amount of drug in the body at steady state.

Single oral dose

The oral route of administration of drugs is so much more convenient than iv injection or indeed than any route requiring injection, and in most circumstances equally effective, that we must examine how these concepts and equations need to be modified to adapt them to this common form of clinical dosing.

Figure 7.17 shows the changes in concentration/time profile that occur when a single dose is input to the compartment by a first order process occurring at different rates but completely (fraction of dose absorbed, $F = 1$).

Notice that as the absorption half-time increases the peak concentration declines, the peak concentration occurs later after dosing and the compartment concentrations at each time after the peak time are larger.

Less obvious from the figure but nevertheless true and useful is the fact that the area under the concentration/time curve is unchanged. This is because the deficit early after the dose due to the delay in absorption is exactly matched by the later excess.

Repeated oral dosing

Repeated oral dosing leads to phasic accumulation of drug somewhere between the smooth ascent of *Figure 7.14a* and the extreme fluctuations of *Figure 7.15*. The average concentration rises asymptotically with a half-time that is usually dominated by the elimination $t_{\frac{1}{2}}$ but may be even longer if the absorption half- time is extreme. In this latter case absorption is also likely to be incomplete because it will be terminated by defaecation.

The C_{avss} attained is determined by the input dose rate ($F \times D/T$) and clearance as in *Equation 7.9*.

The size of the fluctuations is determined by the dose interval and volume of distribution but is more damped as the absorption half-time increases.

Oral loading dose followed by regular maintenance dose

As in *Figure 7.16*, but with the fluctuations damped, the therapeutically required C_{avss} can be established early by administering a loading dose that is larger than the repeated maintenance dose by the factor established in *Equation 7.11* – $t_{\frac{1}{2}}/(0.7 \ T)$.

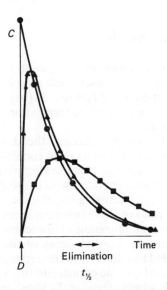

Figure 7.17 Change of concentration (C) with time after administration of a single dose (D) into a one-compartment open model: the effect of altering absorption $t_{\frac{1}{2}}$. ● = absorption $t_{\frac{1}{2}}$ near 0 as with iv bolus; ▲ = absorption $t_{\frac{1}{2}}$ = elimination $t_{\frac{1}{2}}$; ■ = absorption $t_{\frac{1}{2}}$ = 10 × elimination $t_{\frac{1}{2}}$

Summary of pharmacokinetic terms and symbols

Pharmacokineticists who study the processes of drug handling in animals and man have evolved a series of more or less standard terms and symbols.

A (mg) – amount of drug in the body at a particular time

C_{avss} (mg/l) – mean plasma drug concentration when a steady state is attained

C (mg/l) – concentration in main/central/plasma compartment at a particular time after the previous dose

C_0 (mg/l) – concentration at zero time in hypothetical state of complete absorption with no elimination; obtained by back extrapolation

CL (l/h) – drug clearance; volume of fluid (blood, plasma or water) that contains the mass of drug eliminated in unit time

CL_{CR} (l/h) – clearance of endogenous creatinine; useful measure of kidney function that approximates to GFR

D (mg) – dose of drug

F – fraction of dose absorbed from site of administration

k_a (h^{-1}) – absorption rate constant; reciprocally related to the time for 50% absorption

k_{el} (h^{-1}) – elimination rate constant; reciprocally related to the time for 50% elimination

$t_\frac{1}{2}$ (h) – elimination half-time; time for C to fall by one-half or time for 50% elimination

T (h) – interval between doses during a course of drug treatment

V (l) – distribution volume; size of conceptual compartment in which drug is distributed

Two-compartment model

It is common for drugs with significant lipid solubility to show evidence of distribution into more than one compartment after iv injection. Iv injection into the two-compartment model of *Figure 7.24* (page 350) would produce a semilogarithmic central compartment concentration/time curve (analogous to *Figure 7.12b*) like *Figure 7.18*.

Immediately after injection and mixing, the drug is restricted to the central compartment (volume V_1) so its peak concentration is high (D/V_1). The concentration declines not only because elimination clearance is occurring from the central compartment but also because distribution (described by a distribution clearance) is occurring into the second compartment. At a time determined by the ratio of these two clearances, distributional steady state is attained with the minimization of the concentration gradient between the two compartments. Further decay of the central compartment concentration is controlled by elimination clearance and back extrapolation to time zero allows the total volume of distribution ($V_1 + V_2$) to be derived.

When the same drug is administered orally the slowness of the absorptive processes masks the rapid simultaneous distribution processes and the system behaves for all practical purposes like a one-compartment model. Thus in therapeutics a firm grasp of the kinetics of the one-compartment

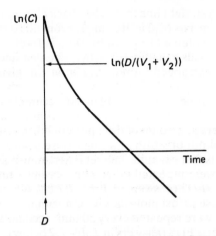

Figure 7.18 The two phases of decay of plasma concentration (logarithmic scale) with time revealing the need for a two-compartment model of drug disposition

open model will allow rational manipulation of the doses and dose intervals of most drugs in most patients. Multicompartment models are needed with high rates of systemic delivery of lipid soluble drugs – iv **thiopentone** in the induction of general anaesthesia (page 352) and inhalational anaesthetic agents (page 357).

Examples

In these examples the dye model has been scaled up to the dimensions that might apply to real drugs used in the treatment of an adult patient.

Table 7.6 Three example sets of concentration/time data following the dose stated at zero time

Dose (time 0 h) Time (h)	A (160 mg)	B (500 μg) Concentration (mg/l)	C (100 mg)
0.5	8.74	–	0.74
1	7.14	–	0.55
2	4.80	–	0.30
4	2.14	–	0.09
6	0.96	0.77	0.03
8	0.45	–	0.01
10	0.19	–	–
12	0.10	0.70	–
24	–	0.56	–
36	–	0.46	–
48	–	0.38	–

Obtain a sheet of two or three cycle semilogarithmic graph paper and plot the concentration data of *Table 7.6*, example A, on the vertical (semilogarithmic) axis against time on the horizontal axis. Alternatively use normal graph paper and plot the $\log_{10}$ of the concentration against time.

The points lie on a straight line that, when back extrapolated to zero time, cuts the concentration axis (C_0) at 10.7 mg/l. From this it can be determined that the distribution volume (V) given by D/C_0 is 160/10.7 or 15 l.

The concentration falls to half in 1.75 h ($t_{\frac{1}{2}}$). The clearance can be found by substituting into a rearranged form of *Equation 7.8*, giving a CL of 0.7 × 15/1.75 or 6 l/h.

If the dose were repeated every 12 h no accumulation would occur. Assuming complete absorption ($F = 1$) the C_{ss} from *Equation 7.9* would be 2.2 mg/l and the average amount of drug present during a dosage interval in the steady state is about one-fifth of a single dose from *Equation 7.11*.

Repeat this exercise for example data set B assuming partial absorption ($F = 0.6$). If the dose were repeated every 24 h, accumulation would occur to what C_{avss} and A_{avss}/FD? (answers in *Table 7.7 below*).

Repeat this exercise for example data set C assuming complete absorption ($F = 1$). If the dose were repeated every 30 min, accumulation would occur to what C_{avss} and A_{avss}/FD? (answers in *Table 7.7 below*). Iv infusion would be a better way of achieving this.

These three examples represent different patterns of drug disposition observed with drugs that have different physicochemical properties (A, page 346, **gentamicin**; B, page 349, **digoxin**; C, page 364, **lignocaine**).

Table 7.7 Answers to examples

	A	B	C
D (given)	160 mg	500 µg	100 mg
C_0	10.7 mg/l	0.84 µg/l	1 mg/l
V (l)	15	350	100
$t_{\frac{1}{2}}$ (h)	1.75	40.8	1.17
CL (l/h)	6	6	60
T (h) (given)	12	24	0.5
F (given)	1	0.6	1
C_{avss}	2.2 mg/l	2.1 µg/l	3.3 mg/l
A_{avss}/FD	0.21	2.4	3.4

Kinetics of zero order elimination

If the elimination of drug is dominated by biotransformation and if the enzymes responsible are saturated by the prevailing concentration, the concentration decays at a rate that is constant and independent of the concentration (a zero-order process). The half-life and other characteristics of first order processes are not constants in this situation but change with concentration or time.

This situation applies to a few drugs in their therapeutic concentration ranges (**phenytoin,** page 354; ethanol, page 356; **aspirin,** page 362) and to many more at toxic concentrations.

Near the foot of the plasma concentration decay curve, where the enzymes responsible for biotransformation are unsaturated, the rate is dependent upon substrate concentration and the characteristic curvature of a first order elimination process is revealed (*Figure 7.19*).

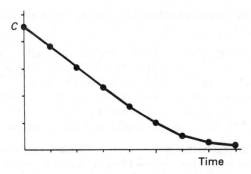

Figure 7.19 Decay of plasma concentration of a drug that displays zero-order kinetics at high concentrations and first-order kinetics at low concentrations

The parameters describing the rate and point of inflection respectively are those of the Michaelis–Menten relationship commonly used in handling saturable phenomena.

$$dC/dt = -V_{max} \, C/(K_m + C)$$

where dC/dt = rate of change of plasma concentration; V_{max} (mg/l)/h = maximal rate of decay of plasma concentration when elimination is saturated; K_m (mg/l) = plasma concentration at which elimination rate is 50% of the maximum.

This can account for the apparent zero-order and first-order phases. At a low serum concentration, when C is very much smaller than K_m, the equation reduces to a form analogous to a first order rate equation. Therefore, the rate of change of concentration is proportional to concentration:

$$dC/dt = -(V_{max}/K_m) \times C = \text{constant} \times \text{concentration}$$

Conversely, at a high serum concentration, when C is very much larger than K_m, the equation reduces to a zero order type of relationship in which the rate of change of concentration is constant:

$$dC/dt = -V_{max} = \text{constant}$$

Drug dosage regimens

The objective of a dosage regimen in therapeutics is to prescribe doses, the size and timing of which will provide the maximum therapeutic benefit at the minimum cost in adverse effects. Most drugs show orderly relationships between the dose rate and both the therapeutic and toxic responses (allergic responses are an obvious exception).

There are two significant boundaries:

(1) that between dose rates that are ineffective and those causing the desired response;

(2) that between dose rates causing the desired response and those causing adverse effects.

One way of defining the therapeutic index, which gives expression to the margin for error in dosing, is the ratio between these boundaries – the multiple by which the just toxic dose rate exceeds the just effective dose rate.

Attempts to determine optimal dose rates from observation or even measurement of therapeutic responses in patients are complicated by the compounding of two sources of variability in the cause/effect chain.

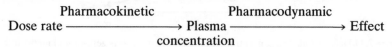

If an orderly relationship (in terms of both intensities of responses and times) holds between plasma concentration of drug and effects (both therapeutic and adverse), optimal dose rates can be determined relatively easily using measurements of plasma drug concentration.

The maximal acceptable toxic and minimal useful effects (*Figure 7.20*) define a therapeutic window in the range of plasma concentrations. The therapeutic objective becomes the prescription of a dosage regimen that ensures the attainment and maintenance of plasma concentrations lying entirely within the therapeutic window.

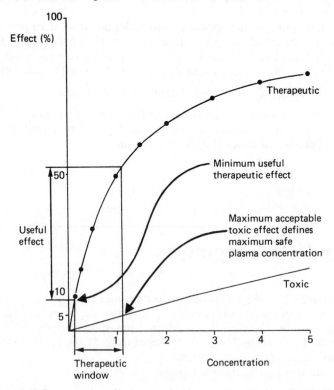

Figure 7.20 Concentration effect curves for therapeutic and toxic effects and the therapeutic window

To determine the dose rate (D/T) that will produce a target steady state plasma concentration (C_{avss}) requires knowledge of the fraction absorbed (F) and elimination clearance (CL) (*equation 7.9*). The clearance can be obtained from a knowledge of the volume of distribution (V) and either elimination half-life $(t_{\frac{1}{2}})$ or elimination rate constant (k_{el}).

To select a dosage regimen that achieves this dose rate within the objectives requires three further considerations, providing that absorption and elimination are first-order exponential processes and that distribution is rapid.

Therapeutic index

If the therapeutic index is high (for example, as with **benzylpenicillin,** page 288), wide variation in dosage is tolerable as are wide fluctuations in concentration stemming from relatively large doses given infrequently relative to the $t_{\frac{1}{2}}$. If it is low however (as with **gentamicin,** page 289; **digoxin,** page 132), the tolerable dosage regimen for an individual patient is narrow and must be achieved by relatively small doses given frequently relative to the $t_{\frac{1}{2}}$ to minimize the fluctuations.

Urgency of onset of effect

A second important consideration is the need for a loading dose. When clinical circumstances demand an immediate drug effect but the drug has a long $t_{\frac{1}{2}}$ it is necessary to give a larger first dose (loading dose; D_0) sufficient to produce a therapeutic concentration after distribution throughout the distribution volume (V). The effect is then sustained by giving, at intervals (T), a smaller maintenance dose (D_m) sufficient to keep pace with clearance (CL).

Elimination half-life

A third consideration is the $t_{\frac{1}{2}}$, which may be short (less than 1 h), moderate (4–24 h) or long (more than 24 h).

Short $t_{\frac{1}{2}}$

If the $t_{\frac{1}{2}}$ is short and the therapeutic index is large (for example, penicillins) a very large dose is given at convenient intervals of 4, 6 or 8 h $(D_0 = D_m)$. The lack of toxicity allows us to compensate for the short $t_{\frac{1}{2}}$ by enlarging the dose – doubling the dose adds one $t_{\frac{1}{2}}$ to the time the plasma concentration spends in the therapeutic window. The effect persists long enough for a therapeutic response although each dose is completely eliminated before the next is given.

When the therapeutic index is small, however, a sustained drug effect can only be attained by small, frequent doses (*soluble insulin* – $t_{\frac{1}{2}}$ less than 9 min – in diabetic ketoacidosis) or, better, by continuous iv infusion (*soluble insulin* as above; *oxytocin* – $t_{\frac{1}{2}}$ several minutes – for induction or augmentation of labour; **lignocaine** for suppression of ventricular ectopic foci after myocardial infarction).

Moderate $t_\frac{1}{2}$

If the $t_\frac{1}{2}$ is moderate it is convenient to give half the initial dose every $t_\frac{1}{2}$ ($D_0 = 2 \times D_m$). Then there is no accumulation (*co-trimoxazole* every 12 h or tetracycline every 8 or 12 h in infections, *see Table 6.5*)

Long $t_\frac{1}{2}$

If the $t_\frac{1}{2}$ is longer than 24 h, a 24 h dosage interval (T) gives much the best patient compliance. The theoretical maintenance dose (D_m) corresponds with the proportion of the loading dose (D_0) that is eliminated during that time (from *equation 7.10*).

A patient receiving **digoxin,** for example, may show a $t_\frac{1}{2}$ of 2 days. 0.7 $T/t_\frac{1}{2}$ = about one-third (from *equation 7.11*). Thus a daily dose of 250 µg would correspond with a loading dose of 750 µg. Even if no loading dose were given the amount in the body would accumulate until the same steady state concentration was attained.

Monitoring of plasma concentrations

Monitoring of plasma concentrations of a drug is of most value as an aid to therapy when the therapeutic effect itself is difficult to quantify over short time periods (**phenytoin** for epilepsy) or when the therapeutic window is narrow (**gentamicin** for serious infections with Gram-negative bacteria, **lithium carbonate** for prophylaxis of manic-depressive psychosis, **lignocaine** for cardiac dysrhythmias). It must be recognized that the therapeutic window is a guide to those plasma concentrations at which benefit generally outweighs hazard. The plasma concentration boundaries will vary between individuals.

Concentration/effect and time/effect relationships

The magnitude of response of an isolated organ to a drug usually exhibits a sigmoidal relationship with log of drug concentration (page 2). The size of drug response in man often shows a similar relationship to log plasma concentration (*Figure 7.21a*). For many drugs the position of the concentration/effect curve during both a rise and fall in concentration will be superimposable, for example during and subsequent to drug infusion. This is seen with neuromuscular blockade produced by **tubocurarine.** After intravenous administration the drug rapidly gains access to the neuromuscular junction and the onset and offset of effect here is rapid.

Some drugs exhibit anticlockwise hysteresis, that is the magnitude of effect for a given plasma concentration is greater during offset than during onset of effect (*Figure 7.21b*). Reasons include:

(1) delay in distribution – site of action is in a deep tissue compartment (for example, peak **digoxin** effect is about 4 h after peak plasma concentration);

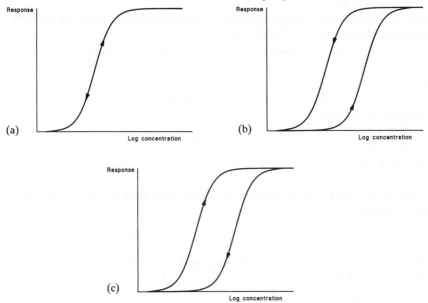

Figure 7.21 Plasma concentration–response relationships:
(a) no hysteresis; (b) anticlockwise hysteresis; (c) clockwise hysteresis

(2) delay in pharmacological response – there is an interval between drug reaching site of action and its measured effect (for example, peak **warfarin** concentrations are followed by rapid inhibition of prothrombin formation but there is a delay of about 1 day before there is a reduction in blood coagulation);

(3) formation of active metabolites (for example, **diazepam** metabolism to several pharmacologically active benzodiazepines).

The opposite phenomenon of clockwise hysteresis can be seen, that is the magnitude of effect for a given plasma concentration is greater during onset than offset of effect (*Figure 7.21c*). Reasons include:

(1) physiological homeostatic mechanisms – these return the perturbed system to normal but there is a delay in their onset (for example, fall in blood pressure with a vasodilator drug countered by reflex tachycardia);

(2) tolerance – the drug effect declines with time. This may occur over minutes, days or even weeks. Tolerance may have a pharmacokinetic basis (for example, increased clearance with *phenobarbitone*) or a pharmacodynamic basis (**morphine**).

Physicochemical groupings of drugs

It is the physicochemical properties, rather than the pharmacological actions of drugs, that determine how they are handled in the body. Five characteristic patterns of drug disposition will be described corresponding with five physicochemical groups (*Table 7.8* and *Figure 7.22*).

Table 7.8 Grouping of drugs by physicochemical properties

Groups	Examples
(1) Water-soluble drugs	**Gentamicin**
(2) Intermediate drugs	**Digoxin**
(3) Lipid-soluble drugs	**Thiopentone, phenytoin,** inhalational anaesthetics
(4) Acidic drugs (pK_a 2–7.4)	Salicylic acid
(5) Basic drugs (pK_a 6–12)	**Lignocaine**

There are two major properties of a drug that determine how it is handled by the body.

The degree of ionization of the drug molecules in solution

This is dependent on the pK_a of the drug and the pH of the fluid in which the drug is dissolved.

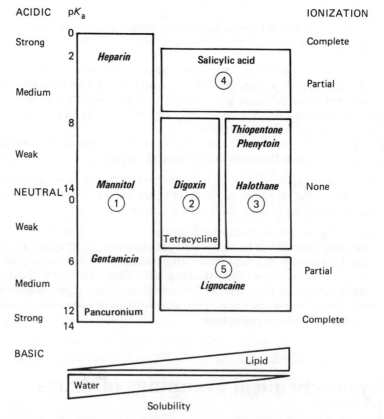

Figure 7.22 Five physicochemical groups of drugs. In this diagram ionization increases when moving up (acidic) or down (basic) from the middle. The lipid solubility of the unionized molecule increases when moving from left to right

The lipid solubility of the unionized drug molecules

This is often measured as the partition coefficient between organic solvents and water.

Water-soluble drugs

Examples

(1) Highly ionized (strong) acids (pK_a less than 2) that are almost 100% ionized in all biological fluids. Drug conjugates – sulphates, glucuronides, glycine conjugates; **sodium cromoglycate.**
(2) Drugs with multiple polar groups. Polyhydric alcohols – *mannitol*, sorbitol; mucopolysaccharides – **heparin;** aminoglycoside antibiotics – **gentamicin,** *streptomycin, neomycin.*
(3) Highly ionized (strong) bases (pK_a more than 12) that are almost 100% ionized in all biological fluids. Quaternary amines ($R_4N^+OH^-$) – **tubocurarine, neostigmine, suxamethonium.**

Characteristic features

All water-soluble drugs are handled by the body in essentially the same way, that is:

(1) absorption from the gastrointestinal tract is negligible and injection is usually necessary for systemic effects;
(2) distribution is restricted to the ECF;
(3) the drugs do not penetrate into CSF or brain;
(4) binding to plasma proteins is not important except for some strong acids;
(5) elimination is mainly by excretion of the unchanged drug in the urine. The drug usually enters the urine by ultrafiltration but many anions and cations are also actively secreted into the urine and the bile. Nonrenal excretion is relatively unimportant for these drugs unless they have a high MW (more than 400 Da) when hepatic excretion becomes important.

The disposition of the aminoglycoside antibiotic **gentamicin** is representative of the group.

Gentamicin

This is a widely used antibiotic that is effective against Gram-negative bacteria including *E. coli* and *Kl. pneumoniae*. It is important to understand how it is handled in the body because it has toxic effects on the inner ear (vestibular function is more impaired than auditory) and on the kidney. The amount of drug required to produce damage is only a little greater than the amount required to treat infection (it has a low therapeutic index).

Chemistry

The antibiotic is a variable mixture of three very similar components giving an average MW of about 480 Da. Each component consists of two sub-stituted amino sugar molecules linked through an amino cyclitol. There are several polar groups on the molecules (chiefly —OH), which make them readily soluble in water and insoluble in lipid or organic solvents.

Absorption

The drug is not absorbed from the gut and must be given by injection if a systemic effect is required. As with other drugs the rate of absorption from the site of injection is proportional to the local blood flow.

Distribution

The water-soluble antibiotic molecules cannot generally penetrate into mammalian cells. Therefore, like inulin, they are restricted to the ECF. The distribution volume (V) is about 15 litres in an adult (see *Figure 7.5*). Penetration across lipid membranes into brain, CSF, inner ear fluid, fetal circulation and sputum is slow.

Elimination

Excretion by the kidney is the major route and the clearance (CL) closely approximates to the GFR or creatinine clearance (CL_{CR}). Since, in general, cells are not penetrated there is little opportunity for contact with in-tracellular enzymes and consequent biotransformation. Again the resem-blance to inulin is strong. An exception to this generalization occurs in the renal tubular cells, some of which take up aminoglycoside antibiotics. This contributes to their nephrotoxicity.

Persistence and accumulation

When kidney function is normal the handling resembles *Figure 7.12a* and the average $t_{\frac{1}{2}}$ is about 2 h. Thus, 8 h after a dose more than 90% (50 + 25 + 12.5 + 6.25) of that dose has been eliminated; the dose can therefore be repeated without accumulation.

Renal impairment produces a very different state however. A reduction in CL causes a proportionate prolongation of $t_{\frac{1}{2}}$. It is then essential to scale down dosage in order to avoid accumulation and toxicity.

Plasma concentration and patient response

Concentration (C) 1 h after dosage must exceed 5 mg/l for a therapeutic effect in septicaemia but can be as high as 12 mg/l without causing toxicity.

Trough concentrations (just before the next dosage) are more relevant to toxicity. Below 2 mg/l there is little risk but above 4 mg/l the risk is high. If the trough concentration is high the tiny but slowly penetrated compartment of the inner ear fluid gradually fills up.

A mean concentration (C_{avss}) of 3–4 mg/l represents a compromise avoiding inadequate peaks and excessive troughs.

Dosage requirements

In renal disease

The daily dosage rate to maintain a desired C_{avss} is a linear function of CL_{CR}. It varies from about 20 mg/day (40 mg every 48 h) in anuric patients (which allows estimation of nonrenal clearance) to 480 mg/day (160 mg every 8 h) in the normal. Thus the daily dosage rate required to produce a given C_{avss} varies over a 24-fold range.

In children

CL_{CR} and **gentamicin** dosage requirements both regress with weight (or surface area) largely irrespective of age. The newborn is a special case, however; he has immature kidneys and CL_{CR} is about one-third of the value appropriate to his size. Since his ECF volume is relatively large the combined effect is a longer $t_{\frac{1}{2}}$ (*equation 7.8*, page 330).

The principle that daily dosage rate for a given C_{avss} parallels CL_{CR} is generally valid for drugs that are not fat soluble (rearrangement of *equation 7.9*, page 331, demonstrates that dose rate per unit concentration has clearance units).

Individualization of the dosage regimen

(1) Estimate the parameters of the pharmacokinetic model (*Figure 7.23, V* and $CL_{gentamicin}$) from patient features (mass, CL_{CR}) and known relationships between these variables for the population.
(2) Determine the dose that should produce a peak concentration in the range 5–12 mg/l and the dosage interval that should produce a trough concentration not greater than 2 mg/l.

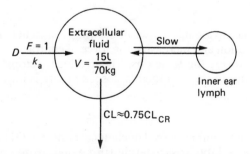

Figure 7.23 One-compartment open dispositional model for **gentamicin**

(3) Start treatment, sample plasma 1 h after a dose and assay for gentamicin concentration.
(4) Deviation from target peak (1 h) concentration represents deviation of this individual's V from the population mean assumed. Adjust dose.
(5) Sample plasma immediately before a dose and assay for gentamicin concentration.
(6) Deviation from target trough concentration represents deviation of this individual's $CL_{gentamicin}$ from the population mean assumed. Adjust interval.

Aids to this process include calculation, tables, nomograms and computer programs.

Drugs with intermediate solubility

Not all drugs have extreme physical properties. Many are intermediate between the highly water-soluble aminoglycoside antibiotics and the highly lipid-soluble iv anaesthetics. Tetracycline is included but **digoxin** has been selected as an important example.

Characteristic features

(1) Absorption from the gut is adequate for clinical use but is often not complete.
(2) Distribution is not restricted to the ECF; the drug penetrates through cell membranes and into the intracellular water.
(3) Protein binding has an influence on the distribution and elimination of the drug.
(4) Elimination is predominantly by excretion of the unchanged drug in the urine; however, a proportion of the drug undergoes biotransformation.

Digoxin

This drug has the invaluable effect of slowing ventricular rate in patients with atrial fibrillation and increasing the force of contraction in heart failure (page 378). However, the toxic dose (heart block, ectopic ventricular activity) is very close to the therapeutic dose, so there is little safety margin.

Chemistry

The relatively lipid-soluble steroid nucleus carrying two OH groups is linked to a highly water-soluble trisaccharide (three digitoxose units) by a glycosidic bond. This structure probably favours concentration at cell surfaces where the drug acts on Na^+/K^+ ATPase. The glycoside (MW 781 Da) dissolves more readily in ethanol than in water or other organic solvents.

Absorption

Digoxin is usually administered by mouth in tablet form. The dissolution standard that tablets are expected to meet is 75% in solution within 1 h. It is absorbed quickly but not completely. The fraction (F) absorbed or bioavailability is about 0.6 mean and rather variable (0.4–1.0). Reduction of particle size in the formulation increases the rate of dissolution and improves bioavailability.

Distribution

Digoxin is distributed throughout body water. It is bound to protein in plasma $(f_b = $ about 0.3) and in tissues. When distribution is complete most of the dose is located in skeletal muscle. **Digoxin** does not enter fat. V is much greater than body weight (about 5 l/kg) because of the high 'capacity' of skeletal muscle. The distribution is best described by a two-compartment model (*Figure 7.24*, page 350, and example B, page 337). The decay of plasma concentration with time is biphasic. The first phase is mainly associated with distribution to tissues and the second phase is a result of elimination.

Elimination

The total CL is greater than for the aminoglycosides but the $t_{\frac{1}{2}}$ is much longer (1–2 days) because of the large V.

Excretion

The renal CL is approximately equal to CL_{CR}: both glomerular filtration and tubular secretion contribute. Seventy per cent of the drug is excreted unchanged in the urine.

Biotransformation

The nonrenal CL is about one-half the renal CL in normal subjects. Sugar molecules are split off and the steroid nucleus is further hydroxylated in the liver.

Persistence and accumulation

About one-third of the dose is excreted per day. **Digoxin** therefore accumulates until the total amount of drug in the body is about three times the single daily dose. This process is 90% complete in about 1 week (3–4 × $t_{\frac{1}{2}}$). Once the steady state has been attained the total amount of **digoxin** in the body fluctuates relatively little during the dosage interval (contrast **gentamicin**).

Plasma concentration and patient response

Absorption is more rapid than distribution so the magnitude of the peak plasma concentration and the time to peak is largely influenced by the rate of absorption. The brief high peak may be associated with nausea via an action on the CTZ but not with cardiac toxicity. The cardiac response parallels the hypothetical concentration in a deeper tissue compartment. C_{avss} is probably the most relevant concentration, which is approximated by C at 6 h.

A concentration of 1–2 µg/l is usually adequate to control the ventricular rate in atrial fibrillation. However a concentration above 2 µg/l is associated with an increased frequency of ventricular ectopic beats. The therapeutic index approaches unity.

Dosage requirements in disease

The rapid attainment of a high therapeutic concentration (2 µg/l) would require iv injection of $2 \times V$ µg or 10 µg/kg. V is approximately halved however in the elderly and in those with severe renal impairment. Both these states are associated with a relatively low skeletal muscle mass. Gradual accumulation is usually preferred.

Daily dosage requirement for C_{avss} of 1–2 µg/l in the adult varies from 62.5 µg (one paediatric/geriatric tablet) in the anuric to 500 µg in the patient with normal kidney function. Dosage requirement approximately parallels CL_{CR}.

Individualization of the dosage regimen

Assay of the plasma concentration of **digoxin** is less useful in dosage individualization (*Figure 7.24* summarizes the pharmacokinetic model) than that of **gentamicin** (page 348).

When **digoxin** is compared with **gentamicin,** dosage individualization is:

(1) more necessary because of the long $t_{\frac{1}{2}}$ and the high incidence and potential for lethality of the cardiac toxicity;
(2) more difficult because there are more sources of variance – bioavailability, V, compliance, nonrenal CL and serum albumin binding.

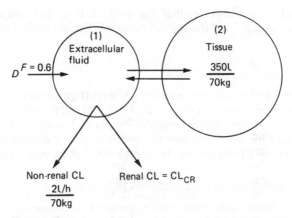

Figure 7.24 Two-compartment dispositional model for **digoxin**

Dosing summary

Decide whether a loading dose is required. Its size is determined from the lean body weight of the patient. Administer it orally or slowly iv.

Determine what maintenance dose is required, from the estimated GFR of the patient. Administer it once, or in two divided doses, daily.

Observe for the slowly developing therapeutic and adverse effects and use them to guide adjustment of the maintenance dose. This is relatively easy in atrial fibrillation, because it is easy to determine whether an appropriate effect (reduction of ventricular rate, loss of pulse deficit) is being produced. It is much harder in congestive heart failure.

Assay of the plasma concentration of **digoxin** is most useful in distinguishing between cardiac disease and **digoxin** toxicity as the source of a patient's cardiac signs and symptoms.

Lipid-soluble drugs

Examples

This group of drugs is large and includes many drugs that act on the CNS. They have in common a high oil (or organic solvent)/water partition coefficient. This group includes:

(1) weakly acidic drugs (pK_a greater than 8) – **phenytoin** and other anticonvulsants;
(2) virtually neutral drugs – **thiopentone** and other iv anaesthetics, many sedatives and inhalational anaesthetics, **glyceryl trinitrate,** steroids (**ethinyloestradiol, norethisterone,** *dexamethasone*).

Characteristic features

(1) Absorption from the gut is usually rapid and complete unless chemically inactivated.
(2) Initial distribution of the drug is very rapid. Characteristically the drugs enter tissues, including brain, at a rate that is limited by the flow of blood, not by the rate of diffusion through the cell membranes.
(3) A large proportion of the drug is bound to plasma proteins and to intracellular proteins and lipids. The concentration of drug molecules free in the body water may be very small indeed.
(4) The concentration of drug in the glomerular filtrate is also very small and the drug molecules are so lipid-soluble that they are reabsorbed from the renal tubule as quickly as the filtered water. Thus the unchanged drug is not effectively excreted in the urine.

(5) Some of the drugs in this group (those that have a high vapour pressure) are excreted unchanged in the expired air.
(6) In the liver, and to a lesser extent in other tissues, drugs of this group are oxidized to more polar metabolites, which may be alcohols or phenols (Phase I, page 324).
(7) Water-soluble metabolites resemble **gentamicin** in their elimination. Many are conjugated with sulphate, glycine or glucuronic acid prior to excretion (Phase II, page 325).

Thiopentone

This very short acting barbiturate is used as the sodium salt – MW (acid) 242 Da; pK_a = 7.6. It is administered iv for the production of complete anaesthesia of short duration or for the induction of sustained anaesthesia.

Distribution

Thiopentone, one of the most lipid-soluble barbiturates, is about 70% bound to serum albumin by 'hydrophobic bonds'. The binding of barbiturates increases with lipid solubility (*Table 7.9*).

Table 7.9 Protein binding of barbiturates to serum albumin is related to lipid-solubility

	CH_2Cl_2/water partition coefficient	Proportion bound
Thiopentone	580	0.75
An intermediate-acting barbiturate	39	0.35
Phenobarbitone	3	0.20

A single iv dose of **thiopentone sodium** can produce almost instantaneous anaesthesia that only lasts for about 5 min. Large doses cause respiratory arrest.

An intermediate-acting barbiturate has a similar potency to **thiopentone** (approximately the same concentration in brain is needed to produce anaesthesia). However, no dose of it will mimic the very short duration of action seen with **thiopentone.** This short duration of action is not due to rapid metabolism but to rapid distribution into skeletal muscle. Only after several hours is a substantial fraction of a single dose located in fatty tissue. Consciousness returns whilst a high proportion of the original dose is still in the body. Repeated doses are cumulative.

Two-compartment dispositional model

The biexponential decay in plasma thiopentone suggests that its pharmacokinetics should be considered in terms of a two-compartment (or more complex) model (page 353, *Figure 7.25*). Entry into various tissues (brain and liver) is so rapid that it appears to be limited solely by the rate of blood flow. Multicompartment 'physiological models' have been devised for thio-

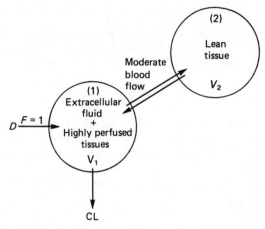

Figure 7.25 Two-compartment dispositional model for **thiopentone**

pentone, which employ known blood flow rates to principal anatomical regions. One relatively simple model of this kind comprises:

(1) highly perfused central compartment or vessel-rich group of organs including brain, liver, myocardium, adrenals, kidneys and receiving about 4 l/min;
(2) lean tissue compartment (mainly skeletal muscle) and receiving about 1 l/min at rest. Adipose tissue is quantitatively less important, receiving about 0.3 l/min.

Metabolism

Thiopentone is 'cleared' exclusively by metabolism from the central vessel-rich compartment; here the clearance concept is equally applicable as to the renal excretion of **gentamicin** or **digoxin.** Less than 1% is excreted unchanged in the urine over 48 h.

Some short-acting **thiopentone** is metabolized to the intermediate-acting pentobarbitone (that is, the S is replaced by O). Both **thiopentone** and its pentobarbitone product are further metabolized by the addition of an OH group to the longer hydrocarbon side-chain. The MFO system is responsible for this metabolism.

Phenytoin

This anticonvulsant is widely used in epilepsy at a daily dose of 200–500 mg. It lacks the pronounced hypnotic action seen with barbiturates.

Chemistry

Phenytoin is mainly used as the sodium salt – MW (acid) = 252 Da; pK_a = 8.3. It is poorly soluble in aqueous solutions (14 mg/l) at pH less than 7.

Distribution

The higher solubility in serum (75 mg/l) is due mainly to extensive protein binding, about 90% being bound to serum proteins *in vivo*. Concentrations in saliva and CSF are about 10% of the serum concentration.

Metabolism

Phenytoin is extensively metabolized by the MFO in the liver, less than 5% appearing in the urine as unchanged drug. The glucuronide conjugate of the para-hydroxylated product is the main metabolite in urine – **phenytoin** exhibits both Phase I and Phase II biotransformations.

Nonlinear kinetics

Generally, a **phenytoin** serum C_{avss} less than 10 mg/l is only partially effective, whereas a C_{avss} more than 30 mg/l is associated with toxic symptoms (ataxia, dysarthria, nystagmus). Monitoring of C_{avss} is desirable, since the relationship between C_{avss} and daily dose is nonlinear. There is a disproportionate rise in C_{avss} with increase in dose rate as a consequence of the distinctive 'dose dependent' pharmacokinetics of this drug. There is an apparent increase in $t_{\frac{1}{2}}$ with dose or C. Therefore the pharmacokinetics cannot be first order. The elimination of **phenytoin** from the body is best described in terms of Michaelis–Menten/enzyme/nonlinear kinetics (page 338) – ethanol and salicylic acid are eliminated similarly.

The C/t curve (*Figure 7.19*) appears to be biphasic: zero order at high C (above 30 mg/l of **phenytoin**), first order (exponential) at low C (below 10 mg/l).

Clinical applications

Progressive but slow (increment every 2–4 weeks) increase in dose rate is appropriate until control of seizures is obtained or further increase is prevented by toxicity. Nonlinear kinetics demands diminishing increments (*Table 7.10*). Reductions in dosage necessitated by mild intoxication require similar adjustments.

Table 7.10 Increments in dose rate producing equal increments in C_{avss} vary inversely with C_{avss}

C_{avss} (mg/l)	Increment in dose rate (mg/day)
Below 5	100
5–10	50
Above 10	25

Individual differences in D_m/T for desired C_{avss} are not accurately predictable. Surface area is the best guide but this only accounts for a part of the variation. Daily dose/surface area (mg/day per m²) is greater in children than adults.

Renal functional impairment reduces the clearance of metabolites of **phenytoin** but does not reduce the rate of biotransformation of unchanged drug. Protein binding is reduced in severe kidney disease and as a result drug is metabolized more rapidly.

Ethanol

Chemistry

In a dispositional sense ethanol (ethyl alcohol, CH_3CH_2OH) belongs to group 3 (*Table 7.8*) but it is not a highly lipid-soluble drug. Its low MW (46 Da) enables the drug to pass readily through the water filled pores of cell membranes and behave as if it were a lipid-soluble drug.

Absorption

Ethanol is rapidly and completely absorbed through the mucosae of stomach and jejunum.

Distribution

Distribution is rapid throughout all aqueous regions of the body. The distribution volume is the total body water. Ethanol equilibrates rapidly across the blood/brain barrier.

Plasma concentration and effect

Progressive increments of plasma concentration (*C*) produce progressive general CNS depression varying from mild sedation to general anaesthesia and fatal respiratory depression. The effect of ethanol on the brain depends not only on *C* (*Table 7.11*) but also on the direction in which *C* is changing. The effect of a given *C* is greater when *C* is rising and less when it is steady or falling. The same is true for other CNS depressant drugs. This is termed acute tolerance.

Table 7.11 Correlation between plasma concentration of ethanol and clinical state

Plasma concentration (mg/l)	Clinical state
500	Mild sedation
800	Legal driving limit
2000	Mild to moderate intoxication
4000	Severe intoxication
5000–8000	Death

Elimination

Metabolism

Hepatic parenchymal cells oxidize 90% to acetaldehyde (by alcohol de-hydrogenase) and then to acetate (by aldehyde dehydrogenase). Disulfiram inhibits the dehydrogenase causing acetaldehyde concentrations to rise. Above a certain C elimination is zero order – independent of C. The average maximum rate equals 10 ml/h or 8 g/h, that is, 200 ml beer or 20 ml whisky/h. $t_{\frac{1}{2}}$ increases with C.

Excretion

Ethanol is reabsorbed from the renal tubule so that the urine concentration is only slightly greater than C. Thus renal plasma clearance about equals the rate of urine flow. After small or moderate doses less than 10% of the dose is eliminated in the urine. Excretion in expired air occurs but represents less than 1% of the dose.

Inhalational anaesthetics

Inhalational anaesthetics are gases or volatile liquids that have a high solubility in lipid at normal atmospheric pressure. The differences in phys-icochemical properties between individual anaesthetics influence the rate of onset of and recovery from anaesthesia and the partial pressures necessary to induce anaesthesia.

Partial pressure

In general the response to a drug is a function of the concentration in the biophase (fluid in intimate contact with receptors). In the case of inhala-tional anaesthetics, it is more convenient to express concentration in terms of partial pressure than mass of gas per unit volume of liquid because diffusion of a gas between phases occurs down a gradient of partial pressure, at a speed proportional to the gradient, until differences in partial pressure are eliminated.

Partial pressure is defined as the individual pressure exerted by a gas in a mixture of gases. In the gas phase the partial pressure of the anaesthetic can also be expressed as a proportion of the total pressure (normally one atmosphere).

Solubility in blood and tissues

Some anaesthetics have a greater affinity for blood than for the gas phase. This affinity is expressed as their solubility in blood.

Henry's law states that:

Mass of gas dissolved by unit volume of liquid =
solubility × partial pressure of the gas at constant temperature

Consequently the amount of anaesthetic that must be dissolved to achieve
a particular partial pressure in blood is proportional to solubility (large mass
for *anaesthetic ether* (diethyl ether), small mass for **nitrous oxide**). Contrast
the soluble diethyl ether (solubility = 12) with the insoluble **nitrous oxide**
(solubility = 0.5) (*Table 7.12*).

The partition coefficient (ratio of solubilities) for the inhalational anaesthetics between most tissues (including the brain) and blood is near unity.
However, the partition coefficient between adipose tissue and blood may be
much greater than unity (**halothane** = 60).

Kinetic models

Since these agents are highly lipid soluble the pharmacokinetics must be
modelled by several compartments (*see Figure 7.26*) as described for **thiopentone sodium.** As in that case, distribution is perfusion- rather than
diffusion-limited:

(0) external air containing gas at a certain concentration;
(1) central, rapidly equilibrating compartment consisting of functional re-
    sidual lung capacity (less dead space) plus blood plus highly perfused
    tissues including the brain;
(2) lean tissue compartment (mainly skeletal muscle);
(3) adipose tissue compartment.

Transfer of anaesthetic into the lean tissue compartment is initially more
significant than into the adipose tissue compartment because of the much
greater blood flow in the former.

An anaesthetic can be considered to be distributed through an apparent

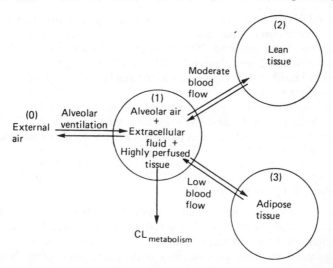

Figure 7.26 Three-compartment dispositional model for gaseous general anaesthetics

volume of distribution (described for solid and liquid drugs with a low vapour pressure on page 318) known as the 'gas equivalent volume'. This volume is the sum of the compartment volumes multiplied by their respective partition coefficients.

Potency

An anaesthetic agent is potent if it produces a given depth of anaesthesia at a low partial pressure in the inspired air. This is expressed as minimal alveolar concentration (MAC) for anaesthesia, which is the proportion (% v/v) of anaesthetic in the inspired air that, at equilibrium, prevents the reflex response to skin incision in 50% of subjects. **Halothane** (MAC = 0.8) is potent whilst **nitrous oxide** (MAC more than 80) is of low potency (*Table 7.12*). The potency of inhalational anaesthetics is positively correlated with lipid solubility (page 4).

Table 7.12 Blood solubilities and potencies of general anaesthetics

Anaesthetic	Solubility (blood/gas)	MAC (% v/v)
Diethyl ether	12	2
Halothane	2.3	0.8
Enflurane	1.9	1.7
Isoflurane	1.4	1.4
Nitrous oxide	0.5	>80

Induction of anaesthesia

The time to induction of anaesthesia is dependent upon the rate of rise of partial pressure of the anaesthetic in the brain. This time is reduced when:

(1) inspired partial pressure is high – consequently use more than one MAC during induction of anaesthesia with subsequent reduction once anaesthesia has been induced. This is equivalent to using a loading dose before a maintenance dose with solid or liquid drugs;
(2) alveolar ventilation is high – this increases transfer of anaesthetic from external air to alveoli;
(3) body weight is small – gas equivalent volume is reduced;
(4) anaesthetic is of low solubility – diethyl ether has a high solubility and induction is slow while **nitrous oxide** has a low solubility and induction is fast (see *Figure 7.27*).

Maintenance of anaesthesia

A near steady state may be reached in which the partial pressure in the brain approaches that in the blood and inspired air. There will still be net transfer of anaesthetic to lean and adipose tissue. Consequently, the mass of anaesthetic dissolved in these sites of loss is proportional to the duration of anaesthesia.

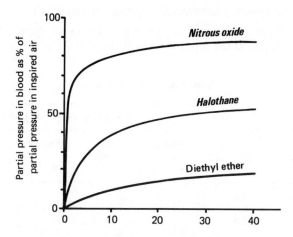

Figure 7.27 Change in partial pressure of three general anaesthetics in blood with time at a constant inspired partial pressure

Recovery

The time from cessation of administration of a general anaesthetic to recovery is dependent on the rate of fall of partial pressure in the central compartment. This time is short when the inspired partial pressure is zero and alveolar ventilation is high, body weight is small, the anaesthetic is poorly soluble and the duration of exposure was short. Unequilibrated muscles represent a sink unless blood flow is impaired by shock. The converse applies – anaesthetic washing out of muscles after long exposure delays recovery. There is some elimination of **halothane** by metabolism.

Acidic drugs

Acidic drugs (pK_a 2–7.4) have similar modes of absorption, distribution and elimination but widely diverse pharmacological actions.

Examples

(1) NSAIDs: **aspirin,** *naproxen.*
(2) Oral anticoagulants: **warfarin.**
(3) Penicillin antibiotics: **benzylpenicillin, ampicillin.**
(4) Sulphonamide antibacterial drugs: sulphamethoxazole.
(5) Oral hypoglycaemic drugs: **tolbutamide.**
(6) Diuretics: **bendrofluazide.**
(7) *Phenobarbitone* is the only common barbiturate with pK_a significantly below 8.

(8) Uricosuric agents: *probenecid, sulphinpyrazone*.

All these drugs are donors of H^+; we can arrange them in order, the strongest (low pK_a) at the top, the weakest (high pK_a) at the bottom (*Table 7.13*).

Table 7.13 Ionization of acids

		Concentration ratio $[A^-] : [HA]^*$			
		Stomach	Urine (acid)	Plasma	Urine (alk)
Drug	pK_a	*pH 3.0*	*pH 5.0*	*pH 7.4*	*pH 8.0*
Benzylpenicillin	2.8				
Salicylic acid	3.0	1:1	10^2:1	2.5×10^4:1	10^5:1
Aspirin	3.6				
	4.0	0.1:1	10:1	2.5×10^3:1	10^4:1
Warfarin	5.0	10^{-2}:1	1:1	2.5×10^2:1	10^3:1
Sulphamethoxazole	5.6				
	6.0	10^{-3}:1	0.1:1	25:1	10^2:1
	7.0	10^{-4}:1	10^{-2}:1	2.5:1	10:1
Phenobarbitone	7.4				

* Calculated from equation 7.1 (page 306)

Characteristic features

(1) Most acidic drugs are present mainly as the uncharged acid (HA) at pH 3. The acid (HA) is the more lipid-soluble form; thus, conditions in the stomach are favourable to absorption but surface area is small.

(2) In the plasma acidic drugs are present to a large extent as the charged anions (A^-). The anions of different acidic drugs compete for a common binding site on plasma albumin and for active secretion into bile and urine.

(3) The plasma clearance (CL) varies inversely with the extent of reabsorption from the renal tubule. If the urine pH is high, the drug in the urine is present mainly as the anion (A^-), nonionic diffusional reabsorption is discouraged and CL is high. Increase in CL causes a corresponding reduction in $t_{\frac{1}{2}}$.

Note:

(1) Urine pH should be controlled when measuring excretion rates of acidic compounds.

(2) The use of alkaline diuresis in acute poisoning by salicylates or *phenobarbitone*.

Salicylic acid

Salicylic acid is used for its analgesic, anti-inflammatory, antiplatelet and antipyretic properties. There are three main use situations: occasional, low dose utilizing the antipyretic and analgesic properties of **aspirin**; chronic low dose utilizing the antiplatelet properties; chronic, high dose utilizing the analgesic and anti-inflammatory properties of **aspirin**. **Aspirin** (acetylsalicylic acid) is rapidly hydrolysed within the body ($t_{\frac{1}{2}}$ 15 min) to give acetate and salicylic acid. **Aspirin** is, therefore, a prodrug although it may exert some therapeutic actions itself.

Physicochemical properties

pK_a 3; soluble in water and organic solvents.

Dosage form and absorption

Drug in solution is rapidly absorbed, primarily from the small intestine. Salicylates are poorly soluble at low pH. Solution of **aspirin** in intestinal fluids is the rate-limiting step in absorption. Simple **aspirin** tablets or dispersible formulations, with consequent rapid dissolution and absorption, are appropriate when rapid onset of effect is required (to treat a headache). For treatment of chronic diseases (joint inflammation), where rapid onset of effect is not required, enteric-coated or other slow-release preparations may be preferred as they minimize the local erosive action on gastric mucosa. Enteric-coated tablets can give erratic and incomplete absorption.

Distribution

Salicylic acid enters cells by diffusion through the lipid membranes. It is distributed throughout total body water and binds to sites on plasma albumin and tissue protein. At high salicylate doses its plasma concentration approaches that of albumin (0.6 mmol/l), binding sites are saturated and there is a disproportionate rise in free drug concentration (*Figure 7.4*). Volume of distribution rises with plasma concentration.

Plasma salicylate and patient response

Below 100 mg/l: therapeutic – antiplatelet, analgesic and antipyretic effects. Side-effects include bleeding from gastric erosions (hypoprothrombinaemia and reduced platelet stickiness may contribute).
150–300 mg/l: therapeutic – anti-inflammatory effects. Adverse effects include tinnitus and deafness at maximum therapeutic concentrations and even bronchospasm (an idiosyncrasy that is not due to allergy but to cyclooxygenase inhibition).
300–750 mg/l: mild to moderate intoxication is manifest as hyperventilation, respiratory alkalosis, sweating, tachycardia, salt and water depletion. Toxicity increases with time: 500 mg/l at 48 h after overdose may represent severe intoxication. Treatment is by correction of salt and water depletion and by alkaline diuresis.
Above 750 mg/l: severe intoxication is manifest as impaired utilization of

pyruvate and lactate, metabolic acidosis, convulsions, circulatory arrest and
renal failure. Haemodialysis may be required.

Metabolism and disposition kinetics (Table 7.14)

Hepatic metabolism is the major mechanism of elimination at low and
moderate plasma concentrations.

Table 7.14 Metabolic fate of aspirin

Fate		Metabolite	Urine (%)
Conjugated (Phase II) with	Glycine	Salicyluric acid	45–55
	Glucuronic acid	Phenolic glucuronide	15–25
	Glucuronic acid	Acyl glucuronide	7–12
Hydroxylated (Phase I)			less than 3
Excreted unchanged (low dose)			5–25

Salicylic acid displays the same nonlinear elimination kinetics as **phenytoin** and ethanol. The process of conjugation to form salicyluric acid and
phenolic glucuronide becomes saturated in the therapeutic dose range.
There is, therefore, an apparent rise in $t_{\frac{1}{2}}$ with dose (*Table 7.15*).

Table 7.15 Zero-order salicylic acid kinetics, dependence of $t_{\frac{1}{2}}$ on dose

Dose (g)	Apparent $t_{\frac{1}{2}}$ (h)
0.3	2.3
1	6
10	19
Overdose	>35 (untreated)

Accumulation kinetics

Within the therapeutic range dosage increase produces a disproportionate
increase in C_{avss} and the time to reach steady state – doubling the dose
(1.5–3 g/day) in one experimental subject produced a 4-fold C_{avss} increase
(30–120 mg/l).

Renal clearance – increases with pH and urine flow

Renal excretion is a minor pathway at low concentration but a major
pathway at high concentration (intoxication) due to saturation of metabolic
elimination. CL increases about 4-fold with each unit rise in urine pH. This
explains the effective use of alkaline diuresis in salicylate intoxication.

Basic drugs

Basic drugs (pK_a 6–12) have similar modes of absorption, distribution and elimination but widely diverse pharmacological actions.

Examples

(1) Opioid analgesics: **morphine.**
(2) Local anaesthetics: **lignocaine.**
(3) Antidysrhythmic drugs: **lignocaine.**
(4) Agonists at nicotinic cholinoceptors: nicotine.
(5) Antagonists at muscarinic cholinoceptors: **atropine.**
(6) ChE inhibitors: *physostigmine.*
(7) Sympathomimetic amines: NA.
(8) Antagonists at adrenoceptors: **phenoxybenzamine, propranolol.**
(9) Antipsychotics: **chlorpromazine.**
(10) Anxiolytics: **diazepam.**
(11) Tricyclic antidepressive drugs: **imipramine.**
(12) Antagonists at histamine receptors: **chlorpheniramine, cimetidine.**
(13) Antiparasitic drugs: **chloroquine,** *piperazine.*
(14) Smooth muscle relaxants: *theophylline*; Ca^{2+} channel blockers – **verapamil, nifedipine.**

All these drugs are acceptors of H^+; we can arrange them in order, the strongest (high pK_a) at the top and the weakest (low pK_a) at the bottom (*Table 7.16*).

Table 7.16 Ionization of bases

Drug	pK_a	Concentration ratio $[B^+H] : [B]$*			
		Stomach pH 3.0	Urine (acid) pH 5.0	Plasma pH 7.4	Urine (alk) pH 8.0
Guanethidine	11.4				
	11.0	10^8:1	10^6:1	4×10^3:1	10^3:1
	10.0	10^7:1	10^5:1	4×10^2:1	10^2:1
Amphetamine (amine group)	9.9				
Atropine, propranolol, imipramine	9.6				
Chlorpromazine, chlorpheniramine	9.3				
	9.0	10^6:1	10^4:1	40:1	10:1
Theophylline	8.6				
Morphine, lignocaine	8.0	10^5:1	10^3:1	4:1	1:1
Hydralazine	7.1				
	7.0	10^4:1	10^2:1	0.4:1	0.1:1
Cimetidine	6.8				

* Calculated from equation 7.2 (page 300)

Characteristic features

(1) Basic drugs exist almost entirely as the nondiffusible cation at pH 3; conditions do not favour absorption from stomach.
(2) Generally in plasma the fraction of bases bound (f_b) to protein is less than the f_b of acids; α_1-acid glycoprotein is involved rather than albumin.
(3) The concentration of total drug (cation plus base) in urine is greatly increased when the urine pH is reduced from 8 to 5 (*Table 7.16*).
(4) When excretion is a major factor in elimination (amphetamine) the plasma concentration $t_{\frac{1}{2}}$ is shortened if the urine is made acid.

Note:

(1) Urine pH should be controlled when measuring excretion rates of basic compounds.
(2) The use of acid diuresis in poisoning by amphetamine.

Lignocaine

This is one of the most widely used antidysrhythmic agents in coronary care units. It has particular value in treatment of ventricular dysrhythmias after myocardial infarction (page 128).

Physicochemical properties

pK_a 8; limited solubility in water (7 mg/l) but very soluble in organic solvents.

Absorption

Absorption is rapid ($t_{\frac{1}{2}}$ about 15 min) and complete from all sites except gut (discussed later). It is more rapid from an alkaline environment and greatest from highly perfused tissues.

Distribution

Fifty per cent of drug in plasma is bound, not to albumin but to α_1-acid glycoprotein. Displacement is an unlikely phenomenon. It is so lipophilic that membranes are no barrier to penetration. The rate of tissue uptake is a function of organ perfusion. This explains the rapid onset (about 1 min) and termination (about 20 min) of CNS and cardiac effects following a therapeutic bolus dose (1 mg/kg). Lipophilicity also explains the size of the 'reservoir' in muscle after prolonged administration. Volume of distribution after distribution is about 120 l/70 kg as the drug lies mainly outside plasma in lung, kidney, brain, muscle and adipose tissue.

The arterial plasma decay curve after an iv bolus is biexponential as with **thiopentone sodium.** The peak concentration in the rapidly equilibrating central compartment is established almost immediately. The initial exponential decay of plasma concentration with time occurs due to distribution into moderately perfused tissues (muscle). The second exponential decay phase is due to metabolism. Distribution into fat is slow (because it is so poorly perfused) and quantitatively less important.

Plasma concentration and effect

Lignocaine is generally ineffective below 1.5 mg/l; frequency and severity of adverse effects (convulsions) increase above 6 mg/l.

Metabolism and disposition kinetics

The hepatic MFO removes one or both ethyl groups (N-dealkylation). Both products are biologically active. Aromatic C-hydroxylation and hydrolysis of the side-chain at the amide position also occur.

Clearance, availability and $t_{\frac{1}{2}}$

Elimination is almost exclusively by hepatic metabolism and is very high (1 l/min/70 kg) approaching liver blood flow (1.5 l/min/70 kg). High hepatic extraction (70%) explains the low bioavailability (30%) of oral **lignocaine.** Metabolites are active so the oral dose is more effective than the low availability suggests. **Lignocaine** has a high hepatic extraction ratio so changes in liver perfusion affect clearance. Consequently dosage requirements are diminished in diseases depressing circulatory function (cardiogenic shock, congestive heart failure) and hepatic metabolism (cirrhosis), where shunting of blood away from damaged areas can occur. **Propranolol,** by reducing cardiac output and hepatic blood flow, reduces the CL of **lignocaine.**

Although CL is high, $t_{\frac{1}{2}}$ is not excessively short (1–2 h) because V is large (example C, page 337). There is a long delay ($3–5 \times t_{\frac{1}{2}}$) between initiation of an infusion and attainment of the plateau concentration. Therefore, a bolus dose is given followed by an infusion to match metabolism.

Renal excretion is a minor pathway of elimination of **lignocaine** due to extensive reabsorption, so urine acidification has no significant influence on its elimination kinetics. This is in marked contrast with amphetamine, the $t_{\frac{1}{2}}$ of which is reduced from 16 h to 5 h by acidification of the urine from pH 7 to pH 5.

8

Clinical pharmacology

Aims

- To provide a stimulus to revision of pharmacological actions and their mechanisms.
- To present information on some *BNF* drugs that are missed by the themes chosen for the bulk of the book.
- To provide insight into the pathophysiology of disease and thus a framework for the rational use of drugs in treatment.
- To introduce more of the language of medicine.
- To satisfy the desire that students of pharmacology express for an understanding of the uses of drugs.

Introduction

Since this is not a textbook of medicine it is neither possible nor desirable to attempt a general coverage of disease.

We have adopted as criteria for the inclusion of disease states and forms of therapy:

(1) a disease state should be a chronic condition of relatively common occurrence;

(2) alternatively or additionally it should be the kind of condition for which community pharmacists are often asked to advise. Since many proprietary preparations are advertised for self medication we have attempted to include some of them so that logical and relevant 'over-the-counter' advice can be given.

Acute poisoning

The problem

In adults acute poisoning is commonly deliberate and self inflicted with the object of harming the patient or manipulating somebody else. It is typically a problem of Western Europe and North America; it is less frequent in countries with a peasant economy and Roman Catholic religion. A small proportion of such patients (less than 20%) have serious psychiatric disease. The annual incidence of hospital admission is about 1:1000 population and annual deaths (England and Wales) about 4000. Eighty per cent of these deaths occur outside hospital – mortality amongst hospital admissions is less than 1%.

In children acute poisoning is an accidental result of oral exploration and is commonest in boys, 1.5–2.5 years, social class IV, with several preschool siblings. There is a high incidence of ingestion (probably similar to adult figures) but poisoning (measurable harmful effects) is uncommon and death is rare (less than 50/year). Some poisoning deaths may however be attributed to other causes.

Drugs involved

Adults: hypnotics, anxiolytics, minor analgesics, antidepressives, anticonvulsants. Medicaments are often combined with each other and with ethanol or carbon monoxide.

Children: a random selection of ingestible items in the environment – anything from iron salts to weed killer, contraceptive tablets to antifreeze.

Principles of management

Note the order of priorities carefully.

(1) Establish and maintain a clear airway: remove debris (vomit, mucus, dentures), suck away secretions, consider the need for an oropharyngeal airway or endotracheal tube.
(2) Ensure adequate ventilation: tidal volume greater than 400 ml and minute volume greater than 4 l/min for adults, by mechanical means if necessary (too little leads to hypoxaemia, too much to alkalosis and hypotension).
(3) Iv fluid therapy has two objectives:
    (a) Expansion of circulating blood volume, restoration of venous return and cardiac output. *Sodium chloride* (0.9% is isotonic with blood) and *glucose* (5%) iv infusion are suitable. Human plasma protein fraction may be needed.
    (b) Water and salt replacement to replace fluid loss and maintain an adequate urine output (more than 15 ml/h).
(4) Decontamination: removal procedures have a low efficiency (only 20–30% of a recent dose is recovered) and a significant morbidity. Gastric lavage 'washes out' the stomach by means of water entering and being emptied via a wide bore rubber tube. It is only of value with most drugs if performed less than 4 h after ingestion. Exceptions are antidepressive drugs (8 h) and salicylates (24 h). *Ipecacuanha* syrup, which

directly stimulates both the medulla and the stomach to induce emesis, is suitable for children and many adults and probably has comparable efficacy to lavage. Avoid in drowsy or unconscious patients because of increased risk of lung aspiration. Activated charcoal 10–30 g in suspension in 100–200 ml water may be introduced to bind unabsorbed drug (**digoxin**, *theophylline*, barbiturates, alkaloids). Other binding agents are more suited to other toxic agents – **desferrioxamine** for iron salts and *Fuller's earth* for paraquat.

(5) Convulsions may be provoked by drug overdose (**aspirin**, *theophylline*, antidepressives) but usually anticonvulsant drugs are not needed.

(6) Identification. Tablet identification may be difficult with old/white/discoloured preparations. The National Poisons Information Service provides useful data on content of household cleaners, bleaches, weed killers, solvents. The hospital biochemistry service can assist with assessment of severity of poisoning by **paracetamol, aspirin**, *theophylline*, **lithium** and iron salts; severity tends to increase with serum drug concentration.

(7) Assisted elimination of the poison is seldom required – if respiration and circulation are adequately supported hepatic metabolism and renal excretion will eliminate the toxic agent without special assistance.

Special cases

Salicylate poisoning in an adult

Alkaline diuresis increases the clearance of salicylate four-fold for each unit of pH rise. High urine pH (above 8.0) may be obtained by iv infusion of *sodium bicarbonate* (1.4% is isotonic). The major principle is alkalinization of the urine with an adequate urine output rather than a forced diuresis.

Specific antagonists are only available for a few drugs (*Table 8.1*).

Table 8.1 Poisons with specific antagonists

Drug	Antagonist	Mechanism
Digoxin	Digoxin-specific antibody fragments	Binding
Iron salts	**Desferrioxamine**	Chelation
Lead salts	*Penicillamine*	Chelation
Mercury salts	Dimercaprol	Chelation
Opioid analgesics (**morphine**)	**Naloxone**	Specific competitive antagonism
Organophosphorus anticholinesterases	**Atropine** and **pralidoxime**	ACh antagonism Cholinesterase reactivation
Paracetamol	*Acetylcysteine*	Reduction of oxidized glutathione

Summary

(1) Progress in the management of acute poisoning has been achieved by the more effective support of vital functions (respiration and circulation). Assisted elimination and drug antagonism have only a limited importance.
(2) Since mortality in hospital is so low, further reduction of total mortality can only be achieved by removal of social causes of self poisoning and by more restricted availability of lethal drugs (for example, barbiturates).
(3) The reduction in the prescribing of benzodiazepines as hypnotics and anxiolytics has helped to reduce the frequency of self poisoning.

Peptic ulceration

Definition

Localized loss of mucosa, submucosa and smooth muscle layers of the oesophagus, stomach (gastric ulcer) or of the duodenum (duodenal ulcer).

Symptoms and diagnosis

Pain in upper part of abdomen, usually midline. Heartburn, nausea and relief of symptoms by food and antacids are common. Poor appetite and weight loss are common in the elderly. Anaemia may be present, the result of chronic bleeding from the ulcer (page 426). Diagnosis requires endoscopy.

Complications

Sudden and severe bleeding. Perforation with leakage of gastric contents into the abdomen causing peritonitis. Fibrotic narrowing of the pyloric outlet of the stomach.

Aetiology

Hydrochloric acid (HCl), pepsin and regurgitated bile are potential mucosal damaging agents. Mucus and sodium bicarbonate secreted by the epithelial cells overlie the mucosa acting as a barrier. Peptic ulceration occurs when the barrier is breached either because of increased attack by secretions (common in duodenal ulcer) or a deficient barrier (common in gastric ulcer). There is a familial component to the causation of duodenal ulceration.

Recently an association has been found between duodenal ulceration and gastritis associated with the microorganism *Helicobacter pylori. Helicobacter* is also present in the altered mucosa surrounding the duodenal ulcer. The precise relationship between organism and ulcer is yet to be determined but a causal relationship seems probable.

Aims of treatment

(1) To relieve symptoms.
(2) To hasten healing.

General therapeutic measures

Determine that a gastric ulcer is not malignant by endoscopic biopsy. Symptoms are reduced by small frequent meals, stopping smoking and avoiding ethanol and any food that makes the symptoms worse. The use of NSAIDs and glucocorticoids should be reduced to a minimum. There is a 40% spontaneous cure rate for gastric and duodenal ulcers but both are also highly likely to recur periodically.

Symptomatic therapy

Antacids may be used intermittently for the symptomatic management of pain. They are weak bases that neutralize HCl so the pH of the luminal contents transiently becomes greater than 4 and pepsin is inactive (*Figure 8.1*). The action of antacids is brief due to their rapid removal from the stomach and duodenum.

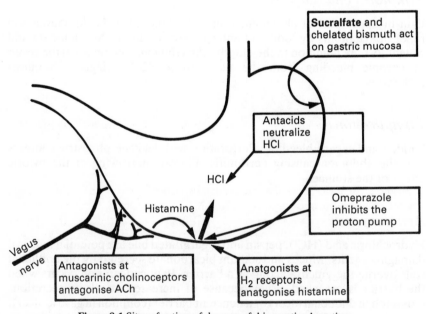

Figure 8.1 Sites of action of drugs useful in peptic ulceration

Sodium bicarbonate can alter ECF pH to give a metabolic alkalosis and alkaline urine. It is not, therefore, suitable for prolonged use.

Magnesium hydroxide and aluminium hydroxide are little absorbed. Mg^{2+} is laxative and Al^{3+} is constipative.

Magnesium trisilicate has a slow onset and relatively prolonged action. On reaction with HCl it forms a hydrated silicic acid that is adsorbent of pepsin.

Therapy that promotes healing

Antagonists at H_2 histamine receptors

Histamine is involved in the final common pathway of stimuli that cause acid and pepsin secretion. **Cimetidine** and *ranitidine* reduce fasting and stimulated acid and pepsin secretion by antagonizing histamine (*Figure 8.1*).

Inhibitors of acid secretion by the parietal cells

The secretion of acid by the parietal cell requires a specific 'proton' pump enzyme (H^+ / K^+ ATPase) located on the luminal membrane of the cell. **Omeprazole** inhibits this pump and virtually abolishes acid secretion. Short-term healing of peptic ulcer is more rapid and effective with this than with other agents. Long-term effects are not yet known.

Improvement of mucosal barrier

Tripotassium dicitratobismuthate, a colloidal bismuth chelate, and *sucralfate*, an aluminium hydroxide complex, appear to act locally at the site of the ulcer, preventing access by acid and pepsin. Both drugs are only partially absorbed but this is sufficient to prevent their long-term use; heavy metal poisoning with aluminium and bismuth respectively, may occur.

The above drugs are equieffective with antagonists at H_2 histamine receptors at short-term ulcer healing. Periodic lapses occur and can be treated with maintenance low doses of antagonists at H_2 histamine receptors.

Surgery

Surgery may be used if medical treatment fails or there are dangerous complications (continued or recurrent haemorrhage). It usually involves selective division of the vagal nerve supply to the antrum of the stomach, thus reducing or abolishing the neural component of acid secretion.

Therapy that reduces relapse of ulcer

Although acid suppression will heal most ulcers, relapse is common. For patients with frequent symptomatic relapses, regular nocturnal therapy with antagonists at H_2 histamine receptors is effective in providing long-term symptom relief.

Relapse also appears to be reduced in patients in whom *Helicobacter pylori* has been eliminated. While the precise aetiological role of *Helicobacter* in ulcer development is yet to be determined, there is now good evidence that eradication of the organism helps to prevent symptomatic relapse. Colloidal bismuth compounds have the ability to kill *Helicobacter* and, when used in combination with antibiotics, particularly **amoxycillin** and **metronidazole,** can achieve eradication of the organism in many patients. Such therapies are likely to become increasingly important in the future.

Inflammatory bowel disease

Definition

Ulcerative colitis is chronic inflammation of the mucosa of the rectum and colon. Crohn's disease is a patchy chronic inflammation that can affect any part of the gastrointestinal tract. The causes are not known.

Symptoms

Ulcerative colitis. Painless bloody diarrhoea is the usual symptom of ulcerative colitis. Persistent disease can lead to malnutrition and anaemia. Dilatation and perforation of the colon may occur.

Crohn's disease. Crohn's disease is associated with similar symptoms to ulcerative colitis but abdominal pain is more frequent, as are mouth ulcers and anal involvement.

General therapeutic measures

Maintain an adequate and balanced diet; parenteral feeding may be required.

Symptomatic treatment

Constipative drugs

Constipative drugs (*see below*) may be used in mild disease but should be avoided in more severe cases since they may mask the development of serious complication.

Glucocorticoids

Glucocorticoids by oral, rectal or intravenous route induce remission by their anti-inflammatory effects but do not remove the underlying cause. Adverse effects limit long-term maintenance therapy.

5-Aminosalicylate (5-ASA) compounds

Sulphasalazine is useful for mild relapses and for maintenance therapy. Its efficacy is due to 5-ASA moiety of the molecule, split from the sulphonamide conjugate by the action of colonic bacteria.

Olsalazine is a 5-ASA dimer split into two active 5-ASA molecules by colonic bacteria, thus avoiding the use of the sulphonamide component of *sulphasalazine*.

Mesalazine is 5-ASA; the drug is usually employed as a delayed release formulation – coated by a resin that delays release until the lower gut is reached.

Immunosuppression

More powerful immunosuppressant drugs (*azathioprine*, *cyclosporin*) may be used in patients with severe disease in whom surgery is contraindicated.

Surgery

Ulcerative colitis. Removal of the affected part including the rectum, with the consequent need for an ileostomy (artificial opening of small intestine through front of abdomen) or construction of an ileoanal anastomosis, enables a return to an active life.

Crohn's disease. Resection should be limited to only severely affected areas. In contrast to ulcerative colitis, the disease can recur.

Gastrointestinal motility disorders

Diarrhoea

Aetiology

In the small intestine the contents are liquid. The small bowel, caecum and the proximal colon absorb Na^+, K^+ and Cl^- and the bulk of the water. The distal colon absorbs Na^+ in exchange for K^+, this process being influenced by aldosterone. Water is absorbed so producing soft but not watery faeces. If the time in the gastrointestinal tract is too short or there is malabsorption of nutrient due to damage to the pancreas or small intestinal mucosa or if there is inflammation resulting in incomplete water absorption then diarrhoea will result.

Causes

(1) Viruses (gastroenteritis) especially in children.
(2) Bacteria (bacterial food poisoning) usually due to heat-stable toxins

(staphylococcal, *E. coli*) but can be infective (*Salmonella*, bacillary dysentery). Superinfection during broad spectrum antibiotic treatment (*Staphylococcus*, *Cl. difficile*).
(3) Fungi, usually *Candida albicans*, by superinfection during ingestion of broad spectrum antibiotic.
(4) Protozoa or metazoa (amoebic dysentery, worm infestation).
(5) Organic disease of colon (Crohn's disease, ulcerative colitis).
(6) Malabsorption syndrome due to small intestinal or pancreatic disease.
(7) Consequence of gut resection.
(8) Drugs – **cimetidine,** diuretics, cytotoxic drugs, **digoxin,** tetracyclines, **ampicillin,** magnesium salts, abuse of purgatives, antagonists at β-adrenoceptors.
(9) Emotion.
(10) Disturbances of endocrine system (hyperthyroidism).

Treatment

The underlying disorder should be diagnosed and treated.

General therapeutic measures

Many episodes of diarrhoea, especially viral and bacterial, are short-lived and self-limiting. Severe diarrhoea (especially infants, elderly people or in tropical climates) may lead to dehydration needing replacement with iv or oral electrolyte therapy. An oral solution containing sugar and NaCl makes use of the linked sodium/glucose absorption mechanism.

Symptomatic treatment

(1) Opioids (*codeine*, **morphine** and **loperamide,** page 234). These drugs reduce secretion, decrease the propulsive intestinal contractions and increase the tone of colonic muscles and sphincters, allowing increased water absorption. **Loperamide** displays slight selectivity for peripheral enteric neural *versus* central actions and may be useful for long-term, noninfective diarrhoea in adults.
(2) Adsorbents (kaolin and chalk). These are said to adsorb bacteria and toxins. They are commonly used with **morphine.**
(3) Bulk-forming agents (*bran* and *methylcellulose*) absorb water so solidifying stools in diarrhoea.
(4) Antibiotics have no place in self-limiting viral or bacterial toxin-induced diarrhoea. Their use can be complicated by bacterial or fungal superinfection (page 292). However *Cl. difficile* infection, usually induced by broad spectrum antibiotics, can be treated by oral *vancomycin*.

Constipation

Aetiology

If the passage of contents through the colon is unduly prolonged there is greater water absorption and therefore constipation.

Causes

(1) Diet containing too little fibre and fermentable carbohydrate.
(2) Prolonged bed rest.
(3) Habitual denial of defaecatory urges.
(4) Organic obstruction of colon (carcinoma, strictures, diverticular disease).
(5) Drug-induced – opioids (page 234), antagonists at muscarinic cholino-ceptors (page 88) or aluminium-containing antacids (page 371).
(6) Endocrine disorders (hypothyroidism).
(7) Neuropathy.

If faeces stagnate and harden, straining may prolapse and thrombose haemorrhoidal veins (piles) or tear the anus. Painful defaecation may make constipation worse.

Specific treatment

The underlying disorder should be diagnosed and treated.

General therapeutic measures

Encourage a well balanced diet with roughage and exercise. Explain that the frequency of defaecation is very variable. Try to establish a habitual time for defaecation.

Symptomatic treatment

Laxatives: chronic use of laxatives may damage the colon and result in an atonic bowel and therefore is contraindicated. Defaecation is promoted by increased colonic or small intestinal propulsive motility and altered electrolyte transport – the exact mechanism of action is unknown for most drugs. One classification is as follows.

Bulk-forming laxatives

Bran and *methylcellulose* swell in water to form a gel, which maintains hydrated, soft faeces. The bulk promotes peristalsis. The onset of action is slow (about 24 h). This group is preferred for long-term use.

Emollient laxatives

These act by direct softening of the faeces. Docusate – a lowering of surface tension may explain its action. *Glycerol* [glycerin] suppositories act by softening faeces.

Osmotic laxatives

Magnesium sulphate is poorly absorbed from the digestive tract and so retains water by osmosis; peristalsis is increased indirectly. There is a fairly rapid onset of action (2–3 h). A *phosphates* enema (sodium phosphate and acid phosphate) acts as an osmotic laxative.

Stimulant laxatives

Their action is to alter water and electrolyte transport as well as stimulation of intestinal motility. The effective dose varies considerably from patient to patient. They act about 8 h after ingestion. Bisacodyl is, in part, absorbed, conjugated in the liver, excreted in the bile and deconjugated by bacteria in the colon to exert its action. Senna is metabolized by bacteria in the colon to the active aglycone.

Congestive heart failure

Definitions

A syndrome resulting from a chronically impaired contractility of the heart (interfering with its efficiency as a pump) and the homeostatic compensations for this.

Pathophysiological

Depression of the (Frank–Starling) curve relating cardiac ventricular performance to the ventricular filling pressure.

Clinical

In clinical practice congestive heart failure is identified by the presence of salt and water retention, an enlarged, tender liver and pulmonary congestion. An inadequate cardiac output causes fatigue, pulmonary congestion causes breathlessness when lying flat or on exertion, and fluid retention causes oedema (ankle swelling).

Aetiology and pathophysiology

Aetiology

There are background causes of impaired contractility on which are usually superimposed precipitating factors bringing about a further impairment and the development of the syndrome. Hypertension, atrial fibrillation, anaemia, hyperthyroidism and the use of salt-retaining drugs are factors, the effects of which can be reversed. Damage to the heart valves (congenital, rheumatic or infective) and the most common cause, coronary vascular obstruction, are more difficult to influence.

Pathophysiology

The slow onset of impaired cardiac pumping allows time for the development of compensatory changes that, to some extent, offset the direct ill effects of low cardiac output but produce their own, different, symptomatology.

The forward features of failure include easy fatiguability (at first on exercise but progressing until present at rest), peripheral cyanosis and salt and water retention – due to underperfusion of muscle, skin and kidney respectively. Patterned vasoconstriction (brain, heart and muscle are spared at the expense of skin, gut and kidney), tachycardia and positive inotropism are the sympathetic responses to decreased output (triggered by baroreceptors). (Antagonists at β-adrenoceptors are contraindicated because cardiac performance is supported through β-adrenoceptors.)

Central venous pressure rises (expanded ECF volume and venoconstriction) and increased atrial priming adds to increased passive ventricular filling bringing about the Frank–Starling improvement in ventricular performance. The ventricles may dilate to the point of stretching the AV ring (functional valvular incompetence) and the ventricular muscle hypertrophies. The liver also becomes congested.

High pressure within pulmonary veins backwards (upstream) from the left ventricle make for stiff lungs (reduced compliance) and breathlessness (at first on exercise but progressing until present at rest).

Renal underperfusion promotes renin release and hence (via the angiotensins) secondary hyperaldosteronism (pages 178 and 191) – distal tubular NaCl and water retention with K^+ and H^+ loss. The exaggerated NaCl and water retention increases the circulating blood volume and also the interstitial fluid volume, which makes oedema inevitable. The raised venous pressure and gravity localize it. These are the backward features of failure. Compensatory processes alleviate the forward features at the expense of aggravating the backward features.

Treatment

General measures include the treatment of precipitating factors, infection (page 282), anaemia (page 424), thyrotoxicosis (page 174), cardiac dysrhythmia (page 124) and fever and avoidance of salt-retaining steroids or NSAIDs.

There are three aims of therapy.

Reduce cardiac work

The patient should rest from physical activity (but this increases the risk of deep vein thrombosis) and, if obese, restrict calorie intake. Treat hypertension (page 380).

Vasodilators

Vasodilators decrease ventricular end-diastolic pressure. Venous dilatation (nitrates), arteriolar dilatation (*hydralazine*), or mixed site vasodilatation (**captopril** or *prazosin*) reduce either the preload or afterload upon the ventricles. Venous dilatation improves the backward features of failure. Tachycardia and postural hypotension are adverse effects with arterial, venous or mixed site dilators but are generally less severe with venous dilators.

Captopril (page 192) and other inhibitors of ACE (*enalapril*) reduce renin secretion and thus arteriolar resistance and also aldosterone production, which decreases sodium and water retention. They are the only drugs in the treatment of heart failure that have been shown to increase longevity.

Arteriolar dilatation allows the ventricles to achieve higher cardiac output at lower working pressures and hence improves the forward features of failure. Tachycardia, postural hypotension and fluid retention (except with **captopril**) are adverse effects.

Nitrates (*see* pages 138, 308 and 388) can be given by the oral, sublingual, buccal, iv or transcutaneous routes.

Decrease pulmonary congestion and peripheral oedema

Diuretic therapy is indicated – start with a thiazide (**bendrofluazide,** page 141), which has a shallow dose/response curve. If the response is inadequate change to a loop diuretic. The response is aided by a moderate reduction in dietary salt intake to about 80 mmol Na$^+$ daily.

Potassium supplements (effervescent potassium salts) may be required (especially in elderly patients) when loop or thiazide diuretics are prescribed for heart failure; the K$^+$-losing action of these diuretics summates with the secondary hyperaldosteronism (contrast with essential hypertension in which potassium salt supplements are rarely needed when a thiazide is prescribed, page 382).

K$^+$-sparing diuretics are **amiloride** and *triamterene* (page 143) and **spironolactone** (an aldosterone antagonist). They have a relatively low clinical efficacy when used alone. **Amiloride** is best used in combination with a loop diuretic in patients in whom it is important to maintain a normal serum K$^+$ concentration. Stop potassium salt supplements when adding **amiloride** or another K$^+$-sparing diuretic. Never use **amiloride** together with another K$^+$-sparing diuretic drug (risk of hyperkalaemia).

Increase cardiac output

Low cardiac output is commonly due to myocardial ischaemia (coronary artery disease). The capacity for increasing the cardiac output (contractility) is greatest with valvular heart disease, atrial fibrillation or hypertensive heart disease.

Digoxin

Digoxin increases myocardial contractility (positive inotropic effect, page 132), which allows the cardiac output to be maintained at a lower ventricular filling pressure.

It slows the ventricular rate in atrial fibrillation thus allowing a longer diastolic filling time, which reduces pulmonary congestion. The ventricular rate should not be depressed below 60/min.

It has a small therapeutic index – the toxic dose (nausea, heart block, ectopic ventricular beats) is very close to the therapeutic dose, especially if there is K^+ depletion. This is another indication for potassium salt supplementation. An oral loading dose of **digoxin** may be given, succeeded by a once daily oral maintenance dose. Dosage reduction is imperative in the elderly and others with renal impairment (page 350).

When **digoxin** therapy has been given for 3 months to patients in sinus rhythm, it is doubtful if continuation is either necessary or beneficial. Prescription should certainly be reviewed regularly and not repeated automatically.

Sympathomimetic agents

By virtue of their agonist action at cardiac β_1-adrenoceptors (page 110), *dopamine* and *dobutamine* can increase the stroke volume of the failing heart. The associated undesirable tachycardia is limited by the admixed agonist action at vascular α_1-adrenoceptors causing vasoconstriction, BP rise, baroreceptor activation and reflex restraint on the cardiac pacemaker.

Dopamine is also an agonist at renal vasodilator dopamine receptors. The $t_{\frac{1}{2}}$ of *dopamine* is 2 min and so it can only effectively be given by iv infusion. A low dose rate (2–5 µg/kg/min) results in an increase in renal perfusion. Higher doses (more than 5 µg/kg/min) increase the cardiac output but the renal effect is lost.

Dobutamine, likewise has a $t_{\frac{1}{2}}$ of only 2 min, hence its administration by iv infusion. A logical treatment of heart failure associated with hypotension (cardiogenic shock) is a combination of *dobutamine* and low dose *dopamine*.

Pulmonary oedema – left ventricular failure

If the left ventricle fails before, or more severely than, the right, the backward features of the failure are localized to the pulmonary vascular circuit.

Pulmonary oedema occurs when the pulmonary capillary pressure exceeds the osmotic pressure exerted by the plasma proteins (principally albumin). Urgent reduction of pulmonary congestion is required. Sit the patient up. Administer 60% oxygen (mask flow rate 6 l/min). Give a loop diuretic (**frusemide,** page 142) for its rapid onset of action, steep dose/response curve and possible direct effect on pulmonary veins before diuretic action. Adverse effects include gastrointestinal upsets, bone marrow depression and, rarely, reversible ototoxicity.

The distress and severe dyspnoea of acute pulmonary oedema can be relieved with **morphine** iv, which also promotes venous pooling and reduction of venous return.

Hypertension and antihypertensive drugs

General principles

Hypertension is the product of many complex physiological interactions. BP shows marked diurnal variations and rises with age. The demarcation between normal and abnormal pressures is an arbitrary one, as BP in a given population is a continuous variable. However, to help decide on treatment, controlled clinical trials have established thresholds of BP above which treatment should bring benefit. Except for patients with severe hypertension (diastolic BP > 130 mmHg) multiple measurements of BP are required to allow for BP variability. The threshold BP taken for entry into treatment trials has been the mean of measurements taken on a patient's third and fourth visits. For adults, adding the diastolic BP to the patient's age provides a threshold for the treatment of systolic BP. Diastolic BP changes less with age; treatment benefits those with diastolic BP averaging above 109 mmHg.

Classification

Hypertension can be classified on the basis of severity or aetiology. The aetiological classification recognizes two basic forms of hypertension – primary and secondary.

(1) Primary or essential hypertension. In 90% of hypertensive patients no obvious cause can be detected. However, family history, obesity, alcohol and cigarette smoking are all risk factors that predispose a patient to hypertension.
(2) Secondary hypertension. In the remaining 10%, a well defined condition causing hypertension can be identified. These include renal parenchymal disease, renal artery stenosis, active adrenal cortical or medullary tumours, drug effect (NSAIDs, oral contraceptive pill), congenital lesions (coarctation of the aorta) and pregnancy.

Hypertension can also be classified, on the basis of severity according to values of diastolic BP obtaining after at least three measurements, into:

(1) mild (90–105 mmHg);
(2) moderate (105–120 mmHg);
(3) severe (<120 mmHg).

Consequences of hypertension

The higher the sustained arterial BP the higher the mortality. The excess mortality is from atheromatous heart disease and stroke. Hypertension may progress to an accelerated or malignant phase characterized by target organ damage involving the kidney and retina leading to albuminuria, retinal haemorrhages and papilloedema (oedema of the optic nerve head). The characteristic pathological lesion is hyalinization and fibrinoid necrosis of arteriolar walls.

Antihypertensive treatment

In patients with secondary hypertension, treatment of the primary condition (as in surgical excision of an adrenal tumour) should produce a cure. Unfortunately, if the BP has been elevated for many years structural narrowing of the resistance vessels may result in the hypertension persisting even when the primary cause has been removed.

The treatment of accelerated or malignant hypertension is life saving as 90% of such patients, if untreated, die within 12–18 months of diagnosis. The beneficial effects of treating 'moderate' essential hypertension are less clear. Reduction of blood pressure to 'normal' levels has been shown to reduce mortality and morbidity from stroke but it does not affect morbidity or mortality from coronary heart disease. In patients with accelerated or malignant hypertension, the advantages of therapy are greater than possible morbidity from drug adverse effects. In those with 'mild' hypertension, however, there is no clear evidence from clinical trials that treatment offers a realistic benefit to a given individual.

Since BP is the product of cardiac output and peripheral resistance, BP reduction can be achieved by reducing cardiac output or peripheral resistance (or both). Cardiac output can be reduced by interfering with the cardiac sympathetic activity or by reducing central venous pressure by venodilatation. Peripheral resistance can be reduced either directly by modifying the contractile biochemistry of resistance blood vessels or indirectly by interfering with the sympathetic vasoconstrictor supply to these vessels.

Antagonists at β_1-adrenoceptors

Antagonists at β-adrenoceptors ('β-blockers', page 113) possess antihypertensive properties yet attempts to define their site of action have yielded no definite answer; each of three sites has some experimental evidence in its favour and a combination of actions seems likely. These are:

(1) a reduction in cardiac output;
(2) inhibition of renin release;
(3) interference with central nervous pathways involved in BP control.

Antagonists at β-adrenoceptors may precipitate cardiac failure in patients with limited cardiac reserve. They may produce bronchospasm (by blocking β_2-adrenoceptors) and cold hands and feet (Raynaud's phenomemon). In insulin-dependent diabetic patients they may promote hypoglycaemic attacks by blocking the sympathetically-mediated sweating and tremor that warn the patient of impending hypoglycaemia. Hepatic glycogenolysis, which is controlled by hepatic β-adrenoceptors, may also be impaired. Lipid soluble drugs (**propranolol**) may produce sleep disturbance marked by vivid dreams; this is less likely with water soluble drugs (**atenolol**).

The antagonists at β-adrenoceptors exert a mild or moderate antihypertensive action and are effective in about 45% of patients. They are widely used, especially in patients with angina and hypertension as they also decrease the frequency of angina attacks. **Propranolol** is metabolized by the liver and has a short plasma $t_{\frac{1}{2}}$. **Atenolol** is excreted by the kidney and has a longer plasma $t_{\frac{1}{2}}$. Antagonists at β-adrenoceptors are often combined with thiazides or vasodilators to produce a greater effect. Postural hypotension is not a problem.

Diuretics

The thiazides (**bendrofluazide**) constitute the major group of diuretics used as antihypertensive agents. These drugs exert an antihypertensive effect not only by reducing ECF volume and sodium depletion but also by nondiuretic mechanisms (vasodilatation, reducing peripheral resistance).

Intravascular volume and total body sodium content are reduced in the first few weeks of treatment; they return to normal over the next month as the renin-angiotensin-aldosterone system compensates but the antihypertensive effect persists. It is thought that the initial diuresis lowers plasma volume and contributes to the fall in BP.

It is likely that the direct vasodilator properties of thiazides are produced by the opening of K^+-channels in vascular smooth muscle, leading to membrane hyperpolarization and relaxation.

Hypokalaemia (plasma K^+ concentration less than 3 mmol/l) is a rare adverse effect of diuretic therapy as the dose employed is, or should be, small. Thiazides are secreted by the same renal tubular mechanism that handles uric acid and hyperuricaemia (gout) can occur. Hyperglycaemia, hyperlipidaemia and impotence are other adverse effects of thiazide diuretics and, much less frequently, bone marrow depression and hypersensitivity reactions.

Thiazides produce a mild antihypertensive action and are effective alone in about 40% of patients. Their antihypertensive effect is achieved at relatively low doses, higher doses make the adverse effects more pronounced. Their frequency of use as antihypertensive agents in clinical practice is declining.

Frusemide has a weak antihypertensive effect except where the hypertension is secondary to salt and water retention in renal disease.

Vasodilators

The vasodilators form the most diverse group of antihypertensive drugs and all reduce peripheral resistance. With most members of this group this results in an initial tachycardia mediated by the baroreceptor reflex. This compensatory response can be blocked by using an antagonist at β-adrenoceptors thereby enhancing the antihypertensive effect. Most of these drugs also cause salt and water retention and are therefore used in combination with a diuretic.

The vasodilators fall into two groups – directly and indirectly acting.

Directly acting vasodilators

These modify the electromechanical properties of the vascular smooth muscle contractile process. They are usually used in combination with diuretics or antagonists at β-adrenoceptors.

Calcium channel blockers

Verapamil and **nifedipine** reduce the influx of Ca^{2+} (page 135) into vascular smooth muscle that occurs during stimulation by vasoconstrictor agents. **Nifedipine** has a greater effect on peripheral vascular smooth muscle while **verapamil** has a greater effect on cardiac conduction tissue. **Nifedipine** causes a reduction in peripheral resistance and a fall in BP. **Verapamil** slows the heart rate and is also useful as an antidysrhythmic agent. It may cause heart block and the concurrent use of antagonists at β-adrenoceptors is best avoided as the combination may cause heart block and/or cardiac failure.

Angiotensin converting enzyme inhibitors

Captopril, *enalapril* and other drugs within this group inhibit the ACE in the lungs and the vascular endothelium (page 191). ACE inhibitors are therefore potentially very useful in lowering diastolic BP. ACE also breaks down the vasodilator peptide, bradykinin and impaired metabolism of this substance may contribute to the fall in BP.

Adverse reactions of proteinuria, neutropenia and rashes occur but their incidence is relatively low. Other potential adverse effects include hyperkalaemia and alteration or loss of taste (ageusia). Patients taking ACE inhibitors may complain of a persistent dry cough. The mechanism of this remains elusive.

ACE inhibitors should be used with caution in patients already on diuretics or who have a constricted circulating blood volume. In such patients the renin–angiotensin system is activated. The introduction of an ACE inhibitor blocks AII production and this can lead to a drop in BP sufficient to impair cerebral or renal blood flow.

Hydralazine

Hydralazine produces direct vasodilatation by an unknown mechanism. It is a reactive molecule that interacts with connective tissue constituents (elastin) and may produce systemic lupus erythematosus (SLE), an autoimmune condition, especially in slow acetylators (page 29) in high doses. The SLE is usually reversible on drug withdrawal.

Minoxidil

Minoxidil is a prodrug. Its active metabolite, minoxidil sulphate, is a potent arteriolar vasodilator drug with many adverse effects (fluid retention, reflex tachycardia, hypertrichosis) and is therefore only used in patients who have not responded to drugs with less adverse effects. *Minoxidil* opens K^+ channels in vascular smooth muscle, leading to membrane hyperpolarization and relaxation.

Indirectly acting vasodilators

These modify the function of noradrenergic mechanisms either in the CNS or in the periphery.

Drugs that act on the cardiovascular control centres

These drugs are thought to act by reducing the frequency of efferent impulses to peripheral noradrenergic nerves. *Methyldopa* is converted to α-methylnoradrenaline, a potent agonist at presynaptic α_2-adrenoceptors on noradrenergic neurone terminals.

Tiredness, lethargy, drowsiness and depression are common adverse effects, probably reflecting reduced noradrenergic transmission elsewhere in the CNS. Postural hypotension may occur, especially with *methyldopa*. Although the use of centrally acting drugs is declining, *methyldopa* is still the drug of choice in hypertension in pregnancy because of its established safety.

Selective antagonists at postsynaptic α_1-adrenoceptors

Prazosin is a selective antagonist at α_1-adrenoceptors. It dilates both arteriolar and venous smooth muscle. Unlike other vasodilators, reflex tachycardia does not seem to be a problem. First dose syncope, in which the patient may develop hypotensive collapse, is thought to be due to the venodilatation. It is circumvented by giving the first dose on retiring to bed. Chronic postural hypotension is not a problem with long-term use. Tachyphylaxis, in which increasing doses are needed to produce the same effect, is sometimes seen. Retrograde ejaculation is a possible side-effect as blockade of α-adrenoceptors relaxes the bladder neck and *prazosin* has been used in the treatment of prostatism. *Prazosin* is also useful, in conjunction with other drugs, in the treatment of refractory hypertension.

Labetolol combines within one molecule antagonism at β- and α-adrenoceptors (page 114). Both effects contribute to its antihypertensive usefulness but also to its pattern of adverse effects.

Selection of an antihypertensive drug

Antihypertensive drug treatment may need to be continued for many years and thus the incidence and severity of adverse effects must be minimized. Patient compliance is improved if it is possible to use a single drug given once daily rather than a multiple drug regimen requiring divided doses at different times of the day.

In the past diuretics and antagonists at β-adrenoceptors were recommended as standard first line therapy for hypertension. However newer agents (calcium channel blockers, ACE inhibitors) that decrease peripheral vascular resistance are being used more often and can be prescribed as first line agents.

Treatment of hypertensive emergencies/hypertensive crises

General

Hypertensive emergencies are rare. However, if diastolic BP is greater than 130 mmHg, or in the conditions eclampsia, hypertensive encephalopathy, acute dissecting aneurysm of the aorta, hypertensive left ventricular failure and phaeochromocytoma in crisis, the BP needs to be lowered urgently. In malignant hypertension it is necessary to reduce BP to a diastolic value of less than 120 mmHg but it is not necessary to do this suddenly. Too rapid a reduction in BP in such cases may lead to reduced cerebral perfusion and even infarction, especially if there is coexisting cerebrovascular disease. A more gradual reduction in BP using oral agents is safer in this situation.

Drug treatment

Drugs can be given parenterally to lower the BP in emergencies but they are rarely needed.

Hydralazine

Hydralazine, administered im, is effective within 10–20 min, reaches maximal response in 1 h and lasts for several hours.

Labetolol

Labetolol, administered iv as an infusion or repeated boluses, reduces BP within 10 min and lasts up to 6 h. Patients should always be kept supine as severe postural hypotension can ensue.

Sodium nitroprusside

Sodium nitroprusside is a nitrovasodilator, which activates soluble guanylate cyclase in both arteries and veins (*see* page 138). Its action is very rapid (1–2 min) and wanes rapidly on cessation of infusion – usually via a constant infusion pump. In the blood, the drug is broken down to CN^-, which is converted to thiocyanate in the liver. It can therefore only be given for up to 12 h before thiocyanate toxicity occurs.

Phaeochromocytoma

This is a tumour of chromaffin cells (usually those in the adrenal medulla) that secretes massive quantities of catecholamines and may cause sudden surges of hypertension, especially when the tumour is being handled during surgical removal. This problem can be avoided by pretreating the patient with oral **phenoxybenzamine** (antagonist at α-adrenoceptors) and by iv infusion of **phentolamine** and **propranolol** to prevent excessive effector stimulation by NA released during handling of the tumour. Oral **phenoxybenzamine** and **propranolol** should be given for 2 weeks before surgery. This drug combination blocks the action of the excess catecholamines thereby controlling the BP and allowing the circulating blood volume to return towards normal. Such pretreatment prevents the catastrophic fall in BP that otherwise occurs when the tumour source of catecholamines (which was maintaining the BP) is suddenly removed at surgery.

Angina of effort

Ischaemic heart disease may manifest itself as acute myocardial infarction, sudden death, unstable angina or stable angina pectoris. The basic underlying pathology of these different clinical syndromes is myocardial ischaemia produced by narrowing of the coronary arteries, usually due to atherosclerosis. This degenerative process can develop in individuals who have a genetic predisposition or who indulge in the modern western life-style characterized by:

(1) cigarette smoking;
(2) overnutrition;
(3) sedentary work and leisure pursuits;
(4) low fibre diet;
(5) stress.

Atherosclerosis is the consequence of the deposition of a lipid material beneath the endothelium of arteries (atheroma), which become thickened, scarred and calcified (sclerotic) and impede the flow of blood (ischaemia). Ischaemia is not an inevitable consequence of coronary atherosclerosis but atheroma is undoubtedly the principal factor underlying myocardial ischaemia. Increased cardiac work or reduced blood O_2 carrying capacity (obesity, hypertension, cardiac dysrhythmias, valvular heart disease and anaemia) are important contributory factors.

Myocardial ischaemia results when the work load on the ventricular myocardium exceeds the metabolic reserve. Cardiac muscle is incapable of operating anaerobically. This concept of supply and demand is demonstrable in atrial pacing experiments. A critical threshold of exercise and therefore of O_2 consumption can be established, above which angina is precipitated.

The rapidity of development of the occlusive process determines the mode of presentation of the patient. Those with fixed or slowly progressive occlusions may present with angina, while those with sudden occlusion may present with sudden death or a myocardial infarction. An intermediate stage of unstable angina occurs in the case of haemorrhage, oedema or thromboses on a pre-existing plaque of atheroma.

The characteristic symptom of angina of effort is a crushing pain in the chest (retrosternal) precipitated by exertion and relieved by rest. It may radiate to the left arm, neck or jaw. Patients commonly present with pain in atypical sites and may even present to the dentist with an ache in the lower jaw.

There is a variant form of angina pectoris (Prinzmetal's angina) in which the ischaemia results from a reflex spasm of a coronary artery in response to such stimuli as a heavy meal or a chill wind on the face and neck; it thus lacks the characteristic association with exercise. Some patients have a combination of the two kinds.

Myocardial work

The work and O_2 consumption of the heart are directly related to:

(1) heart rate;
(2) peripheral resistance (and BP);
(3) ventricular end diastolic filling pressure ('venous return');
(4) cardiac contractility;
(5) plasma free fatty acid concentrations.

Cardiac work may be increased when no external physical work is performed (watching television or arguing). Increased sympathetic activity can increase heart rate and BP separately or together. Such adrenergic (sympathoadrenal) stress may precipitate angina at rest in susceptible patients and these attacks last 5–15 min. In contrast, angina of effort rarely lasts longer than 3 min if the exertion is lessened or stopped.

Coronary perfusion

The major resistance to flow through the terminal branches of the coronary arteries as they penetrate the myocardium is provided by the tension in the ventricle walls. This tension is a reflection of the ventricular pressure. Little or no flow occurs during systole and therefore mean flow is reduced if the total time in diastole falls (when the heart rate is high). In addition, flow is reduced if left ventricular end diastolic pressure is raised (increased preload).

Treatment

The aim of treatment is to reduce myocardial oxygen demand or improve blood flow.

Prevention of coronary atherosclerosis – avoid risk factors

(1) Do not smoke cigarettes.
(2) Nutrition:
    (a) avoid obesity;
    (b) take high fibre diet;
    (c) treat severe hyperlipidaemia.
(3) Maintain physical fitness.

Prophylaxis of angina

(1) Remove contributory factors – anaemia, hypertension, heart failure, obesity, thyrotoxicosis.

(2) Reduce cardiac work.

Three groups of drugs are useful in the treatment of angina pectoris:

(1) organic nitrates;
(2) antagonists at β-adrenoceptors;
(3) calcium channel blockers.

Organic nitrates

Ischaemia is a most potent stimulus for increasing tissue perfusion, and atherosclerotic arteries are not capable of dilatation, so that capillary beds supplied by atherosclerotic arteries are likely to be fully dilated already. Coronary blood flow is unchanged or reduced by **glyceryl trinitrate** given for angina. Vasodilatation of capacitance veins and resistance vessels other than in the coronary circulation accounts for the therapeutic efficacy. Cardiac preload (ventricular end diastolic filling pressure) and afterload (diastolic BP) are lowered by increased venous capacity and reduced peripheral resistance respectively. Cardiac work and myocardial O_2 consumption are decreased despite a reflex rise in heart rate. The reduction in ventricular end diastolic filling pressure also reduces resistance in the coronary circulation, allowing perfusion to begin earlier in diastole. The smooth muscle relaxation is also helpful in patients with coronary artery spasm.

Peripheral vasodilatation accounts for the principal adverse effects of nitrate therapy (headache, light headedness, fainting attacks). Nitrates undergo extensive first pass metabolism and are best given by the sublingual route if a rapid onset of action is required.

Glyceryl trinitrate:

(1) is the drug of choice for treating angina of effort;
(2) has an onset of action within 2 min if the chewed tablets are kept under the tongue or an aerosol spray is used;
(3) has a duration of action up to 20 min.

Isosorbide dinitrate and *isosorbide mononitrate* are long acting formulations, resistant to degradation in the gut and liver. They are useful in the prophylaxis of angina. However, development of tolerance with continuous long-term use occurs to these preparations that can be avoided by ensuring drug-free periods (most conveniently, several hours during the night) in order to regain effectiveness. **Glyceryl trinitrate** can also be administered for longer lasting effect as a buccal or oral sustained release tablet, an ointment or a 'patch' for transdermal diffusion.

Antagonists at β-adrenoceptors

Heart rate, cardiac contractility and BP rise during exercise and stress. **Propranolol** and other antagonists at β-adrenoceptors (page 113) prevent increases in these determinants of myocardial O_2 consumption and are most effective prophylactic agents in angina with up to 70% of patients gaining benefit. As the bulk of coronary perfusion occurs during diastole, slowing the heart increases the total time the heart is in diastole and allows increased coronary flow. Therapeutic efficacy is related to antagonism at cardiac β-adrenoceptors and not to the *quinidine*-like activity (page 130) or the intrinsic sympathomimetic (partial agonist) activity possessed by some antagonists at β-adrenoceptors. The dose of **propranolol** should be increased until relief is obtained or until the resting heart rate is reduced to 50–60 beats per min. Twice daily administration has proved satisfactory.

In patients with congestive heart failure, antagonists at β-adrenoceptors can precipitate severe cardiac failure. In patients with asthma **propranolol** can precipitate bronchospasm (page 394). This risk is diminished but not abolished if cardioselective antagonists are used (**atenolol**).

Lipid soluble drugs (**propranolol**) are more likely to cause visual disturbances, vivid dreams and hypnagogic hallucinations as they cross the blood brain barrier readily. Water soluble drugs (**atenolol**) have the advantage of once daily dosage and hence encourage compliance. Sustained release preparations of the shorter acting preparations are also available but are more expensive.

Calcium channel blockers

This is a group of drugs that interfere with Ca^{2+} movement across muscle cell membranes (page 134), reducing the amount of Ca^{2+} available to the contractile mechanism. In the heart, this reduces the force of contraction and therefore reduces the oxygen demand. On peripheral resistance and capacitance vessels, impaired Ca^{2+} entry causes relaxation and consequently vasodilatation that reduces both preload (capacitance vessels) and afterload (resistance vessels).

Calcium channel blockers are also useful in the treatment of angina due to coronary artery spasm.

Verapamil acts mainly on the heart and also has antidysrhythmic properties (page 131).

Verapamil may precipitate bradycardia and cardiac failure, especially if used parenterally in conjunction with β-adrenoceptor antagonists.

The principal adverse effects are headache, flushing and ankle oedema due to vasodilatation in the case of **nifedipine** and bradycardia and heart failure with **verapamil.**

Nifedipine has little action on the heart. It relieves angina primarily by virtue of its vasodilating action. The reduction in afterload considerably reduces the risk of cardiac failure.

Asthma

Definition

The current clinical definition of asthma is a 'syndrome of widespread narrowing of peripheral airways in the lung, varying in severity over short periods of time either spontaneously or as a result of treatment'. A more useful clinical definition of asthma comprises a symptom complex of shortness of breath, wheeze or chest tightness that:

(1) often wakes the patient at night;
(2) persists in the early morning for more than 1 h if untreated;
(3) involves bronchial irritability to a variety of nonspecific stimuli (exercise and the inhalation of cold air, smoky atmospheres, diesel fumes, perfumes, hair and paint sprays).

A major underlying abnormality of asthma is bronchial hyper-reactivity. This is defined as an increased responsiveness of the airways to a variety of nonspecific bronchoconstrictor stimuli including inhalation of nonisotonic solutions, allergens and chemicals (histamine, methacholine, PGs). Inhalation of antigen (for example, pollen or house dust mite) produces an early, immediate response in sensitized asthmatic subjects. However, in 50% of these, it produces a dual response characterized by both the early reaction and also a late bronchoconstrictor response with onset some 8 h after inhalation of allergen. It is now thought that this late response correlates most closely pathogenetically with clinical asthma.

Pathologically, asthma may be defined as a chronic inflammatory disease of the airways, which is often disproportionate to asthma symptoms. Mild clinical disease may be accompanied by marked pathological changes including smooth muscle hypertrophy, airways constriction and mucus hypersecretion with formation of luminal plugs. A chronic infiltration of the lung by inflammatory cells also occurs. This initially comprises neutrophils and eosinophils but macrophages are recruited later. Shedding of the airways epithelium occurs even in mildly asthmatic subjects.

Epidemiology

Asthma is a common disease and its prevalence in western populations appears to be increasing. Asthma may affect up to 10% of the childhood and adult populations. However, most general practitioners surmise that only 3% of their patients have asthma. Thus asthma is under-diagnosed and therefore under-treated in the community.

Asthma is not only increasing in prevalence but also in severity. Up to 2000 people die from asthma each year in England and Wales and in young males there is a 5% increase in mortality per annum. A retrospective analysis of deaths from asthma identified avoidable factors in 80% of cases, including a failure to diagnose asthma (10%) and a lack of appreciation of the severity of the attack of asthma by the patients, their relatives and medical practitioners. Such factors cause delays in seeking medical attention, referral to hospital and institution of glucocorticoid therapy.

Investigation

During an exacerbation of asthma, pulmonary function tests demonstrate airflow obstruction with a diminished forced expiratory volume in 1 s

(FEV$_1$) together with a low FEV$_1$/forced vital capacity (FVC) ratio and a low peak expiratory flow rate (PEFR). Administration of a bronchodilator drug could demonstrate reversible airflow obstruction. However, when many asthmatic patients are seen by their general practitioners, complaining of episodic breathlessness, their peak expiratory flow rates are normal.

In addition to an accurate history, a diagnosis of asthma may be made by use of a peak expiratory flow meter (these are prescribable), asking suspected patients to record their PEFR throughout the 24 h period and particularly at times when they become breathless or wheezy. Based on the day-to-day patterns of airflow obstruction, there are three kinds of asthmatic patient:

(1) the brittle one who exhibits frequent and pronounced fluctuations in peak expiratory flow;
(2) the early morning 'dipper', characterized by nocturnal or early morning wheeze;
(3) the 'irreversible' asthmatic patient who shows little or no variation in airflow obstruction and yet responds to glucocorticoid therapy in the absence of response to other bronchodilator drugs. Patients in this subgroup may be mislabelled as having chronic obstructive bronchitis, particularly if they smoke. Thus a trial of glucocorticoid therapy in patients with severe airflow obstruction is indicated, even when the patient presents with a clinical pattern that is not typical of asthma.

Domiciliary peak flow monitoring can also be used to give an indication of the severity of asthma. Patients with 50% variability in peak flow over a 24 h period are at an increased risk of sudden death from asthma.

Additional investigation of asthmatic subjects might include a blood eosinophil count and measurement of plasma IgE concentration. These are often elevated in asthma. On occasion, skin testing for responsiveness to a variety of allergens is a useful diagnostic aid. Up to 80% of asthmatic subjects are atopic (*see* page 25) compared to 30% of a control population.

Basic mechanisms

The mechanism underlying bronchial hyper-reactivity, which appears to be fundamental to the pathogenesis of asthma, is not known. Pathophysiological disturbances at various levels may contribute to the development of bronchial hyper-reactivity. These include abnormalities of:

(1) the noradrenergic innervation of the airways and/or the sympathoadrenal release of catecholamines;
(2) the cholinergic control of the airways at the level of muscarinic cholinoceptors;
(3) the nonadrenergic, noncholinergic (peptidergic) inhibitory innervation of the airways;
(4) the permeability of the airway mucosa allowing increased penetration of causal agents;
(5) the synthesis and release of inflammatory mediators, hormones and neurotransmitters derived from mast cells, eosinophils, basophils and macrophages.

It is likely that regulation of the airways is not achieved through a single system but rather through an integration of several of these mechanisms.

The mast cell

By virtue of its capacity to release inflammatory mediators, the mast cell has classically been thought the pivotal cell in the pathogenesis of asthma. Mast cells have been observed lying free in the lumen in human bronchi, intraepithelially (usually adjacent to the basement membrane) and submucosally (beneath the basement membrane). In allergic (atopic, extrinsic) asthma, luminal mast cells may initiate the bronchoconstrictor response, since mediator release might be expected to affect the integrity of epithelial tight junctions, permitting penetration of antigen to mast cells situated deeper within the airway epithelium.

Human lung mast cells contain approximately 130 000 receptors for the C4 domain of the Fc fragment of IgE. IgE-dependent activation of mast cells occurs through the triggering of cell surface IgE by specific antigen with subsequent cross-linking of IgE Fc receptors. This stimulates the production of inositol trisphosphate (IP_3) from membrane phospholipids, thereby triggering the release of intracellular calcium. This, in turn, leads to the aggregation of microtubules with movement of granules containing preformed mediators to the plasmalemma and their subsequent extrusion.

The preformed mediators include histamine, tryptase, heparin and various factors chemotactic for white cells (eosinophils, neutrophils), which recruit inflammatory cells locally into the airway. Membrane phospholipids also provide substrate for phospholipase A_2 (PLA_2) yielding arachidonic acid. This may be metabolized along either the cyclo-oxygenase pathway to generate PGs, or the lipoxygenase pathway to generate LTs.

Such mediators have the potential to produce the pathophysiological abnormalities characteristic as asthma:

(1) contraction of bronchial smooth muscle (for example, histamine, PGD_2, $PGF_{2\alpha}$);
(2) secretion of mucus from bronchial mucosal glands;
(3) local vasodilatation (for example, prostacyclin (PGI_2));
(4) increased protein permeability of mucosal capillaries and oedema;
(5) leucocyte infiltration, especially eosinophils;
(6) irritation of sensory nerve endings.

The mast cell is not unique in its production of inflammatory mediators. Sputum eosinophilia has long been recognized as a hallmark of asthma. However, the important pathogenetic role of the eosinophil in asthma has only been recognized quite recently. The eosinophil, upon activation, releases platelet activating factor (PAF) from its membrane. This is an extremely potent bronchoconstrictor substance and increases nonspecific bronchial hyper-reactivity in man. PAF is also an eosinophil chemotactic factor and causes activation of eosinophils, producing a positive feedback loop. Eosinophils also release major basic protein, which has been shown to cause shedding of the airway epithelium.

Available medications that inhibit mediator release or action

Sodium cromoglycate is inhaled either as a finely divided powder using an insufflator (Spinhaler^R) or as an aerosol. It suppresses the release of mediators from sensitized mast cells challenged with allergen. It is of no value when administered after the challenge but is useful when given 30 min before exercise in exercise-induced asthma. Side-effects are minor and seen only with the cheaper powder formulation – cough, transient bronchoconstriction and throat irritation.

Anti-inflammatory glucocorticoids

Oral **prednisolone** or inhaled *beclomethasone* provide very effective prophylaxis (onset of action 3–7 days) but can produce serious systemic adverse effects (page 180); therefore, use as low a dose as possible, change from oral to inhaled steroid as soon as possible and try alternate morning steroid therapy (allows normal growth in children and avoids pituitary-adrenal cortical suppression.

Selective agonists at β₂-adrenoceptors

Salbutamol (page 111) and *terbutaline* are long acting because they are not metabolized by COMT. These agents are more effective against the early rather than the late phase of airway narrowing in an attack of asthma. Side-effects (tremor, nervous tension, tachycardia) are rare with low doses administered by aerosol but common with the larger doses used orally and by nebulization.

Methylxanthines

Theophylline (page 136) in a sustained release formulation is given twice daily and both absorption and metabolism vary with smoking and dietary habits and in liver and heart disease. The therapeutic window is 5–15 mg/l and plasma or saliva assay is advisable to develop a dosage regimen.

Theophylline is complexed to increase water solubility as *aminophylline* for iv injection. Adverse effects (nausea, vomiting, headache, faintness, tachycardia, cardiac dysrhythmias, convulsions) are related to blood concentration and dose.

Quaternary ammonium antagonist at muscarinic cholinoceptors

Ipratropium inhibits reflex bronchoconstriction (page 88). It is inhaled as an aerosol. Therefore it has a local action with delayed onset (30–60 min).

Properties of an ideal bronchodilator drug

The ideal bronchodilator drug should fulfil certain criteria, particularly if it is to be used on a long-term regular basis:

(1) it should be effective in producing its therapeutic effect with a satisfactory onset and duration of action;

(2) it should be convenient to take;
(3) it should have a low toxicity;
(4) it should have an additive or synergistic effect with other bronchodilators;
(5) drug tolerance should not develop.

Preferred route of administration

The inhaled route of administration confers may advantages over the oral one. Administration of drugs by the inhaled route results in the production of a high concentration of drugs locally in the airways, thereby minimizing unwanted systemic effects. In addition, the inhaled route of administration results in rapid bronchodilatation when using an agonist at β_2-adrenoceptors.

The major objection to inhaled therapy, observed particularly in children and the elderly, is difficulty in synchronizing inhalation with activation of the inhaler (50% of asthmatic patients fail to derive maximum benefit from their inhalers). However, with the introduction of new inhaler devices, poor inhalation technique may be circumvented without having to resort to oral therapy. There are various devices available:

(1) dry powder inhalers (for example, the Turbohaler^R for inhaled *terbutaline* and *budesonide*);
(2) the Diskhaler^R or Rotahaler^R for inhalation of **salbutamol** and *beclomethasone*;
(3) spacing devices (for example, the Nebuhaler^R for *terbutaline* and *budesonide* and the Volumatic^R for **salbutamol** and *beclomethasone*).

It is essential that inhaler technique be checked in each asthmatic patient, who should be supplied with a device that he or she can use effectively.

Management of chronic persistent asthma

Avoidance of triggering factors

Where certain drug triggers (for example, antagonists at β-adrenoceptors, **aspirin,** NSAIDs) or particular allergens (for example, pets, bedding material, moulds and food) are identified, or occupational asthma is diagnosed, such triggers should be avoided if possible. Antagonists at β-adrenoceptors are dangerous even as eye drops and extreme caution must guide the use of even selective antagonists at β_1-adrenoceptors (page 114) in patients with asthma. There is no role for immunotherapy in the form of desensitization of asthmatic patients to specific allergens.

Bronchodilators

A selective agonist at β_2-adrenoceptors (for example, **salbutamol** 100–200 µg or *terbutaline* 250–500 µg) should be used on an 'as required' rather than regular basis. In this way, patients can use their frequency of inhalation of β_2-adrenoceptor agonist as a monitor of their asthma severity by using it as a 'rescue inhaler'. Two new agonists at β_2-adrenoceptors have been developed, formoterol and salmeterol. These have a much longer duration of action, up to 12 h. They may have a role in the management of severe nocturnal asthma. The exclusive use of agonists at β_2-adrenoceptors in the management of asthma should be reserved for patients who have no sleep disturbance, normal lung function and infrequent symptoms.

Inhaled anti-inflammatory agents

Patients who require to use their bronchodilator (β_2-adrenoceptor agonist) inhaler more than once daily or who are awoken at night by symptoms, require regular, inhaled anti-inflammatory treatment. The treatment options include:

(1) inhaled glucocorticoids;
(2) inhaled **sodium cromoglycate** or *nedocromil sodium*.

Inhaled glucocorticoids are the treatment of choice and should be instituted at a dose of 100–400 µg twice daily every day. In patients who fail to respond in terms of symptoms and peak flow monitoring, inhaler technique should be rechecked and, if satisfactory, the inhaled glucocorticoids can be used in higher doses or more frequently, up to four times daily. Rinsing the mouth after an inhalation of glucocorticoid helps to circumvent the problems of oral thrush and occasional hoarseness of speech (dysphonia). Once symptoms are controlled, the dose of inhaled glucocorticoid should be reduced to the minimum required to maintain this control.

For patients with persistent nocturnal asthma despite inhaled glucocorticoid treatment, either a nocturnal sustained release agonist at β_2-adrenoceptors or nocturnal sustained release *theophylline* might be tried to good therapeutic effect.

Inhaled **sodium cromoglycate** and *nedocromil* are used infrequently in adult patients but may benefit a few. In children **sodium cromoglycate** is the treatment of choice initially but the use of inhaled glucocorticoid therapy is increasing in importance in the paediatric age group.

Oral glucocorticoids

Maintenance, long-term oral **prednisolone** should only be used if adequate control cannot be achieved on maximum doses of inhaled glucocorticoids together with bronchodilators. High dose inhaled glucocorticoids should always be continued in patients receiving oral glucocorticoid treatment.

High dose inhaled bronchodilator therapy

In patients with chronic severe asthma, further benefit may be derived by administering both bronchodilator and anti-inflammatory agents via a nebulizer. Agonists at β_2-adrenoceptors and antagonists at muscarinic cholinoceptors can be delivered from prediluted vials through a nebulizer (for example, **salbutamol** up to 5 mg, *terbutaline* up to 10 mg and *ipratropium* up to 500 µg) but ideally this should be supervised through a hospital. In addition, both *budesonide* and *beclomethasone* can be administered as nebulizer solutions. Rarely, patients who do not derive benefit from nebulizer therapy do respond to 6 hourly administration by im injection of an agonist at β_2-adrenoceptors (for example, *terbutaline* 1–3 mg four times daily).

The commonest cause of poorly controlled asthma is noncompliance with treatment and to overcome this, it is essential that the difference between the inhaled agonists at β_2-adrenoceptors (reliever/rescue inhaler) and inhaled anti-inflammatory drug (preventer) is emphasized to the patient. Compliance with glucocorticoid inhalation is often poor because such explanation is not given and patients find that inhalation of an agonist at β_2-adrenoceptors works best at times when they are wheezy!

Indications for oral glucocorticoids (short course)

(1) Deteriorating asthma with recent onset of sleep disturbance and deteriorating peak expiratory flow rate.
(2) Whenever emergency nebulized or injected bronchodilators are necessary.
(3) Acute severe asthma.
(4) As a trial of reversibility in chronic severe airflow obstruction.

Management of acute severe asthma

Acute severe asthma (previously called status asthmaticus) is a life-threatening medical emergency. Patients presenting to casualty departments need to seen quickly by an experienced doctor. Patients should ideally always be admitted to hospital even if there is an apparent 'good response' in the accident and emergency room to nebulized bronchodilator therapy.

The three cardinal physical signs of severe asthma that should be rapidly assessed are:

(1) tachycardia > 120 beats/min (take into account any previous administration of bronchodilator drugs with positive chronotropic effects);
(2) pulsus paradoxus (an exaggeration of the normal systolic BP swings with respiration) measured using a sphygmomanometer;
(3) cyanosis.

The objective assessment must at least include:

(1) chest X-ray (to exclude other causes of severe breathlessness – pulmonary oedema or pneumothorax). All that wheezes is not asthma!
(2) arterial blood gas analysis. During an attack of acute severe asthma, low arterial PaO_2 (hypoxaemia) and low $PaCO_2$ (hypocapnoea) usually occur. A normal or high $PaCO_2$ in a patient with acute severe asthma indicates an extremely severe attack.
(3) peak expiratory flow rate.

Treatment

Oxygen

Oxygen should be administered in high concentration (for example, 60%) using either an Edinburgh or MC mask. This contrasts sharply with the controlled oxygen therapy (<28%) of patients with chronic airflow obstruction, who may be reliant on hypoxaemic drive.

Bronchodilators

Agonists at β_2-adrenoceptors should be administered, ideally by the nebulized route, which permits high doses to be administered locally to the airways. **Salbutamol** and *terbutaline* are both available as nebulizer solutions in break-off nebule form. Rarely, agonists at β_2-adrenoceptors are administered by the iv route but this is no more efficacious than nebulization and produces more side-effects (tremor, tachycardia).

Glucocorticoids

Glucocorticoids should be administered both orally and by the iv route. For the first 24 h, the patient should receive *hydrocortisone* 200 mg 6 hourly iv and a suggested oral regimen would be **prednisolone** 40 mg daily for 5 days, 30 mg daily for a further 5 days and then the oral course can be stopped. In patients taking maintenance glucocorticoids, doses up to 80 mg daily are advised.

Intravenous fluids

Patients with acute severe asthma are dehydrated at the time of admission and should receive *sodium chloride* 0.9% iv for the first 24 h (for example, 4 litres).

Antibiotics

These should not be routinely administered, since acute severe asthma is not usually triggered by bacterial infection. Green sputum during an exacerbation usually indicates sputum eosinophilia rather than bacterial infection. However, if the patient is febrile, or the blood white cell count is elevated, or pathogens can be cultured from sputum, then the appropriate antibiotic may be administered.

Assisted ventilation

Rarely, nowadays, is it necessary to ventilate patients with acute severe asthma. However, the decision whether or not to ventilate must be made by a doctor experienced in the management of such patients. The indications may be purely the appearance of the patient from the end of the bed on the grounds of impaired speech and gross exhaustion. Deteriorating blood gas tensions are an obvious indication but in many cases the indication to ventilate may be present prior to obvious worsening of hypoxaemia or hypercapnoea. Close cooperation with doctors in intensive care is vital and often it may be advisable to request placement of the patient in the intensive care unit before the need for assisted ventilation is apparent.

Drugs that are contraindicated

Respiratory depressants, opioids and sedatives (benzodiazepines) can kill asthmatic patients if administered during an acute attack and they must not be given.

Only in exceptional cases should iv *aminophylline* or nebulized *ipratropium bromide* be instituted. Although iv *aminophylline* is a bronchodilator of similar efficacy to a nebulized agonist at β_2-adrenoceptors, it is a relatively toxic agent and, in patients being managed in the manner suggested, *aminophylline* confers no extra advantage but does produce many adverse effects. Iv *aminophylline* is contraindicated in patients currently receiving an oral *theophylline* preparation. If *aminophylline* is administered it must be monitored by plasma concentration assay as soon as possible.

Patient improvement should be monitored by regular PEFR measurements (in addition to clinical assessment) and special attention must be paid to any who persist in early morning dipping or marked bronchial lability (more than 50% variability in peak flow over 24 h periods).

All patients, having been admitted to hospital with acute severe asthma, should be discharged on an inhaled glucocorticoid.

Sudden onset – life threatening asthma

Rarely, asthma may become severe within minutes in spite of little instability of asthma in the preceding days. Such patients are at great risk of sudden death. Although loan of a domiciliary nebulizer for inhalation of a high dose of an agonist at β_2-adrenoceptors may help, many physicians educate such patients in the self-administration im of a preloaded syringe (Min-I-Jet^R) containing 0.5 mg of *adrenaline*.

Coughs and colds

Cough

This is a powerful reflex initiated through irritation of receptors in the mucosa of the upper respiratory tract. These receptors are sensitive to stimulation by the mediators of inflammation associated with allergy or infection, by chemicals (sulphur dioxide, cigarette smoke) or by particles, foreign bodies and secretions. They are also responsive to distortions, or changes in the calibre, of the airways. Stimulation of these receptors discharges afferent impulses to the cough centre in the brain stem. From here efferent impulses are carried along somatic motor pathways to the diaphragm and the intercostal and abdominal muscles. Convulsive contraction of these muscles causes a rapid expulsion of air from the lungs in an attempt to remove any irritating particles or mucus from the respiratory tract. The secretion of mucus by the goblet cells is increased by the reflex.

A cough may be one of two kinds:

(1) productive cough – the act of coughing removes from the lungs and respiratory tract mucus that might otherwise act as a site of infection and disturb gaseous exchange;
(2) nonproductive cough – this is usually a dry, irritating or tickly cough that does not produce mucus. It may be present after the common cold and in chronic bronchitis. Such a cough may be initiated by the dripping of mucus from the postnasal space onto the pharynx and trachea, or by oedema of the pharyngeal mucosa after a sore throat.

If the cough is the main complaint of the patient the rational treatment is to suppress a nonproductive cough. A productive cough should not be suppressed (it is attempting to clear the airways) but the clearance may be improved by altering the consistency of the mucus. A cough that persists may indicate a more serious disease (bronchitis, tuberculosis, cancer) and should be investigated accordingly.

Expectorants

Normal bronchial mucosa has ciliated columnar cells with few goblet cells. Mucus is also secreted by submucous glands, which receive vagal innervation. The cilia beat rhythmically and move upwards a layer of fluid on which the mucus floats. This is then usually swallowed. (The bronchial mucosa of smokers has many more goblet cells and fewer ciliated cells than normal. The daily coughing up of mucus is indicative of chronic bronchitis.)

The aim of expectorants is to aid the clearance of mucus from the lungs. This is achieved by increased bronchial secretions and the production of mucus that is less viscous and therefore coughed up more easily. Clearance of mucus can be assessed by measuring the rate of removal of inhaled radioactive microspheres from the lungs.

Expectorants are claimed to act by irritation of the gastric mucosa that reflexly stimulates bronchial mucus secretion. There is doubt as to their effectiveness. Unfortunately many preparations containing expectorants also contain a cough suppressant (*see below*): these preparations should be avoided.

Inhalation of steam aids expectoration. The warm water vapour hydrates the bronchial tree and increases the secretion of mucus that is less viscous and can more easily be removed by coughing. Additions (menthol, eucalyptus oil) probably exert no additional effect on secretion but may encourage deep inhalation of the steam.

Mucolytics

These reduce the viscosity of the mucus by changing the structure of its components. Acetylcysteine breaks disulphide bonds in proteins in the mucus. Despite these effects on the viscosity of mucus (which can be assessed by measuring sputum viscosity at different shear rates) there is no clear evidence that the majority of patients experience any beneficial effects from the use of mucolytics. Fragmentation of the mucus may interfere with ciliary movement and therefore clearance of the airways.

Cough suppressants

A nonproductive cough causing sleep loss may be suppressed by drugs acting at some stage of the cough reflex. Cough suppressants can be assessed by their ability to suppress cough induced by a citric acid aerosol. The most effective cough suppressants are the opioids (page 233), which act at the cough centre and reduce impulses in the efferent pathways to the muscles involved in the act of coughing. *Diamorphine* is the most potent but because of abuse potential both it and *methadone* are used only in painful cough associated with terminal illness. In other situations opiate derivatives showing cough suppression at subanalgesic doses (**codeine,** pholcodine) or selective antitussives (**dextromethorphan**) are used. *Codeine* linctus is liable to abuse. Preparations offered for the treatment of cough that contain the irrational combination of a cough suppressant and an expectorant should not be used.

Antagonists at H_1 histamine receptors may suppress coughing by acting at receptors in the bronchial mucosa that are involved in initiating the reflex. The antagonistic activity at muscarinic cholinoceptors also possessed by many of these compounds reduces the secretion of mucus; however, such antihistamines are offered inappropriately combined with expectorants.

Coryza – the common cold

The common cold is a viral infection resulting in an inflammatory reaction of the lining of the upper respiratory tract, particularly the nasal mucosa. This is manifested as local vasodilatation, increased blood flow, oedema and a watery discharge from the nose. As the infection is a viral one, only symptomatic treatment is available. An antipyretic analgesic (**aspirin, paracetamol**) relieves any associated fever or headache (page 402) and a decongestant reduces the nasal symptoms.

Production of mucus by the nasal mucosa may be reduced by antagonists at muscarinic cholinoceptors, most often as antagonists at H_1 histamine receptors with antimuscarinic activity (**chlorpheniramine**). These are liable to cause sedation and antimuscarinic side-effects including dry mouth, disturbed accommodation and mydriasis (a danger in patients predisposed to closed angle glaucoma).

Decongestants

Decongestants directly or indirectly activate α_1-adrenoceptors, resulting in constriction of the blood vessels in the nasal mucous membranes. Both oral and topical preparations are used. With oral preparations (*ephedrine*) the possibility of serious systemic adverse effects or interaction with other drugs

(MAO inhibitors, tricyclic antidepressives, page 100) exists. They are best avoided at night or their stimulant effect of the CNS may prevent sleep. Oral decongestants are usually formulated with other components (cough suppressants, analgesics, antihistamines).

Local application of decongestants to the nasal mucosa is made by sprays or drops containing *ephedrine* or phenylephrine. The risks of systemic effects are small. The most common problem with these drugs is local reactive hyperaemia through overenthusiastic and prolonged use.

Sinusitis

The air sinuses within the face bones and communicating with the nose may become inflamed in coryza and constant nose blowing forces nasal discharge into them. Decongestants shrink the mucosa and aid drainage from here. If the sinuses become blocked with infected material antibiotic treatment may be necessary.

Allergic rhinitis

This occurs as a result of exposure to allergens. It can be seasonal (pollen) or perennial (house dust mite). Symptoms are similar to a cold but the conjunctivae may also be involved.

Antagonists at H_1 histamine receptors (page 195) administered systemically are of doubtful value, result in sedation and are often associated with adverse effects due to blockade of muscarinic cholinoceptors. Newer compounds (*terfenadine*) that do not readily cross the blood brain barrier, are claimed to cause very little sedation, psychomotor impairment or antimuscarinic effects.

Prophylactic intranasal and eye drop use of **sodium cromoglycate** (page 196) may prevent attacks and nasal application of a glucocorticoid (*beclomethasone*, page 207) is also helpful.

Some patients may benefit from a course of hyposensitizing injections of allergen extracts if the responsible allergen can be identified.

Headache and migraine

Headache

Headache is a common symptom and is usually due to:

(1) muscular spasm – the tension headache;
(2) referred pain – from cervical spondylosis (arthritis), sinusitis, glaucoma, or errors of refraction. Within the cranium, only large blood vessels and

the lining of the inside of the skull have receptors for pain, the brain itself does not. The tissues of the scalp (blood vessels) are sensitive to pain;

(3) vasodilatation – responsible for the headache associated with migraine, histamine, **glyceryl trinitrate** and systemic infections.

Contrary to popular belief headache is not a feature of essential hypertension.

Treatment

Wherever possible the underlying cause should be identified so that specific and effective therapy can be instituted (for meningitis, cerebral tumour, depression). If intracranial pathology is suspected opioid analgesics should not be given because the associated respiratory depression raises intracranial pressure via hypercapnoea and may disturb consciousness. Simple analgesics should be the first treatment for headache. Proprietary, over-the-counter preparations usually contain **aspirin, paracetamol** or **codeine.** Singly or in combination, these drugs are adequate for all kinds of moderate headache. Double-blind controlled trials have shown that 500–1000 mg of **paracetamol** and **aspirin** are equipotent as antipyretics and analgesics and are as effective as **codeine** (30 mg), *dihydrocodeine* (30 mg) and *dextropropoxyphene* (65 mg). Increasing the dose of these drugs does not provide further analgesia but should prolong the duration of action at the expense of increased toxicity – gastric irritation with **aspirin,** constipation and drowsiness with opioids. The short-term use of an anxiolytic (**diazepam**) may occasionally be warranted if stress is an important causative factor. Which analgesic a doctor or a patient chooses is usually based on habit rather than on recognized prescribing considerations (apart from the risk of gastric mucosal ulceration with salicylates, although modern formulations of dispersible **aspirin** are much less hazardous, and avoidance of **aspirin** in children under 12 years of age, *see* page 242). In the UK frequently prescribed compound analgesics are co-proxamol (paracetamol and dextropropoxyphene) and co-dydramol (paracetamol and dihydrocodeine) although such preparations rarely have any advantage and complicate the treatment of overdosage.

Migraine

Migraine is a familial disorder characterized by recurrent attacks of headache widely variable in intensity, frequency and duration and is often associated with neurological disturbances. The classic syndrome comprises:

(1) a prodromal phase, in which visual disturbances are common – blind spot (scotoma), hemianopia, scintillating lines – accompanied by drowsiness, nausea and vomiting, thought to be due to intracerebral vasoconstriction;

(2) the headache, which is usually unilateral and throbbing, due to vasodilatation of extracerebral vessels.

All the above characteristics are not present in each attack or in each patient.

The mechanism of the instability of intracranial and extracranial blood vessels is unknown. This abnormality of vasomotor control is of pharmacological interest because 5-HT has been implicated in its pathogenesis and drugs that mimic or antagonize 5-HT are of value in the prophylaxis of migraine. The effects of 5-HT on the cardiovascular system are complex but intracarotid infusion causes constriction of the temporal artery and scalp pallor, both of which occur in the prodromal phase of migraine.

Normally, 5-HT is confined to platelets but during an attack a factor in the plasma activates the release of 5-HT from platelets. Tyramine-containing foods precipitate attacks in susceptible patients and the headache associated with ingestion of these foods by patients on MAO inhibitors shows features of migraine. A higher premenstrual incidence of migraine in women may be related to a decrease of platelet MAO activity after ovulation. PGs released from activated platelets promote aggregation, the further release of 5-HT and a lowering of the pain threshold in vessel walls. The lateralization of many migrainous headaches is unexplained.

Therapy

Based on the above considerations, a number of approaches might prove of value in the prophylaxis of migraine and in the treatment of an acute attack.

Prophylaxis

(1) Remove factors triggering the disorder, for example, avoid stressful situations – psychotherapy, anxiolysis (**diazepam** or better **propranolol,** which can also reduce the effects of increased sympathetic activity); withdraw offending foodstuffs and ethanol. Inhibit ovulation.
(2) *Pizotifen* [pizotyline] is an antagonist at $5-HT_2$, H_1 histamine and muscarinic cholinoceptors. Whilst effective, the predictable side-effects are impairment of motor coordination, increased sedation with ethanol and dry mouth.
(3) Tricyclic antidepressive agents (**amitriptyline**) at night.
(4) Inhibition of PG synthesis with **aspirin** (600 mg twice daily) has been shown to reduce the frequency of headache in migrainous patients by more than 75%.

Treatment of the acute attack

It would appear rational to use agents that can cause vasoconstriction of scalp vessels to treat the headache.

(1) **Ergotamine** is the most reliable agent for relief but to be maximally effective it must be given parenterally (0.25 mg im or sc) before the vasodilator phase. **Ergotamine** suppositories are also used (formulated with *caffeine*, which may enhance absorption). To overcome the erratic

absorption from the gut a pressurized aerosol delivering a metered dose of micronized **ergotamine** is available. A maximum of six doses in 1 day has been recommended. The drug is highly toxic, causing vomiting and diarrhoea, convulsions and severe vasoconstriction, leading to paraesthesiae and gangrene (*cf.* St Anthony's fire of ergot poisoning due to fungal contamination of rye). For this reason a treatment course is restricted to 12 doses in a week, with a break of at least 4 days between courses. It is contraindicated in patients with vascular disease, thrombophlebitis, hepatic or renal disease and during pregnancy.

(2) Analgesics (**paracetamol, aspirin, codeine**) have some palliative effect if taken early in the vasoconstrictor phase.

(3) For nausea and vomiting an antiemetic (by suppository to ensure its absorption) – *prochlorperazine, metoclopramide* (page 231). If nausea and vomiting are frequent features of recurrent attacks, their oral use together with simple analgesics during the vasoconstrictor phase may be effective.

(4) If drowsiness is a problem *caffeine* is a weak cerebral stimulant and is often a constituent of compound analgesic preparations. In excessive doses or on withdrawal, *caffeine* may itself cause headache.

Trigeminal neuralgia

This consists of excruciating pain that shoots across the cheek, chin and lips. Attacks last for a few seconds but can recur frequently. Attacks can be precipitated by the lightest of touches to a defined trigger zone.

The electrophysiological defect of trigeminal neuralgia must be related to that in epilepsy since anticonvulsant drugs are effective. Amongst these **carbamazepine** is the drug of choice. **Carbamazepine** has no other analgesic activity.

Drugs and mental disorders

Aims

For each of anxiety neurosis, depressive illness and schizophrenia to elucidate the:

(1) nature of the disease;
(2) rational selection and use of drugs;
(3) role of drug therapy in the context of other therapies.

Anxiety neurosis

Anxiety is being troubled in mind about some uncertain event. It is the natural psychological reaction to social and physical problems. There should be no temptation to prescribe for anxiety unless it is part of the illness – anxiety neurosis.

Neurosis is the result of the action of stressful events on the personality – enough to be regarded as a 'disease' by the doctor, patient or the patient's social contacts. A neurosis is usually recognizable as an exaggeration of a normal behavioural pattern (an anxious or depressed state) but may occasionally be severe, as in panic disorder, agoraphobia, obsessional-compulsive disorder and cardiac hypochondriasis. Environmental factors are often causative, and patterns of neurotic behaviour are easily learned in childhood. Stress can push each of us into these behaviour patterns (for example, examination anxiety, bereavement depression). The neurotic patient has a lower threshold for, and a longer persistence of, this behaviour.

Symptoms of anxiety neurosis

Psychological

A sense of fearful anticipation, irritability, sensitivity to noise, feeling of restlessness, impaired concentration, and disturbed sleep.

Physical

Resulting in part from autonomic overactivity. Palpitations, dry mouth, sweating, diarrhoea, frequency of micturition and impotence or frigidity.

Caused by overactive skeletal muscles. Headaches and aching in the back or neck.

Caused by hyperventilation. Dizziness, paraesthesiae, faintness and palpitations.

Natural history and prognosis of anxiety neurosis

Rapid spontaneous resolution is to be expected in a sound personality with a short-lived stress.

Objectives of treatment

The patient is encouraged to learn to cope with prolonged stress and to adjust his/her life style to live within their limitations. If the patient is young and well motivated to change an unsound personality these objectives may be attainable. Drugs may be used for a few weeks to suppress symptoms while a psychological technique is being taught.

Treatment of anxiety neurosis

A combination of treatments is aimed at changing aetiological factors amenable to change.

Psychological

Simple psychotherapy sometimes suffices. Listen carefully to the patient's account of his/her symptoms and anxieties. Demonstrate that you recognize these as part of a common illness. Explain the nature of the illness and its likely causes. Reassure the patient that a more feared illness is not present and that treatment, which the doctor will supervise, will be effective. Provide relaxation training and teach behavioural and cognitive procedures for controlling anxious thoughts. Specialist psychotherapy may be needed.

Anxiolytics

Today the benzodiazepines are the principal anxiolytic drugs (page 247) in use, having replaced barbiturates, which are much more sedative and dangerous in overdose. In the 1960s the advertising strategy of the pharmaceutical industry promoted a syndrome to the medical profession and to the public. The typical patient was an over-anxious housewife with young children, unable to cope with her lot, exhibiting physical manifestations of sympathoadrenal overactivity. This syndrome was alleged to respond dramatically to the first benzodiazepine, chlordiazepoxide – 'a sedative anticonvulsant with marked taming effects in vicious animals'. Anxiety neurosis became respectable, chlordiazepoxide fashionable, and more potent analogues were introduced (**diazepam,** *lorazepam*). Controlled trials reveal a high rate of spontaneous remission in anxiety neuroses with only small additional effects of benzodiazepines. These additional benefits are short-lived. Physical dependence and withdrawal anxiety develop rapidly.

Selection of a benzodiazepine

Each benzodiazepine possesses all the properties of the group with only minor differences in relative potency. Some effects are readily demonstrable in people – sedation, suppression of paradoxical sleep, safety in overdosage and anterograde amnesia. Others (appetite stimulation and relaxation of voluntary muscle – an effect mediated by depression of spinal synaptic transmission) are less so. The clinical use of individual drugs is determined to some extent by the marketing strategy of the manufacturers – *nitrazepam* is promoted as a sedative, *clonazepam* as an anticonvulsant.

Most benzodiazepines have an active metabolite with a prolonged elimination phase ($t_\frac{1}{2}$ more than 24 h). Administration once daily is therefore appropriate, preferably at night to prevent insomnia due to anxiety, but they are often given thrice daily and accumulate. In the elderly, elimination is less efficient ($t_\frac{1}{2}$ up to 90 h) with cumulation leading to confusion, ataxia, drowsiness and incontinence. A few (*lorazepam, oxazepam,* **temazepam**) show a shorter elimination $t_\frac{1}{2}$.

Anxiolytic drug therapy should not be continued for more than 1 month. There are however many patients who have received benzodiazepines daily for many years. Withdrawal then becomes very difficult and requires strong motivation and support.

CSM advice on the use of benzodiazepines

Benzodiazepines are indicated for the short-term relief (2–4 weeks only) of anxiety that is severe, disabling or subjecting the individual to unacceptable distress, occurring alone or in association with insomnia or short-term psychosomatic, organic or psychotic illness.

The use of benzodiazepines to treat short-term 'mild' anxiety is inappropriate and unsuitable.

Disadvantages of benzodiazepines

Delay psychological adjustment. Their use diverts attention from the provision of more effective aid.

Adverse effects. Sedation – drowsiness, ataxia, impaired judgement, prolonged reaction time, unfitness for driving or operation of machinery, hostility, aggression, antisocial acts, confusion and summation with alcohol.

Drugs of dependence. Tolerance, psychological and physical dependence that is worse in alcoholism, drug abuse or personality disorder. It occurs after long, high dose exposure. Withdrawal gives insomnia, apprehension, anorexia, tremor, sweating, disordered perception, confusion and convulsions after an onset time of about 24 h after short-acting drugs and 3–10 days after long-acting ones. This withdrawal syndrome lasts 8–10 days.

Managing withdrawal from benzodiazepines

In 75% of patients a tapering regimen (reduce dose by one-quarter weekly) is successful if agreed with the patient. If sleep is disrupted, advise against catnapping.

In 25% of patients withdrawal symptoms are unavoidable; transfer from a short- to a long-acting benzodiazepine, substitute **propranolol** and again taper the dose of benzodiazepine. Interpret the occurrence of the problem as a signal to use an alternative strategy in managing anxiety.

Other anxiolytics

Antagonists at β-adrenoceptors (**propranolol**) leave untouched the primary psychological symptoms of worry, tension and fear. They do reduce the somatic adrenergic symptoms of palpitations, sweating and tremor and the secondary psychological symptoms that arise from them.

The anxiolytic effect of *buspirone* shows a slow (2 week) onset. It does not substitute for benzodiazepines in their withdrawal syndrome.

Depressive illness

Symptoms of depressive illness

Anxiety symptoms

Worrying and/or nervous tension, hypochondriasis, headache and other tension pains, restlessness and/or agitation, panic attacks and phobias and/or obsessional symptoms.

Cognitive symptoms

Self-deprecation, loss of self-confidence, ideas of guilt and/or worthlessness, impaired concentration, loss of interest and inefficient thinking.

Mood changes

Depressed mood, hopelessness and suicidal ideas and/or plans.

Biological symptoms

Disturbed sleep pattern, loss of libido, loss of energy and/or fatigue, appetite/weight loss, diurnal variation of mood and psychomotor retardation.

Psychotic symptoms

Depressive delusions and depressive hallucinations.

Natural history of depressive illness

Depressive illness is common. It represents 3.5% of all male patients and 7.5% of all female ones presenting to general practitioners. In one-quarter it shows a rapid recovery, in half it fluctuates over a period of about 1 year and in the remaining quarter it becomes a chronic problem.

Treatment of depressive illness

A combination of treatments is aimed at changing the aetiological factors amenable to change.

Psychological

An opportunity to explore difficulties may be of more benefit than drugs in mild depression. Cognitive therapy. Help in dealing with the problems of social isolation, employment, money and children.

Physical

Physical forms of treatment are needed in moderate and severe depressive illness.
Drugs – tricyclic antidepressive and related drugs, 70% respond (35% respond to placebo); MAO inhibitors or, where depression is part of manic-depressive illness, lithium salts.
Electroconvulsive therapy (ECT).

Antidepressive drug selection

The biochemical basis of depression may be related to a functional loss of monoamines in the brain (page 212) or to disturbance of presynaptic receptor function. Early treatment used amphetamine-like agents for mild depression and electroconvulsive therapy for severe depression. Important developments in treatment stemmed from observations of mood elevation in patients receiving drugs for other illnesses:

(1) with the antitubercular drug **isoniazid,** which was shown to be due to inhibition of MAO. The dietary restrictions and adverse drug interactions of the MAO inhibitors (page 102) are disadvantages. **Phenelzine** is most used because of acute stimulant effects and least tendency amongst MAO inhibitors to cause serious adverse effects.
(2) with **imipramine** – a tricyclic compound – (on trial as an antipsychotic drug in schizophrenia), which was later shown to inhibit reuptake of NA (page 104) and 5-HT.

More selective reuptake blockers were developed (dothiepin, maprotiline, *lofepramine*) that selectively inhibit the uptake of NA. More recently drugs that have highly selective actions on the 5-HT uptake have been developed (*fluvoxamine, fluoxetine*).

Mianserin and *trazodone* have minimal effects on amine uptake and their mechanism of action is obscure. They may enhance NA release by blocking presynaptic α-receptors that inhibit NA release. They also block postsynaptic 5-HT receptors.

Selection is based on considerations of safety in use, adverse effects, length of experience and cost. More sedative drugs (**amitriptyline,** *mianserin*) are prescribed at night for the more agitated or anxious patient. Less sedative drugs (**imipramine**) are preferred for the withdrawn, apathetic patient.

Safety in overdosage is an important consideration given the hazard of a suicide attempt. Tricyclic antidepressive drugs are less safe than either *mianserin* or MAO inhibitors. Patients should be provided with only a small supply of the drug. A relative should be made aware of the dangers associated with the drug.

Adverse effects (*see below*) will deter the patient from taking the drug. Patient compliance can be improved by building up the dose over 1 week and informing the patient about side-effects. This is important because the onset of antidepressive effect is delayed for some 1–2 weeks after the start of treatment.

Suicidal tendencies necessitate admission to hospital because of the delay in therapeutic effect.

Imipramine is commonly used in severe depression but electroconvulsive therapy may occasionally be needed for a rapid effect. **Amitriptyline** is more sedative and is suitable if agitation or insomnia are problems. Recent pharmacokinetic studies have shown that once daily administration is adequate. The sedative effect is turned to advantage by taking the drug at night and dose-related antimuscarinic adverse effects (dry mouth, blurred vision) do not obtrude during sleep.

The selective reuptake blockers (*see above*) have fewer peripheral antimuscarinic adverse effects and are less likely to affect the cardiovascular system (page 224). They are useful in treating depression in patients suffering from heart disease. They are less sedative than nonselective reuptake blockers.

The selective 5-HT uptake blockers (*fluvoxamine, fluoxetine*) are the only antidepressive drugs that do not cause weight gain. They are especially effective in obsessional-compulsive disorder.

The atypical antidepressive drugs *mianserin* and *trazodone* are strongly sedative but safe because their lack of cardiotoxicity and anticholinergic effects.

Adverse effects and cautions with antidepressive drugs

Sedation (**amitriptyline,** *mianserin*) and respiratory depression in overdose.

Inhibition of neuronal NA uptake (tricyclic antidepressive drugs more than *mianserin*) leads to cardiotoxicity, dysrhythmias and conduction defects, which are especially dangerous after a recent myocardial infarction and in the elderly.

Antagonism at muscarinic cholinoceptors (tricyclic antidepressive drugs more than *mianserin*) produces dry mouth, impaired vision, constipation, difficulty of micturition, glaucoma and urinary retention. These effects are worst in the elderly.

Postural hypotension also occurs and there is a reduction in convulsive threshold. Blood dyscrasia occurs in about 1:10 000 with *mianserin*.

Life events on the prescribing of tricyclic antidepressive drugs

In pregnancy there is some danger of neonatal toxicity but too little is secreted in milk to be harmful to the breast-fed child. Dosage reduction is required in renal and liver impairment.

In elderly patients lower (halve) the dose. The prescribing problem is greater because: depressive illness is commoner, other disease is often present, heart disease is usually present, there is a greater susceptibility to side-effects and an interacting drug is likely to be in use.

Response to tricyclic antidepressive drugs and relatives

Improvement occurs early in insomnia and anxiety and after 10–14 days in other symptoms but can take up to 6 weeks.

If no improvement occurs (15% of patients) increase the dose or change to another form of physical treatment. In patients successfully treated, withdrawal of the drugs produces relapse in less than 6 months in 50%, while 50% remain symptom free. Maintenance therapy improves these figures to 20% and 80% respectively. Treatment should therefore be maintained for 4 months and then tailed off over 6 weeks.

Lithium carbonate

Severe depression (so-called 'unipolar' illness) may be one pole of the bipolar manic/depressive psychosis and recovery from depression may be followed by pathological elevation of mood with acute mania. Suppression of such swings of mood can be achieved with **lithium carbonate.** Its acute toxicity can be avoided by regular monitoring of blood concentrations and by the use of slow-release preparations.

Serum concentration should be 0.6–1.2 mEq/l at 12 h after dosage. Dosage adjustment is aided by further serum lithium concentration assays at 3–4 days, 1 week and then at 4 weekly intervals. At concentrations within the therapeutic window lithium:

(1) regulates the mood in mania;
(2) reduces the incidence and severity of recurrent bipolar or unipolar depressive illness. (So too do prophylactic antidepressive drugs but in bipolar disease they tend to accentuate the mania element.)

Toxicity of lithium salts

CNS – tremor, ataxia, dysarthria, nystagmus and convulsions. Kidney – impaired function. Toxicity is treated by withdrawal of lithium salts and administration of salt and water.

Schizophrenia

Psychosis is a qualitative abnormality of mental functions. It is recognized by the doctor, patient or the patient's social contacts as 'madness'. There is disordered thought and loss of contact with reality. A delusion is an unshakeable false belief regarding an objective thing. An illusion is a sensory misinterpretation giving rise to a false belief. A hallucination is an apparent perception of an absent external object.

First rank symptoms of schizophrenia

Thought insertion (experience of thoughts being put into one's mind). Thought broadcasting (experience of one's thoughts being known to others). Feelings of passivity (experience of emotions, or specific bodily movements or specific sensations being caused by an external agency or being under some external control). Voices discussing one's thoughts or behaviour, as they occur, sometimes forming a running commentary. Voices discussing or arguing about one, referring to 'he/she'. Voices repeating one's thoughts out loud or anticipating one's thoughts.

Primary delusions, 'primary' meaning arising inexplicably from perceptions that in themselves are normal (for example, the traffic lights change and this is taken to mean that a message is being conveyed by the colours to the patient).

Treatment of schizophrenia

Admission to hospital is often required, to protect both the patient and his/her family. Usually this is voluntary but compulsory admission is sometimes necessary. The role of antipsychotic drugs is to relieve the thought disorder, hallucinations and delusions (though the memory of these events is unaffected) and to prevent relapse.

Acute phase (first month). For the florid, acute, positive and disturbed patient a sedative antipsychotic drug is indicated (*Table 8.2*). For the withdrawn, negative and inactive patient a less sedative drug (low dose *sulpiride*) is better.

Table 8.2 Selection of antipsychotic drugs

	Sedation	Anti-cholinergic effects	Extra-pyramidal effects
Short-acting preparations			
Phenothiazines			
Group 1 (**chlorpromazine**)	+++	++	++
Group 2 (*thioridazine*)	++	+++	+
Group 3 (*trifluoperazine*)	+	+	+++
Butyrophenones (*haloperidol*)	++	+	+++(+)
Diphenylbutylpiperidines (*pimozide*)	+	+	+++
Sulpiride	−		
Long-acting depot preparations			
Thioxanthines (*flupenthixol decanoate*)	+	+	+++(+)
Phenothiazines (fluphenazine decanoate)	+	+	+++(+)
Butyrophenones (haloperidol decanoate)	++	+	++++

Medium term (1–3 months). Exert effort to avoid the rejection of the patient by his family, workmates and employer. Depot im antipsychotic drug (every 2 weeks at first, then monthly) can return patient behaviour nearly back to normal.

Long term. Continue with maintenance antipsychotic drug treatment. Rehabilitation involves finding the optimum balance between patient initiative and planned help. The patient will need to seek work less ambitious than he held down before the onset of illness.

Antipsychotic drug selection

On first administration of a depot formulation of antipsychotic drug it is wise to administer a test dose. The route is deep im injection and extrapyramidal reactions are usually present a few hours – 2 days after each dose.

Adverse effects of phenothiazines

Antagonists at muscarinic cholinoceptors – dry mouth, constipation, difficult micturition and blurred vision.

Antagonists at α-adrenoceptors – hypotension and tachycardia.

Antagonists at D_2 dopamine receptors –

(1) Parkinsonism (hypokinesia, rigidity, tremor) is dose-related and more common with the potent antipsychotic drugs (*haloperidol, pimozide*). Patients who need high doses and show these effects also require treatment with *procyclidine* or *benzhexol* (note peripheral antimuscarinic side-effects).

(2) Acute dystonic responses occur in the young on first exposure to the

drug and may be mistaken for tetanus. They require treatment with oral or iv anticholinergics (*procyclidine, benzhexol*).

(3) Akathisia is restlessness of the legs and may cause continuous pacing and an inability to sit still. Anticholinergics sometimes help.

(4) Tardive dyskinesia occurs in patients chronically taking antipsychotic drugs. It is of delayed onset (tardive) and may be irreversible. The disorder involves buccolingual masticatory movements and, less commonly, jerky and bizarre movements (dyskinesia) of the limbs, trunk or head and neck. The cause is not understood although proliferation of dopamine receptors following prolonged blockade (upregulation) has been suggested.

Tardive dyskinesia occurs after many months of treatment in 15–20% of patients (long duration of treatment, high dose and old age of patient seem to be risk factors). It is difficult to manage – the best policy seems to be gradual reduction of antipsychotic drug over 1–2 years, perhaps with drug holidays.

Temperature regulation is disturbed – hypothermia (occasionally pyrexia).

Sedatives – feeling uneasy, mental fatigue and lethargy.

Hypersensitivity – skin rashes, photosensitivity, jaundice (intrahepatic obstruction), agranulocytosis, aplastic anaemia. Purplish pigmentation skin, cornea, conjunctiva, retina, corneal and lens opacities.

Life events on the prescribing of antipsychotic drugs

Do not stop the drugs in pregnancy. Too little is secreted in milk to be harmful to the breast-fed child. Dosage reduction is required in renal and liver impairment.

In elderly patients lower the dose. Select drugs showing less sedation, extrapyramidal symptoms and hypothermia (for example Group 2 phenothiazines – *thioridazine*).

Prognosis

In patients successfully treated for a first attack of acute schizophrenia, withdrawal of the drugs produces relapse in 75%, while 25% remain symptom free. Maintenance therapy improves these figures to 33% and 67% respectively. Treatment should therefore be maintained for 4 months and then tailed off over 6 weeks.

Duration of treatment

Maintenance treatment is effective but associated with adverse effects. The danger of relapse (present over several weeks) with its social consequences make continuation a preferable strategy to withdrawal. Withdrawal should only occur with specialist approval, when the patient is in a stable social environment, when there have been no psychotic symptoms for 6 months and the patient has the insight to recognize early signs of relapse and respond by returning for resumption of therapy. Abrupt withdrawal produces a syndrome lasting a few weeks resembling cholinergic overactivity plus insomnia and dyskinesias. Dosage should instead be reduced over several months.

Epilepsy

The characteristic feature is a sudden and brief interruption of consciousness or 'seizure'. About one person in 50 will experience a seizure at sometime during his/her life and the prevalence of people who experience repeated seizures or who need drugs to prevent them is almost 1:100. Thus epilepsy is the commonest serious neurological disorder.

During the seizure there is a rapid and synchronous discharge from cerebral neurones. This can arise in the normal brain if the destabilizing stimulus (for example, hypocalcaemia or hypoglycaemia) is sufficient but in epilepsy either the threshold for starting a seizure is low throughout the brain or there is a locally damaged area from which the seizure starts.

Classification of seizures

Generalized seizures

The abnormal neuronal discharge involves the whole of the cerebrum. It is primary when it arises simultaneously in all parts.

(1) Generalized tonic/clonic (grand mal): consciousness is lost suddenly and all skeletal muscle contracts, first continuously (tonic) and then rhythmically (clonic). Falls and injury are common. Recovery is slow and often requires sleep.
(2) Myoclonic jerks are brief muscle contractions without loss of consciousness.
(3) Absences (petit mal): the patient (usually a child) is vacant for a few seconds whilst the electroencephalogram (EEG) shows a generalized 3 Hz spike and wave discharge. There may be flickering eye movements but the patient does not fall and recovers instantly.

Partial seizures

Only a part of the cerebrum is involved but consciousness can be lost (complex).

(1) Simple: depending on the part affected these may be autonomic (skin pallor, piloerection), sensory (abnormal smell or sound; tingling or 'swelling'), motor (twitching of face or limb) or psychic (*deja vu* or fear).
(2) Complex (temporal lobe): stereotyped movements often involving

hands or mouth. There may be fumbling with clothing or objects. The patient may wander into danger or do familiar tasks without purpose or recall (automatism).

The seizure may start simple ('warning') and become complex. A motor seizure may spread from hand or face to the whole of one side (Jacksonian progression). Similarly any partial seizure may progress to tonic/clonic (secondary generalization). Conversely drug treatment that suppresses tonic/clonic events may reveal previously unrecognized partial seizures.

Serial seizures

A series of seizures can arise particularly if administration of CNS depressant drugs (antiepileptics, alcohol) is suddenly stopped. Status epilepticus arises when consciousness is not recovered between seizures. Convulsive status can cause lasting brain damage if not treated promptly.

Causes of epilepsy

Every pathology that affects the brain (vascular malformation, abscess, injury including surgery, tumour, haemorrhage, ischaemia or infarction) can be manifest as partial and secondary generalized epilepsy. Primary generalized epilepsy can have a genetic basis; for example, juvenile myoclonic epilepsy is associated with an abnormality in the HLA region of chromosome 6.

Precipitating factors

In a predisposed person, a seizure can be precipitated by a variety of stimuli (drug withdrawal, excitement, fever, flashing lights – photoconvulsive epilepsy, over-breathing, sleep lack). It is not uncommon however for a seizure to occur without any obvious precipitant.

Epileptiform activity in the EEG is accentuated during sleep and by iv drugs used for anaesthesia. Antidepressive, corticosteroid and antipsychotic drugs can increase the likelihood of seizures when used at conventional doses in predisposed patients. Salicylates cause seizures when taken in overdose.

Seizures can occur when organ failure (kidney or liver) causes serious metabolic disturbance and when disease states (eclampsia, severe hypertension) cause cerebral oedema.

Electrophysiology

Hughlings Jackson (born 1835) defined a seizure as 'a sudden, excessive, rapid and local discharge in the grey matter of the brain'.

Multispike discharges can be observed in the surface EEG of some patients and with intracranial electrodes the origin can be traced to a particular area, often the anteromedial part of one temporal lobe. Surgical removal of that area is sometimes practicable and curative. Histology has revealed a deficiency of GABAergic neurones and neurophysiological studies on slices give some insight into the nature and properties of the epileptic focus. It is possible that future treatments will include the implantation of fetal neuroblasts that will develop into inhibitory neurones. Experimental epileptic foci in animals can be induced with aluminium chloride and used to study the effects of excitatory amino acids (aspartate and glutamate) that act at the *N*-methyl-D-aspartate (NMDA) receptor, and inhibitory agents, that act at the GABA receptor complex.

The focus probably generates continuous abnormal discharges but for a clinical (partial) seizure the amount of normal grey matter around the focus that becomes excited must exceed a 'critical mass'. Precipitating factors may act by reducing, and antiepileptic drugs by increasing, the threshold for excitation of this surrounding tissue. The antiepileptic drugs do not extinguish the focus.

Antiepileptic drugs

The most widely used are **carbamazepine, sodium valproate** and **phenytoin**; comparative trials show equal efficacy against generalized tonic/clonic and complex partial seizures. *Phenobarbitone* and *primidone* (active metabolites include phenobarbitone) are more sedative at equieffective doses and use in the developed world has therefore waned. Only *ethosuximide* and **sodium valproate** prevent absence seizures.

There was a gap of 15 years from **sodium valproate** (1975) to the introduction of the next major antiepileptic drug (*vigabatrin*) but it is likely that several other new drugs will get product licences in the next few years.

Carbamazepine is chemically related to tricyclic antidepressives. It is effective against tonic/clonic and partial seizures but patients with absence or myoclonic seizures are not helped. It may be of particular help in patients with psychotic features complicating epilepsy. Dose related adverse effects include double vision and unsteadiness. The drug induces hepatic MFO, thereby shortening its own $t_{\frac{1}{2}}$ and interacting with other drugs as described under 'Adverse drug interactions' (page 41). Inappropriate ADH secretion shows itself as hyponatraemia; recurrent cough or sore throat suggests white cell suppression (leucopenia); an allergic skin rash is produced in about 5% of patients but despite these problems **carbamazepine** is now the most popular antiepileptic drug in the UK. It is generally well tolerated and has less adverse effect on mental concentration and memory than **phenytoin.**

Sodium valproate is effective against primary generalized seizures including absences and myoclonic jerks; it is the drug of choice in juvenile myoclonic epilepsy. Adverse effects include weight gain, hair loss and tremor but they are generally mild. Nausea and heartburn have been overcome by enteric coating of the tablets (page 308). A biochemical abnormality may underlie the rare but life-threatening liver toxicity that is almost confined to handicapped children aged below 3 years. In contrast to **carbamazepine** and **phenytoin, sodium valproate** does not induce, but rather inhibits, MFO and tends to raise the plasma concentrations of other antiepileptic drugs.

Phenytoin, once the most popular of these drugs, is now less used. It is no less effective than **carbamazepine** against tonic/clonic and partial seizures but adverse effects and awkward pharmacokinetic properties (page 354) discourage its use. Gum overgrowth, acne and increased facial hair can be disfiguring and memory and mental acuity can be impaired; headache, double vision, slurred speech and unsteadiness are symptoms of excessive plasma concentration and can be corrected without loss of effectiveness by dosage adjustment that follows the pharmacokinetic principles described earlier. Excessive concentrations are sometimes caused not by increase in dose but by concurrent treatment with a drug that inhibits MFO (for example, **cimetidine**).

Vigabatrin is a close structural analogue of GABA that produces selective, irreversible inhibition of the aminotransferase that inactivates GABA. In combination with one of the established drugs it can further reduce the frequency of partial and generalized tonic/clonic seizures. Adverse effects include drowsiness, dizziness, confusion and even psychosis in predisposed patients. There is no evidence in human tissue post mortem of the intramyelinic oedema observed in the white matter of rat and dog brain. If current clinical trials confirm the efficacy of single drug treatment with *vigabatrin* and postmarketing surveillance (page 51) detects no long-term neurotoxicity, it is likely to be used in the treatment of newly diagnosed epilepsy. Its use in pregnancy is not at present authorized.

Ethosuximide is used primarily for the treatment of absence seizures particularly in early childhood, where the risk of hepatotoxicity with **sodium valproate** is greatest. Adverse effects include nausea, vomiting, tiredness and unsteadiness. They can usually be prevented by dosage reduction.

Benzodiazepines suppress myoclonic jerks, partial seizures and generalized tonic/clonic seizures. Entry into brain is rapid with immediate onset of antiepileptic action but effectiveness wanes with continued use (tolerance: page 251). CNS depression is manifest as drowsiness and lack of concentration but seldom as depression of respiration. These properties make benzodiazepines very suitable for emergency use and for intermittent use. A series of tonic/clonic seizures can often be stopped by **diazepam** as rectal solution; this acts more quickly than tablet or suppository and can be given by relatives or carers not able to give iv injections. For intermittent use, the 1-5 benzodiazepine, *clobazam* is preferred to the other more sedative (1-4) members of the group (for example, *clonazepam*). It may be taken orally by the patient to prevent seizures during a special social occasion, over a high risk time (the week before the menstrual period) or whilst experiencing a cluster of partial seizures. Once the special indication has passed the drug is stopped and held in reserve until the next time.

Paraldehyde is a cyclic trimer of acetaldehyde. It is used in solution as an alternative to rectal **diazepam.** Unlike **diazepam** it is also effective by im injection. It becomes oxidized if stored too long, is incompatible with plastic syringes on more than brief contact and gives an unpleasant smell to the expired air. Despite these drawbacks it is safe and effective.

Acetazolamide may raise the threshold to seizures by reducing salt and water retention (for example, premenstrually) and by raising brain PCO_2. Tolerance develops within a few weeks making the drug more suited to intermittent treatment.

Development of new drugs

There is need for more effective drugs with less toxicity. Antiepileptic activity is demonstrated by prevention of experimental (electrical or drug-induced) seizures in animals and freedom from short-term adverse effects is demonstrated in healthy volunteers. Therapeutic efficacy can, however, only be established in patients with epilepsy. It would not be ethical to expose new patients to an unproven agent nor to alter treatment when an established drug had given complete control of seizures. Early clinical trials must therefore rely on volunteers from that small proportion of patients whose epilepsy responds poorly to established drugs. This gives an inevitable bias against the new drug.

Management of epilepsy

The history from the patient and a description of the supposed epileptic events from an observer will often give the diagnosis. Cardiovascular causes for syncope must be excluded and the search for an underlying cause pursued.

With drug treatment 70–80% of newly diagnosed patients will become free from seizures. If only one seizure has occurred and there was a clear precipitant (for example, severe sleep deprivation), it may be proper to give no drug but the likelihood of chronic epilepsy is increased in proportion to the number of seizures experienced before drug treatment is started.

Choice of drug

Since **carbamazepine, sodium valproate** and **phenytoin** are broadly equieffective the choice is often based on the relevance to the individual patient of the common adverse effects described earlier. With any of the drugs, drowsiness, dizziness and lack of concentration are often experienced at the start of treatment but these fade as tolerance develops; the drug is therefore best started at a low dose, which is increased slowly according to the clinical response.

A diary of epileptic events kept by the patient or relatives is essential. Benefit means fewer seizures per month, reduced duration or severity of seizures (less secondary generalization) or an increase in seizure-free days. This is weighed against cost in adverse effects; the aim is not freedom from seizures at any price but preservation of function with maximum realization of individual potential.

Guided by the response and by the plasma drug concentration, the daily dose is adjusted until the optimum for the individual is found. In this process the recommended ranges (*Table 8.3*) are interpreted flexibly. Big variation in concentration without change in dose indicates poor compliance. This should be discussed with the patient who may be troubled by adverse effects or simply forgetful. Reduction of dose or simplification of treatment may give more consistent concentrations.

Table 8.3 Recommended antiepileptic drug concentration

Drug	mg/l
Carbamazepine	6–12
Sodium valproate	50–100
Phenytoin	10–20
Ethosuximide	40–100
Phenobarbitone	10–30

Pharmacokinetic factors

All the antiepileptic drugs listed above remain effective when given as two spaced doses per day. The necessary persistence of effect is based on slow decay of plasma drug concentration (**phenytoin,** *phenobarbitone*), active metabolites (carbamazepine epoxide, *N*-desmethyl clobazam) and long-lasting inhibition of enzymes (carbonic anhydrase, GABA aminotransferase). This removes the need to take medicines to school or work for a mid-day dose. Young children have a shorter $t_\frac{1}{2}$ and may sometimes need three spaced doses each day.

The saturable nature of **phenytoin** metabolism demands small dosage increments when approaching the recommended concentration range. Failure to appreciate this can cause the concentration to overshoot into the toxic range.

Drug combinations

Treatment with one drug alone is the ideal. If the first drug does not work well, a second is introduced and the dose built up until it is safe to withdraw the first; the response to the second drug in isolation is then assessed. When strict monotherapy fails, a satisfactory result may still be obtained by adding a second drug (*clobazam* or less commonly *acetazolamide*) on an intermittent basis as described for benzodiazepines above. In more severe cases with multiple kinds of seizure, combinations of two or even three major antiepileptic drugs are sometimes unavoidable.

Drug withdrawal

When a patient on drug treatment has been free from epileptic events for 2 years it is right to question whether the drug is still needed. One option is to withdraw the drug by small reductions in dosage at intervals of 1 month or more to avoid precipitating withdrawal seizures. In the case of **phenytoin,** the early reductions must correspond with the smallest available dosage form (25 mg capsule). The patient has another option however; he is now eligible to hold a UK driving licence, but if he selects this option, no reduction in dosage is permissible so long as he continues to drive.

Pregnancy

Congenital malformations have been reported in association with each of the major drugs and none can be considered entirely safe; on the other hand poor seizure control can also harm the fetus. The best compromise is probably to adjust treatment to a moderate dose of a single drug before conception occurs. The aetiology of congenital malformations is multifactorial (page 35), thus avoidance of alcohol and smoking, provision of a balanced diet and prevention of folate deficiency are all relevant. Neural tube defects should be excluded before the pregnancy is too far advanced for termination.

In mid and late pregnancy it is often necessary to increase daily dosage to offset the tendency for increased liver metabolism to lower the plasma drug concentration. Allowance must however be made for the reduction in plasma albumin concentration, which increases the proportion of drug in the free state. After delivery, antiepileptic drug therapy does not prevent breast feeding except when high concentrations of *phenobarbitone* are present. It is necessary, however, to reduce dosage gradually to the prepregnant rate as liver metabolism returns to normal.

Drugs and fertility

Choice of family planning method

Reasons for family planning include the desire to:

(1) temporarily prevent pregnancy;
(2) increase the interval between births;
(3) permanently prevent pregnancy when the required family size is achieved.

Decision on whether to use family planning and which method is influenced by the above and:

(1) political, cultural and religious background, including whether family planning is accepted as a male or female prerogative;
(2) efficacy (*Table 8.4*) – less efficient methods may become acceptable as fertility declines with age;
(3) acceptability;
(4) availability;
(5) cost.

Family planning has had a major influence on individual families but none on the populations of countries unless accompanied by socioeconomic development.

Contraception

'Natural' methods

Lactational amenorrhoea

During lactation, suckling reflexly induces prolactin secretion, which acts upon the ovary to inhibit follicular development. Consequently, the first ovulation post partum is delayed (by about 30 weeks) and subsequent ovulations are less frequent. Therefore, the interbirth interval is on average increased. This method has a major influence on family size in developing countries. Its reliability for individual women is unpredictable.

Withdrawal

Coitus interruptus describes withdrawal of the penis from the vagina before ejaculation. This method is widely used but of doubtful reliability.

Rhythm methods

The knowledge that ovulation occurs about 14 days before the next menstrual period and that sperm can survive up to 3 days and ova 1 day in the female reproductive tract allows prediction of 'safe' times for intercourse. The time of ovulation may be calculated from the date of onset of the last menstrual period or identified by keeping a daily early morning temperature record, as body temperature rises following ovulation. Alternatively the cervical mucus can be sampled; the mucus changes from a watery consistency to thick and extendable at ovulation. A disadvantage of these methods is the difficulty in predicting the time of ovulation with any accuracy. Domestic urinary hormone assay methods can detect the surge of LH 24–36 h before ovulation.

Mechanical methods

Condom

This method is widely used and with correct use family size, on average, may be reduced to 2–3 children. The 'method' failure rate is low but the 'user' failure rate is higher. There are no adverse effects and no medical involvement. Condoms may be impregnated with spermicide and may also offer protection from sexually transmitted diseases.

Diaphragm and cap

These block the entry of sperm into the cervix. Supplementation with spermicidal preparations makes them moderately effective. There are no adverse effects and, following a preliminary training session, no medical involvement. These methods were widely used until oral contraceptives and intrauterine devices (IUDs) became available.

Intrauterine devices

With an IUD (a plastic loop or coil) in place the blastocyst probably still develops but implantation does not occur. The exact mechanism of action is unknown. It does not prevent ectopic pregnancies. An IUD is also effective if inserted within 72 h postcoitally. Once fitted it usually remains in the uterus for several years. Occasional problems are expulsion, perforation, prolonged uterine bleeding and pelvic inflammatory disease. The efficacy is slightly improved and adverse effects reduced if copper wire is wound around the IUD; the mechanism of action of the copper is unknown. Generally undesirable for nulliparous women, it is an effective safe method in older women.

Chemical methods

Spermicides

Spermicides lower surface tension and so kill sperm by destroying their cell membranes. They are formulated as creams, gels, foams and pessaries and are not very effective by themselves. Sponges are impregnated with spermicide and absorb sperm but do not present a barrier; their efficacy is still being evaluated. They are active for up to 24 h, unlike unsupported spermicides, which lose activity after 2–4 h *in situ*. Evidence suggests that spermicides will kill the biological vectors of sexually transmitted diseases including the AIDS virus.

Hormonal methods

For mechanisms of action *see* page 167.

Combined oral contraceptive tablets. This is the most popular systemic contraceptive, widely used in developed countries. It has a negligible failure rate; any reported failures are likely to be due to missed tablets.

Epidemiological studies suggest caution in their use in women over 35 or in heavy smokers and obese women due to a higher incidence of cardiovascular disease compared with nonusers.

Progestogen-only contraception. This may be achieved by depot injection or tablets. Depot injection of *medroxyprogesterone acetate* lasts 3–6 months. Regular injection causes disturbance and eventually absence of menstrual cycles and a delay in the return to fertility on cessation. Consequently it is a very effective contraceptive. The method is popular in developing countries, especially as it does not affect lactation and rigid compliance is not required. In developed countries it is mainly used after rubella vaccination or before vasectomy becomes effective. An association with breast tumours has been claimed.

Tablets of a 19-nortestosterone derivative. **Norethisterone** is administered continuously. The efficacy is lower than that of the combined oral contraceptive. It is useful in women during breast feeding or where the combined oral contraceptive tablet is contraindicated due to high cardiovascular risk (older patients). Compliance is important, efficacy is lost even if the tablet is taken 3 h late.

High dose combined oral contraceptives. These are effective postcoitally if given within 72 h of intercourse but are not recommended for routine use. Two tablets containing the maximum oestrogen dose (50 μg) are given, followed by another two 12 h later. Contraception is achieved by effects upon the Fallopian tube, endometrium and ovary. Considerable nausea and vomiting occurs at this oestrogen dose. The long-term use of oestrogens is associated with cardiovascular disease therefore this method should serve only as an occasional measure.

Surgical methods

These methods are sought by 20–30% of couples after completion of their families. They are essentially permanent.

Vasectomy

The vas deferens is divided and the ends occluded. This is minor surgery usually done as an outpatient procedure under local anaesthesia. Sperm continue to be produced in the testis but do not reach the ejaculate. Fertility may be restored in a small proportion of cases using microsurgery.

Table 8.4 Approximate failure rates of contraceptive methods

Method	Pregnancy rate per 100 woman years*
Oviductal occlusion	About 0.02
Vasectomy	About 0.02
Combined oral contraceptive tablets	0.03–0.10
Progestogen-only depot injection	About 0.5
Progestogen-only contraceptive tablets	1.5–3.0
Intrauterine device	1.5–3.0
Lactational amenorrhoea	3–5
Condom	4–28
Diaphragm	4–35
Spermicides	4–38
Rhythm	8–40
No contraception	About 80

* 100 women treated for 1 year

Oviductal occlusion

Access to the oviducts may be gained by abdominal, transvaginal or transcervical routes. They are either tied or sealed by cautery, clips or bands.

Usually it is performed as an inpatient procedure. Very occasional recanalizations and subsequent pregnancies occur. The operation is expensive in medical resources.

Abortion

The distinction between a method of contraception (requiring precoital action) and a method of abortion (requiring postcoital action) is not always clear (pages 168 and 422).

It is estimated there are 125 million live births, 40 million spontaneous abortions and 30 million induced abortions annually in the world. In some countries abortion on demand is available as a contraceptive measure. The hazards of abortion increase with gestational and maternal age.

Surgical methods

Vacuum aspiration

Up to about 4 weeks' gestation it is possible to remove the uterine contents by suction with a syringe using a plastic cannula. At this time it will not be certain that the woman is pregnant. After 6 weeks' gestation cervical dilatation is usually required first. These are outpatient procedures.

Dilatation and curettage

Following cervical dilatation, uterine contents can be removed by scraping (curettage) and suction. This method is used from about 9 to 12 weeks' gestation. There is evidence that forced cervical dilatation is followed by a higher subsequent spontaneous miscarriage rate, so cervical softening should be produced first by local application of *dinoprostone* (PGE_2).

Chemical injection methods

Chemical methods are used in the second trimester (about 13–26 weeks' gestation). Extra-amniotic injection of *dinoprostone* is used to induce abortion. It probably acts by a combination of a direct contractile action on the myometrium and a reduction in the placental endocrine support of pregnancy. Vomiting and diarrhoea are frequent adverse effects.

Haematinic drugs and the cellular elements of blood

Anaemia

Anaemia (lit. 'lack of blood') means deficiency of haemoglobin. It usually has an insidious onset and is asymptomatic. If very severe or of a more rapid onset the anaemic patient may have some of the following symptoms: listlessness, tiring easily, palpitations, muscle aches and pains, 'blackouts'; angina pectoris, intermittent claudication, breathlessness on exertion (high output cardiac failure).

The major clinical feature is pallor, better sought in the mucous membranes rather than skin. This feature is unreliable, however, as it correlates poorly with blood haemoglobin content. Definitive recognition requires measurement of blood haemoglobin content (normally 14 g/dl men; 12 g/dl women). The haemoglobin content and red cell (erythrocyte) count of blood are closely linked.

There are two general ways in which erythrocytes are reduced in number. Formation may be impaired or destruction accelerated.

Impaired formation of erythrocytes arises from defects of:

(1) haemoglobin synthesis – the functional erythrocyte mass is selectively reduced in iron deficiency anaemia;
(2) DNA synthesis – erythrocytes, granulocytes and platelets are all affected in megaloblastic anaemias (large peripheral blood cell parent cells in the bone marrow);
(3) cell synthesis – all three cellular elements are again deficient in aplastic anaemia.

Accelerated destruction or loss of erythrocytes arises from:

(1) chronic blood loss, which leads to iron deficiency anaemia;
(2) haemolysis, which leads to a macrocytic anaemia (abnormally large erythrocytes in the peripheral blood).

Drugs used to correct these disorders are known as haematinics.

Iron deficiency anaemia

Normal iron balance

Dietary iron (present in most foods) is absorbed best in the first part of the small intestine – proximal duodenum. Since no excretion mechanism exists, the efficiency of absorption is modulated to maintain iron balance; absorption falls when stores are full and rises in iron deficiency.

Transferrin is the serum iron transport protein and is measured as 'total iron binding capacity'. It is synthesized in the liver at a rate inversely proportional to the state of the iron stores. Ferritin is the normal storage form of iron in gut mucosa, liver, spleen and bone marrow.

Figure 8.2 shows the pools of iron and their turnover. Iron is essential for haem synthesis.

Causes

It is essential to find an underlying cause as specific therapy is curative.

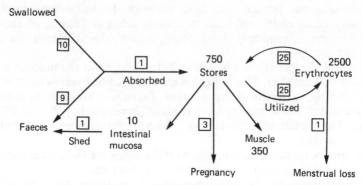

Figure 8.2 The amount of iron (in mg) in key locations and the average daily movements (boxed figures, in mg)

(1) Inadequate intake:
   (a) absolute – old poor living alone, infants over 6 months of age fed exclusively on milk;
   (b) relative to a high need – pregnant women, premature or twin babies and infants delivered by Caesarean section.
(2) Inadequate absorption – gastrointestinal surgery, malabsorption syndrome.
(3) Excessive loss – apparent or occult bleeding:
   (a) gastropathy from irritant drugs:
       NSAIDs (10–15% of patients with rheumatoid arthritis on 900 mg of **aspirin** four times daily lose more than 10 ml a day from gastric erosions); ethanol;
   (b) peptic ulceration;
   (c) gastrointestinal neoplasm;
   (d) heavy menstrual bleeding.

Clinical features

Iron deficiency produces anaemia, inflamed corners of mouth, smooth shiny tongue (sore when eating) and longitudinally ridged, flat (even concave) nails.

Tests

The blood film shows hypochromic, microcytic cells that vary in size and shape. Evidence is sought for depletion of iron stores (serum ferritin concentration is low, bone marrow cellular iron is absent and serum total iron binding capacity is increased) and for lack of iron immediately available for haemoglobin synthesis (serum iron concentration and total iron binding capacity saturation is low).

Treatment

The cause, the iron deficiency and the anaemia may need treatment.

Oral iron

Ferrous sulphate dried 200 mg supplies 60 mg of iron.
Ferrous fumarate 200 mg supplies 65 mg of iron.
Ferrous glycine sulphate 225 mg supplies 40 mg of iron.

About 10% of swallowed iron is absorbed from a normal diet. This
increases in iron deficiency to about 25%. Swallowing more iron increases
the amount but reduces the percentage of the dose absorbed. An erythrocyte has a life span of about 100 days, so the 1% replaced each day needs 25
mg of iron. In severe deficiency at least 100 mg of iron must be swallowed
daily for about 5 months for restitution of haemoglobin and stores.

Gastrointestinal adverse effects of the therapeutic dose are common:
nausea and epigastric pain are dose-related, diarrhoea and constipation are
less so. If they are troublesome the following manoeuvres may alleviate
them and aid continued compliance: take the dose after a meal, try other
salts and add ascorbic acid, which increases absorption.

Parenteral iron

The indications for parenteral iron are noncompliance or malabsorption.
Iron dextran or *iron sorbitol*, by deep im injection, may cause pain and local
staining and a significant incidence of hypersensitivity reactions (higher and
more severe with the iv route – *iron dextran* only). Guard against severe
reactions by a test dose experiment.

Response to treatment

A brisk reticulocytosis (appearance of newly formed erythrocytes in the
peripheral blood) occurs within 1 week. Haemoglobin should then rise by
about 0.15 g/dl daily. Failure to respond suggests a wrong diagnosis, continuing blood loss or that the prescribed iron is not being taken.

Prophylaxis

The high requirement for iron in pregnancy is commonly met by the prescription of 100 mg daily of oral iron as a salt.

Vitamin B_{12} deficiency megaloblastic anaemia

Normal vitamin B_{12} balance

Dietary (meat, eggs, milk) vitamin B_{12} combines with a glycoprotein, intrinsic factor, secreted into the lumen by the parietal cells of the gastric
mucosa. It is absorbed by a carrier-mediated process in the terminal ileum.
Sufficient stores are maintained in the liver for about 3 years' supply of the
daily requirement of about 3 μg.

Vitamin B_{12} is essential for the conversion of methylmalonate to succinate. When the former accumulates, abnormal fatty acids are formed and
incorporated into neuronal cell membranes. Vitamin B_{12} is also essential for
the formation of tetrahydrofolate from the stored form, methyl-tetrahydro-
folate. Therefore deficiency of vitamin B_{12} resembles that of folate in so far

as both cause megaloblastic anaemia. However, it is essential to distinguish between them as an attempt to treat vitamin B_{12} deficiency with folate could result in the neurological defect being precipitated or aggravated and it may become irreversible.

Causes

(1) Low intake occurs rarely – vegans.
(2) Impaired absorption:
    (a) cessation of intrinsic factor secretion occurs with gastrectomy and in pernicious anaemia, an autoimmune gastritis, which typically begins at over 40 years of age and has an annual incidence of 9 per 10^5. Other gastric mucosal secretory functions are also lost – achlorhydria.
    (b) damage to, or bypass of, the terminal ileum – ileal surgery, fistula, inflammatory disease or stasis in a blind loop.

Clinical features

Vitamin B_{12} deficiency produces anaemia, sore mouth and tongue, sterility and neuropathy and spinal cord degeneration.

Tests

The blood film shows large oval erythrocytes, hypersegmented nuclei in polymorphonuclear leucocytes and large platelets. The bone marrow shows large stem cells of these three peripheral blood cells. There is a high unconjugated bilirubin (due to shortened cell life) and low vitamin B_{12} concentration in serum. Absorption without and with addition of hog intrinsic factor can be assessed using ^{57}Co-labelled cyanocobalamin.

Treatment

Hydroxocobalamin is the form of vitamin B_{12} with the best retention characteristics after injection. The dose is 1 mg im five times over 2 weeks to replenish stores; about 30% is retained. In patients with impaired absorption (*see* Causes above) treatment will need to be life-long; 1 mg every 3 months is adequate. Potassium salt supplements may be needed at first as new cell formation occurs so fast.

Response to treatment

The bone marrow becomes normal in 2 days. Reticulocytosis is obvious within 1 week and there is complete correction of the anaemia within 2 months.

Folic acid deficiency megaloblastic anaemia

Normal folate balance

Dietary folate complexes (yeast, liver, green vegetables) are hydrolysed to folic acid in the brush border of the mucosa of the proximal jejunum and then absorbed there. Stores are limited; most body folate is in metabolic use. Folate is needed for the production of an essential cofactor in the biosynthetic processes involving single carbon units that occur in purine and deoxythymidylate synthesis – both essential to DNA synthesis.

Causes

(1) Inadequate intake – commonest (alcoholic, food fadist, psychotic, mentally defective, old poor living alone).
(2) Increased utilization combined with poor diet. This occurs during pregnancy (incidence 1:200) particularly in the last trimester.
(3) Malabsorption – rare (gluten-sensitive enteropathy).
(4) Drugs:
   (a) anticonvulsants (**phenytoin,** *phenobarbitone, primidone*) interfere with absorption;
   (b) **methotrexate** (folinic acid is needed to overcome inhibition), pyrimethamine, *proguanil* and **trimethoprim** interfere with utilization.

Clinical features

Folate deficiency shows similar clinical features and blood picture to that of vitamin B_{12} except there is no neurological disturbance. It must be distinguished by history and tests from vitamin B_{12} deficiency as an attempt to treat vitamin B_{12} deficiency with folate can precipitate the neuropathy.

Tests

There is a low erythrocyte folate concentration.

Treatment

Folic acid 5 mg daily by mouth for 4 months.

Prophylaxis

In pregnancy routine prophylaxis employs iron and folic acid tablets that contain 100 mg and 350 µg respectively.

Transfusion – iron overload

If any anaemia needs correction more urgently than can be achieved with haematinics, packed red cells may be slowly transfused. The danger is of circulatory overload and precipitation of cardiac failure.

If many transfusions are needed in treating any anaemia, surplus Fe^{2+} (iron overload) can be chelated with **desferrioxamine.**

Drugs in joint disease

Arthritis

Arthritis is a term used to describe joint inflammation, which occurs in a variety of diseases. The anti-inflammatory analgesic drugs are of value principally for symptomatic relief.

Infective arthritis is uncommon but very important to recognize, requiring prompt treatment with appropriate antibacterial drugs.

Rheumatism is an ill-defined term covering a variety of painful musculoskeletal disorders, both nonarticular and articular.

Rheumatic fever is an inflammatory disease of autoimmune origin, which can follow a pharyngeal infection with group A β-haemolytic streptococci. The heart, joints, skin and CNS can be involved. Bed-rest, **aspirin** and a penicillin (for both eradication of the throat infection and prophylaxis against further episodes) are the mainstays of treatment.

The commonest forms of arthritis are osteoarthritis and rheumatoid arthritis.

Osteoarthritis (sometimes referred to as osteoarthrosis) is generally regarded as a degenerative disease due to wear and tear, although there can be a secondary inflammatory component. It can be either primary (idiopathic) or secondary (occurring as a late result of a number of joint problems, e.g. injury). It particularly affects those over the age of 50 years in their weight bearing joints (spine, hip, knee). Movement may be limited with loss of function. Pain is variable. Weight loss, physiotherapy and local measures (for example, collar, walking stick) are often helpful. The simple analgesic **paracetamol** may relieve pain and only if this is inadequately effective should an NSAID (*ibuprofen*) be additionally prescribed.

Rheumatoid arthritis has a higher incidence in women than men (ratio 3:1) with a usual age of onset 35–60 years. The cause of the disease is unknown but it is associated with the production of abnormal antibodies. In the classic form of the disease joint involvement is symmetrical, with early involvement of the small joints of the hand. Morning stiffness is a common complaint. The disease has a remitting course with acute exacerbations followed by quiescent periods. In severe cases deformity occurs and all joints can be affected.

Treatment of rheumatoid arthritis

General therapeutic measures are:

(1) rest affected joints, with splinting, during acute exacerbations;

(2) physiotherapy;
(3) occupational therapy;
(4) patient education and encouragement to come to terms with a disease likely to be chronic.

NSAID group

This group of agents (**aspirin,** *ibuprofen, indomethacin, naproxen*) exerts its therapeutic effects by inhibiting cyclo-oxygenase activity, and thereby PG synthesis and the inflammatory response, in a variety of tissues (page 206). They are the first line of treatment in rheumatoid arthritis. Symptomatic relief can be obtained from any of these drugs, and by adjusting the dose almost the same effect can be obtained from each, although the response to each varies between individuals. The toxicity, as well as the beneficial effect, is dose related and determines the biggest dose of an individual drug that can be used. Most adverse effects are probably related to PG depletion and include gastric mucosal damage (erosions, ulcers, gastrointestinal bleeding – the acidic nature of the drug contributes), decreased platelet aggregation, salt and water retention, nephrotoxicity, asthma (diversion of PG-substrate to LT synthesis may contribute).

A large number of NSAIDs is now available but all share similar adverse effects. Suppository preparations may be useful in minimizing gastrointestinal side-effects.

Disease-suppressing or second-line drugs

These drugs modify disease activity in rheumatoid arthritis and are used in progressive disease not controlled by NSAIDs. Their mechanisms of action are poorly understood. Onset of action is slow and a beneficial effect of treatment may not be apparent for several months. The patient should continue on NSAID treatment in addition to disease-suppressing therapy as long as symptoms are troublesome. All disease-suppressing agents have potentially serious adverse effects.

(1) *Penicillamine* (page 208) can cause renal and bone marrow toxicity (leucopenia, thrombocytopenia, occasionally aplastic anaemia), rashes and other adverse effects. The blood haemoglobin concentration, white cell and platelet counts and urine (presence of protein and blood) must be monitored throughout treatment. The maintenance dose should be as low as is compatible with control of disease activity.
(2) Gold compounds (page 208) are usually administered by deep im injection (*sodium aurothiomalate*) but an oral preparation (*auranofin*) is available. Adverse effects on the kidney, bone marrow and skin occur, and a full blood count and urinalysis must be performed before each gold injection or monthly with oral treatment.
(3) *Chloroquine* (page 208) can cause retinal damage and regular (3–6 monthly) ophthalmic monitoring is essential.
(4) *Sulphasalazine* is often associated with gastrointestinal side-effects, malaise and headache. Serious adverse effects are unusual, although leucopenia and hepatotoxicity can occur. Patients should discontinue use of soft contact lenses as these may be discoloured.

(5) Immunosuppressant drugs (*azathioprine*, **cyclophosphamide, metho-trexate**) may be indicated in patients with severe, aggressive articular disease who have not responded to, or who do not tolerate, other disease-suppressing treatment, or in patients with life-threatening systemic disease. Adverse effects (page 299) are frequent and serious.

(6) Glucocorticoids (page 207). Although very effective in reducing inflammation and providing symptomatic relief, systemic glucocorticoids should be avoided if possible because of the adverse effects (page 180) associated with the long-term use of the doses needed to suppress symptoms. Exacerbation of symptoms on withdrawal makes dosage reduction difficult. Nevertheless patients with severe systemic disease may require high dose systemic glucocorticoids. Intra-articular injection of a glucocorticoid is useful in suppressing inflammation in a severely affected joint provided there is no infection.

Surgery may be indicated to relieve pain or improve function.

Gout

Gout is a disease featuring recurrent attacks of acute arthritis, which is at first usually monoarticular, typically affecting the metatarsophalangeal joint of the big toe, although several joints may be involved. It is a disorder of purine metabolism characterized by a raised blood urate concentration (more than 0.4 mmol/l). Either overproduction or underexcretion of uric acid (or a combination of both) may be responsible. Gout may result from:

(1) hereditary predisposition;
(2) drugs (some diuretics, low dose salicylate, lactate accumulation due to ethanol);
(3) excessive cell breakdown (for example, myeloproliferative and lymphoproliferative disorders);
(4) renal failure;
(5) ketoacidosis and starvation.

The deposition of urate crystals is responsible for the clinical manifestations. This causes arthritis when in and around joints and renal damage when in the kidney.

Renal handling of urate is complex. Urate is:

(1) filtered at the glomerulus;
(2) absorbed in the proximal tubule;
(3) secreted in the loop and distal tubule;
(4) reabsorbed in the distal tubule.

Net urate excretion depends on the balance of these processes. Drugs used to enhance urate excretion (uricosurics – *probenecid, sulphinpyrazone*) disturb this balance but only at high doses is excretion increased.

An alternative way to lower blood urate concentration is to inhibit xanthine oxidase, which catalyses the metabolism of purines to urate (via hypoxanthine and xanthine), with **allopurinol.**

Treatment of the acute attack of gout

Symptomatic treatment is with a NSAID (*indomethacin, naproxen* but not **aspirin,** which is contraindicated), initially at high dose, which can then be quickly reduced as symptoms permit.

An alternative, now seldom used, is *colchicine*, an antimitotic agent, which often causes profuse diarrhoea.

Prophylaxis of acute gout attacks

General therapeutic measures include:

(1) avoid excessive consumption of ethanol and food rich in nucleic acids;
(2) reduce weight;
(3) withdraw or replace any drug (for example, diuretic) precipitating the attacks.

Prophylactic drug therapy should be initiated once the acute attack has settled. Treatment should be continued indefinitely.

Inhibition of uric acid synthesis

Allopurinol is particularly useful in patients in whom uric acid is overproduced.

Uricosuric agents

These agents (*probenecid, sulphinpyrazone*) should not be used if there is renal impairment or a history of renal stones.

Fluid intake should be increased to prevent crystallization of urate in the urine. During the first weeks of treatment with either **allopurinol** or a uricosuric agent, a NSAID should be prescribed concomitantly, as an acute attack may be precipitated.

Drugs and the skin

Infections

Infestations have been dealt with on page 269 and fungal infections on page 280.

Bacterial infections

Many antibacterial drugs are formulated for topical application to the skin but their use is often not necessary. Washing and other hygienic practices are usually adequate. Not all skin complaints are manifestations of infection. Antibiotics can themselves cause sensitivity reactions in the skin (page 436).

Staphylococcus aureus

A carbuncle is a coalescence of deep boils and needs to be treated with systemic antibiotic.

Impetigo is a spreading superficial infection of the skin. Because it is superficial, topical antiseptics are effective (*cetrimide*, *chlorhexidine* and *hexachlorophane*; *sodium hypochlorite*, *povidone-iodine*). *Chlortetracycline* can be applied topically.

If impetigo is widespread on the body then a systemic antibiotic (**flucloxacillin**) should be used. To minimize the development of resistant microorganisms the drugs used topically and systemically should be different.

Streptococcus pyogenes

Erysipelas is differentiated from impetigo by an advancing, raised, sharply demarcated edge, thin seropurulent discharge from ruptured vesicles and lymphatic spread. One per cent of cases suffer allergic acute glomerulonephritis 1–3 weeks later. Treat erysipelas promptly with systemic **benzylpenicillin.**

Viral infections

Herpes simplex (cold sore) – crystal violet prevents superinfection, **acyclovir** or *idoxuridine* treat the cause but treatment needs to be started at the onset of sore development (page 294).

Herpes zoster (shingles). When immunity wanes latent chicken pox virus in the posterior root ganglia spreads down the sensory nerves to invade the dermal segment supplied. Management – early **acyclovir,** analgesics, *idoxuridine* for ocular involvement.

Human papilloma virus (warts) is self-limiting – 5–20% regress spontaneously within 6 months, therefore treatments that are painful or leave scars are not appropriate. *Salicylic acid* collodion paint, local soaking with formaldehyde or glutaraldehyde, or *podophyllum resin* paint are chemical alternatives to curettage under local anaesthesia or cryotherapy. They are irritant to normal skin.

Acne

Cause

The hair follicle sebaceous glands produce too much sebum and their necks too much keratin that is too cohesive. The incidence is 90% in teenagers, declining to 15% at about 25 years; there is a familial tendency. Local sensitivity to androgens determines the pathophysiology. In females the functional antagonism of androgens by oestrogens is revealed by the exacerbation of acne premenstrually when plasma oestrogen concentration is minimal (page 159).

Clinical features

The pilosebaceous canal is obstructed by a comedone (blackhead). Sebum excessively secreted behind this obstruction blows up the gland. Bacterial colonization by the commensal anaerobe *Propionobacterium acnes* and breakdown by its lipases lead to a further increase in volume. Rupture into the dermis initiates an inflammatory response.

Self-management

Sunlight (short of burning) is beneficial in increasing keratin turnover. The commensal skin flora are reduced by skin cleaning with antiseptic detergents (*cetrimide*).

Treatments

Local

UV irradiation. Keratolytics (benzoyl peroxide, *tretinoin*) produce a plug of loosely packed horny cells that unseats the existing comedone.

Systemic

Antibacterial agents (**erythromycin,** *tetracycline*) in small doses for weeks or even months, are accumulated in sebum.

In females severe acne may respond to **ethinyloestradiol** and **cyproterone** – the antagonist at testosterone receptors. This preparation is also contraceptive.

Seborrhoeic dermatitis

Cause

Excessive sebum secretion (greasy skin), fungal infection with the yeast form of *Pityrosporum ovale* plus low-grade bacterial infection.

Clinical features

A recurrent dermatitis with characteristic distribution; the scalp shows scaling and hair loss (cradle cap in a baby), in and behind the external ears, eyebrows, nasolabial fold, over the sternum, between the shoulder blades, axillae, pubis and groins.

Management

Regular cleaning with antiseptic detergent shampoo (*cetrimide, hexachlorophane*). The imidazoles (*ketoconazole* shampoo) are very effective in clearing the fungal infection. Inflammation may be severe enough to warrant glucocorticoids.

Contact dermatitis

Two very different causes operate – (1) irritation, and (2) sensitization.

Irritant contact dermatitis

Causes – alkali cleaners, abrasives, solvents. Nappy rash is an irritant dermatitis to the ammonia formed by bacterial breakdown of urea. Ensure adequate frequency of nappy changing, cleaning of nappy if not disposable kind and use barrier cream.

Sensitization contact dermatitis

Causes

A delayed (type IV) hypersensitivity reaction to cutaneous allergens or haptens:

(1) vehicles – lanolin (wool fat, wax and alcohol used as emulsifiers in ointments, creams and cosmetics) and parabens (alkylhydroxy-benzoates used as preservatives in creams, lotions and cosmetics);
(2) antibiotics locally applied – penicillins (especially **ampicillin**), aminoglycosides, *chloramphenicol* and sulphonamides are all common causes; *fusidic acid* is an infrequent cause and *chlortetracycline* a rare one;
(3) antiseptics – *iodine* and *hexachlorophane*; occasionally hydroxyquinolines, rarely *chlorhexidine* and *benzoyl peroxide*;
(4) local anaesthetics – all are liable to sensitize the skin when locally applied but **lignocaine** least so;
(5) antagonists at H_1 histamine receptors – all are liable to sensitize the skin when locally applied;
(6) adhesives – colophony and rubber chemicals but not acrylate monomer;
(7) elastic, nickel, rubber, plants.

Incidence

Up to 10% of all patients with dermatitis have allergic contact dermatitis; 1–2% of those with eczema are allergic to lanolin (rare in those with normal skin).

Clinical features

Previous contact with skin is essential for the development of sensitization. Once developed, the whole skin is abnormally reactive, both to skin contact and blood-borne allergen. The condition persists for years and is specific to close chemical analogues of the sensitizer. It occurs more commonly in adults than children and more commonly with damaged skin. The rash is symmetrically distributed. A detailed history of temporal associations suggests the agent, which may then be identifiable by patch testing.

Treatment

Specific – identify the cause and exclude it. The latter is not always a practical option for the patient. Symptomatic – *see* page 438.

Atopic eczema

Eczema means little more than dermatitis of unknown cause. It is one of the diseases of atopy (page 25). There is (incidence 1–3%) a heritable tendency to low itch threshold, deficient sweat and sebum secretion and ready vasodilatation. Scratching produces most of the damage to skin (excoriation, thickening, reddening, exudation, soreness).

Clinical features

In infants it begins (at 2–3 months) on the face then becomes generalized and a dietary origin is relatively common. In childhood (1.5–7 years) flexures are most affected and inhaled allergen is commoner. It tends to decline in steps, at the onset of puberty and at 18 years.

Treatment

Avoid any demonstrable cause. Symptomatic treatment – *see* page 438.

Psoriasis

A genetically transmitted tendency to a ten-times faster than normal epithelial cell proliferation rate. Cell life becomes 4, instead of 28 days. The surface layer shows poor differentiation towards a keratinized corneum.

Incidence

Two to three per cent of the population show psoriasis, beginning in the age range 25–60 years. It fluctuates, is triggered by normal stimuli to cell multiplication and is commonly subject to spontaneous remissions and recurrences.

Clinical features

Well defined plaques of red thickened skin covered with loose silvery scales. Commonest sites – scalp, elbows, knees and knuckles.

Management

Local

Sunlight (the 280–320 nm band) is beneficial.

The mainstay is the local application of drugs that depress mitosis. Various irritants have been found empirically to hasten remission: *coal tar* (0.5–5%) is effective but messy. Irritant preparations for addition to the bath water have little effect.

The standard treatment in this irritant group is the application to the lesion of **dithranol** [anthralin] 0.1–2%. It is applied daily (to thick) or twice a week (to thin plaques) and accurately, in amount just sufficient to cause a feeling of local warmth. The area is covered for 1 h and then the application is washed off; a red-brown staining of the skin occurs. Treatment is continued until the skin is clear as judged by appearance, feel and lack of scale on scratching. Applications should cease if soreness or weeping develops.

Glucocorticoids should be avoided as tachyphylaxis may occur and local pustules emerge.

Systemic

Some dermatology clinics offer PUVA – the combination of long wave ultraviolet, UV-A, irradiation (320–400 nm) with an oral psoralen (methoxsalen; chemicals, naturally-occurring in some plant saps, that interact with skin and sunlight to produce phototoxic dermatitis) which, when activated by UV, binds to DNA.

Severe resistant cases may be treated orally with **methotrexate** in low dosage or *etretinate*.

Symptomatic management of dermatitis

The symptomatic treatment of dermatitides depends less on the cause of the dermatitis or the distribution of or name given to the rash and more on the stage of skin inflammation and patient complaints.

Acute weeping stage

Astringents for the weeping, soothing wet dressings for the soreness, local anti-inflammatory glucocorticoids (page 439) if unbearable and antibacterial drugs if secondarily infected, may be required. Dressings wetted (replaced so area never dries) with lotions of aluminium acetate or *potassium permanganate*, which are both astringent – precipitate proteins and reduce the serous oozing. *Potassium permanganate* is also antiseptic.

Subacute stage

When weeping stops the lesions can be protected by a thickly spread paste (*zinc compound paste*) twice daily.

Dry fissured and scaly stage

Washing the lesions with soap irritates and defats – emulsifying ointment is useful as a soap substitute. An emollient (*aqueous cream*) soothes, smooths and hydrates the epidermis, thus allaying irritation. Zinc oxide (an astringent) and *calamine* (an antipruritic) are often incorporated.

Chronic stage

This is characterized by marked thickening of the skin and pronounced scaling. Keratolytics (*salicylic acid, coal tar* – the look and smell of which make it unpopular) increase the rate of loss of surface scale. They must be avoided or discontinued on broken or acutely inflamed skin.

Topical glucocorticoids

These are nonspecifically anti-inflammatory and patients with dermatitis, eczema and psoriasis frequently demand them having heard of their efficacy from other patients. *Hydrocortisone* cream (0.1 and 1%) and ointment (1%) are available from retail pharmacists without prescription.

For maximum effect (3–10% of applied dose can enter the skin) the vehicle and diluent are critical; a soft white paraffin-based ointment is the simplest satisfactory base; creams, lotions and propylene glycol diluents all interfere with activity.

The intensity of the anti-inflammatory effect obtained depends on the potency and efficacy of the glucocorticoid drug used and the dose rate of application to the skin – to avoid adverse effects the least intensity that will control the disease should be used. Preparations producing four intensities of effect are recognized:

I the highest: preparations are available but their use is usually ill-advised;
II *fluocinolone acetonide* 0.025%, *betamethasone valerate* 0.1% and *hydrocortisone butyrate* 0.1% are equieffective;
III *fluocinolone acetonide* 0.01% and *clobetasone butyrate* 0.05% are equieffective;
IV the lowest: *hydrocortisone* 1%.

Florid inflammatory skin lesions can be brought under control by systemic **prednisolone** or a high intensity local glucocorticoid. As soon as control is achieved continued treatment should be local and with the minimum intensity of glucocorticoid that will retain control of the lesions.

These are so effective (though only providing symptomatic relief) and so widely used that an appreciation of their limitations is essential.

Local complications

Glucocorticoids are contraindicated in any infected condition (whether fungal or bacterial) because they mask the inflammatory response to, and therefore the signs of, infection.

As well as masking the signs of infection, they predispose to infection. They also cause skin atrophy (both dermal and epidermal), telangiectasia (groups of visible dilated small blood vessels), purpura and striae. These effects are maximal with more intensely active preparations, used on the face, in the younger patients and for long treatment times.

Systemic complications

Toxicity identical to that of systemic glucocorticoids (page 180), due to systemic absorption, is uncommon but seen with extensive application, to permeable skin and/or under occlusive dressings.

Sunlight

Sunscreens

The normal skin is burnt by ultraviolet (UV) radiation of wavelength 290–320 nm. Sensitive skins may react to the same wavelengths as normal skins, or to longer wavelengths. Skin can be shielded by an opaque, reflective layer of titanium dioxide paste but this is thick and greasy and is not often acceptable to the patient. Lotion formulations are more acceptable. They contain sunscreens (*aminobenzoic acid*, *padimate O*) that, if generously and frequently applied, effectively absorb a proportion of the harmful rays.

Suggested further reading

ALBERT, A. (1979). *Selective Toxicity: Physico-chemical Basis of Therapy*, 6th edition. London: Chapman and Hall

BOWMAN, W. C. and RAND, M. J. (1980). *Textbook of Pharmacology*, 2nd edition. Oxford: Blackwell

BRADLE, P. B. (1989). *Introduction to Neuropharmacology*. Oxford: Butterworth-Heinemann

British National Formulary. London: British Medical Association and Royal Pharmaceutical Society of Great Britain

CARPENTER, J. (1988). *Pharmacology from A to Z*. Manchester: Manchester University Press

COOPER, J. R., BLOOM, F. E. and ROTH, R. H. (1982). *The Biochemical Basis of Neuropharmacology*, 4th edition. New York: Oxford University Press

DAY, M. D. (1979). *Autonomic Pharmacology: Experimental and Clinical Aspects*. Edinburgh: Churchill Livingstone

Drug and Therapeutic Bulletin. Hereford: Consumer's Association

FRANKLIN, T. J. and SNOW, G. A. (1989). *Biochemistry of Antimicrobial Action*, 4th edition. London: Chapman and Hall

GARROD, L. P., LAMBERT, H. P. and O'GRADY, F. (1981). *Antibiotic and Chemotherapy*, 5th edition. Edinburgh: Churchill Livingstone

GILMAN, A. G., GOODMAN, L. S., RALL, T. W. and MURAD, F. (1985). Goodman and Gilman's *The Pharmacological Basis of Therapeutics*, 7th edition. New York: Macmillan

GOLDSTEIN, A., ARONOW, L. and KALMAN, S. M. (1974). *Principles of Drug Action: The Basis of Pharmacology*, 2nd edition. New York: Wiley

HALL, R., ANDERSON, J., SMART, G. A. and BESSER, M. (1981). *Fundamentals of Clinical Endocrinology*, 3rd edition. London: Pitman Medical

KATZUNG, B. G. (1989). *Basic and Clinical Pharmacology*, 4th edition. Norwalk, CT: Appleton and Lange

KATZUNG, B. G. and TREVOR, A. J. (1989). *Pharmacology: Examination and Board Review*, 2nd edition. Norwalk, CT: Appleton and Lange

KRUK, Z. L. and PYCOCK, C. J. (1983). *Neurotransmitters and Drugs*, 2nd edition. London: Croom Helm

LAURENCE, D. R. and BENNETT, P. N. (1987). *Clinical Pharmacology*, 6th edition. Edinburgh: Churchill Livingstone

LEE, J. and LAYCOCK, J. F. (1983). *Essential Endocrinology*, 2nd edition. Oxford: Oxford Medical Publications

NEAL, M. J. (1989). *Medical Pharmacology at a Glance*. Oxford: Blackwell.

NOGRADY, T. (1988). *Medicinal Chemistry. A Biochemical Approach*, 2nd edition. New York: Oxford University Press

Prescriber's Journal, Hannibal House, Elephant and Castle, London

RANG, H. P. and DALE, M. M. (1991). *Pharmacology*, 2nd edition. Edinburgh: Churchill Livingstone

ROWLAND, M. and TOZER, T. N. (1989). *Clinical Pharmacokinetics: Concepts and Applications*, 2nd edition. Philadelphia: Lea and Febiger

RYALL, R. W. (1989). *Mechanisms of Drug Action on the Nervous System*, 2nd edition. Cambridge: Cambridge University Press

TAUSK, M. (1977). *Pharmacology of Hormones*. Chicago: Year Book Medical Publishers

WHO EXPERT COMMITTEE. (1977). Technical Report Series, 615, *The Selection of Essential Drugs*. Geneva: WHO

WINGARO, L. B., BRODY, T. M. CARNER, J. and SCHWARTZ, A. (1991). *Human Pharmacology: Molecular to Clinical*. London: Wolfe

Index